Black Lung

W9-BYQ-177

23.96

Purchased by:_____

BLACK LUNG

Also by Alan Derickson:

Workers' Health, Workers' Democracy:
The Western Miners' Struggle, 1891–1925

BLACK LUNG

ANATOMY OF A PUBLIC

HEALTH DISASTER

ALAN DERICKSON

CORNELL UNIVERSITY PRESS

ITHACA AND LONDON

First published 1998 by Cornell University Press.

Printed in the United States of America.

Cornell University Press strives to use environmentally responsible suppliers and materials to the fullest extent possible in the publishing of its books. Such materials include vegetable-based, low-VOC inks and acid-free papers that are recycled, totally chlorine-free, or partly composed of nonwood fibers.

Library of Congress Cataloging-in-Publication Data

Derickson, Alan.
Black lung : anatomy of a public health disaster / Alan Derickson.
p.   cm.
Includes index.
ISBN 0-8014-3186-7 (cloth : alk. paper).
1. Lungs—Dust diseases—United States—History.   2. Coal miners—
United States—Health and hygiene.   3. Coal miners—Legal status,
laws, etc.—United States.   I. Title.
RC733.D44   1998
616.2'44—dc21   98-13612

Cloth printing   10   9   8   7   6   5   4   3   2   1

To my parents

CONTENTS

ILLUSTRATIONS

PREFACE

Richard Nixon could not face the widows. The president fully intended to veto the coal mine health and safety legislation passed by Congress on December 18, 1969. Although he could tolerate the disagreeable prospect of federal intervention to regulate conditions in this most hazardous industry, Nixon could not accept the wholly unprecedented plan to compensate victims of work-induced respiratory disease. With a series of warnings that the cost of federal benefits would be exorbitant and that the states properly had jurisdiction over workers' compensation, representatives of his administration laid the groundwork for killing this sweeping reform measure.[1]

On December 29, 1969, a delegation of seven women whose husbands had died a year earlier in a mine explosion in Farmington, West Virginia, arrived at the White House to demand passage of the health and safety bill. On the same day, protest strikes broke out in the coalfields. Rather than chance a disruptive, nationwide strike and an unpleasant encounter with the widows, the president gave in. Nixon refused to meet with the women, but sent word that he would approve the mining bill. The following day, without public ceremony, he signed the Federal Coal Mine Health and Safety Act, which included the highly objectionable Black Lung Benefits Program. After Nixon had slipped away, the women received a tour of the White House. In the empty Oval Office they picked up pens used in signing the bill, souvenirs that the president left lying on his desk. Looking past the snub, Sara Kaznoski, the leader of the group, declared it "a wonderful day for all miners."[2]

That day came after almost a century of controversy. Misunderstanding of the nature and extent of dust-induced lung disorders had long forestalled compensatory and preventive measures for coal workers. Although from our contemporary vantage point the danger in inhaling dense concentrations of mineral particles for up to two thousand hours a year for twenty years or more might seem uncontroversial, it took a protracted campaign to convince mine owners, health professionals, and political leaders of the risks of such exposure. For much of the twentieth century, many in positions of authority held that breathing coal mine dust was harmless, or even beneficial, to human health. As one stalwart agitator for recognition of this occupational disease put it in 1970, "ill-informed complacency has had a stultifying effect on the entire medical profession, mining engineers, compensation attorneys, legislators, and mine operators." In this critical view, the failure to identify and control pneumoconiosis among coal miners "constitutes what may be labeled in the future as the greatest disgrace in the history of American medicine." Although this assertion was perhaps hyperbolic, it is clear in retrospect that denial of the dangers of mine dust shortened the lives of hundreds of thousands of anthracite and bituminous workers.[3]

The ascendance of the "ill-informed complacency" that dominated the half century up to 1969 was preceded by almost a half century during which coal miners' dust disease was accepted, in both lay and professional circles, as a major form of industrial disease. Complacency settled in only after a concerted effort to discredit and supplant established ideas.

The defeat of complacency depended upon forceful advocacy as well as cogent science. The thesis of this book is that social movements, more than any of the other forces operating on this problem, fostered advances in recognition of coal workers' lung disorders. The turn-of-the-century miners' union, social medicine activists at mid-century, and the black lung insurgents of the late sixties each played decisive roles in giving this issue broader visibility. At critical junctures in the political contest over medical ideas, confrontational collective action accomplished what careful scientific investigation and subtle private negotiation could not. Especially when miners and their professional allies promoted accessible vernacular conceptions of disease—"miners' asthma" or "black lung"—the fog of mystifying scientific jargon lifted to reveal masses of breathless, displaced old men, destroyed by their work.

I wrote this book for three main reasons. As a strictly historical exercise, it sheds harsh light on the enormous human cost of producing the basic energy source used to make the United States the world's preeminent industrial nation. This book also offers a broader perspective on two contemporary issues. First, it demonstrates that the battles of the 1960s and the resulting legislation did not politicize the definition of miners' respiratory diseases: the biomedical science bearing on this subject had already been entangled with the political economy of the coal industry for many decades. Second, the tragedy of black lung is not that a federal benefit program can be difficult and expensive to administer. This book reveals the real tragedy: that this human-made condition could have been prevented at the turn of the century. Preventive action would have saved more than the thirty billion dollars spent thus far on the Black Lung Benefits Program.[4] It would have saved millions of years of lost life and diminished quality of life for coal workers and their families.

It is a pleasure to acknowledge those who enabled me to complete this project. Many archivists and librarians graciously guided me to research material. I thank the patient staff at the National Archives, the Library of Congress, the National Library of Medicine, the Pennsylvania State Archives, the Birmingham Public Library, the Catherwood Library at Cornell University, the West Virginia University Library, the Bancroft Library at the University of California, the King Library at the University of Kentucky, the Butler Library at Columbia University, the Pattee Library at the Pennsylvania State University, the Stapleton Library at Indiana University of Pennsylvania, and the Illinois Historical Survey Library at the University of Illinois. Maier Fox provided expert guidance to the records of the United Mine Workers of America during the time when the union held its own historical records. Other exceptionally helpful archival workers whom I must thank individually are Denise Conklin, Peter Gottlieb, and Diana Shenk.

Several individuals gave me access either to their own personal papers and libraries or to those of deceased family members. I thank Sara Anderson, Leslie Falk, Louis Friedman, Ken Hechler, and Murray Hunter for granting me this privilege. Many people gave me access to their memories. I want to express my appreciation to all those who participated in my oral history interviews.

In its various incarnations, this work benefited from the exertions of numerous careful critics. Helpful readings of all or part of the manuscript came from Robert Asher, Allan Brandt, Martin Cherniack, Paul Clark, Tom Dublin, Elizabeth Fee, Maier Fox, the late Lorin Kerr, Dan Letwin, Robert Proctor, Donald Rasmussen, David Rosner, Kitty Sklar, Mark Wardell, and Jim Weeks. I took some, but probably not enough, of their suggestions. Peter Agree played the part of the canny editor, offering a seemingly endless supply of smart advice. Grey Osterud's copyediting improved the manuscript in many ways.

Generous assistance from Pennsylvania State University included a sabbatical leave and two research grants. The university also made available the services of four very able research assistants: Deirdre Curristin, Sharon Litchkowski, Jennifer Stewart, and Lynn Vacca. Funds from the National Institute for Occupational Safety and Health enabled me to conduct a valuable series of oral history interviews.

My family handled this lengthy expedition with a mixture of stoicism and good humor. My daughters, Elizabeth and Katherine, lifted my spirits and even took on a few editorial chores. My wife, Peg, offered not only moral support but medical wisdom and editorial sense as well. I am very grateful to them for all their help.

ALAN DERICKSON

University Park, Pennsylvania

ABBREVIATIONS

AALL	American Association for Labor Legislation
ACGIH	American Conference of Governmental Industrial Hygienists
ACSC	U.S. Anthracite Coal Strike Commission
ADMW	Association of Disabled Miners and Widows
BLA	West Virginia Black Lung Association
BLS	U.S. Bureau of Labor Statistics
BOM	U.S. Bureau of Mines
CWP	coal workers' pneumoconiosis
HEW	U.S. Department of Health, Education, and Welfare
HRFA	United Mine Workers of America Health and Retirement Funds Archives
ILO	International Labor Organization
MRC	Medical Research Council
NCLC	National Child Labor Committee
PHS	U.S. Public Health Service
RG	Record Group
TCI	Tennessee Coal, Iron and Railroad Company
UMW	United Mine Workers of America
UMWJ	*United Mine Workers Journal*
VISTA	Volunteers in Service to America
WRF	United Mine Workers of America Welfare and Retirement Fund

BLACK LUNG

CHAPTER ONE

THEY SPIT A
BLACK SUBSTANCE

●n September 14, 1881, H. A. Lemen, professor of medicine at the University of Denver and president of the Colorado State Medical Society, presented a paper at the society's annual meeting. Lemen offered for his colleagues' edification the case of his patient James McKeever, for thirty years a coal miner in Scotland, England, and Pennsylvania. He noted McKeever's "harassing cough," "care-worn expression," and other non-specific symptoms. In contrast to such vague indications of chronic respiratory disease, he also announced the less ambiguous finding that this patient sometimes expectorated more than a pint of black liquid in a day. After commenting on the "decidedly inky appearance" of the substance, the Denver physician made this disclosure: "The sentence I am reading was written with this fluid. The pen used has never been in ink." The impact of this stratagem on its immediate audience remains unknown. But it is evident from the inclusion of Lemen's case report in the state medical society's program that by the 1880s physicians in Colorado had developed some curiosity about the health consequences of mining coal.[1]

As pneumoconiosis made its first appearance in coal-mining districts across the United States, medical practitioners like Lemen struggled to understand its causes and effects. They achieved a degree of success. Clinical and pathological studies managed to illuminate a discrete clinical entity well before the turn of the twentieth century. The state helped clarify the nature, if not the full extent, of this disorder. By 1900, investigators

had brought forth compelling evidence of the existence of a debilitating occupational disease, known most commonly in biomedical discourse as anthracosis and in lay parlance as miners' asthma.

Early initiatives to recognize dust-induced respiratory disease in the
coalfields had to surmount considerable obstacles. The enormous toll ex-
acted by traumatic injuries served to obscure anthracosis. In the 1890s,
occupational injuries killed more than 1,000 coal diggers per year. In
particular, frequent spectacular disasters diverted attention from the less
spectacular phenomenon of chronic disease. When, for instance, the Avon-
dale mine near Wilkes-Barre, Pennsylvania, caught fire on September 6,
1869, taking 108 lives, the nation was momentarily transfixed.[2] The histo-
riography of nineteenth-century working conditions in coal has tended to
reinforce the view that injury, not illness, constituted the only important
type of risk to miners. This chapter shows that miners' repiratory illness
became a significant problem even in the nineteenth century and, further,
that it was identified as such at the time. Indeed, this account will demonstrate that anthracosis stood out as one of the leading occupational diseases of the industrializing era.[3]

The lack of historical research on the emergence of coal workers' disease
is, unfortunately, hardly unique. There have been very few in-depth studies of occupational diseases, except lead poisoning, for the period before
1900. Carey McCord's review of the nineteenth-century medical literature
demonstrated that considerable interest surrounded work-induced illness.
Reacting to the assertion that U.S. investigators published only about
twenty reports on occupational disease before 1900, McCord compiled
a bibliography of more than two hundred entries on diverse acute and
chronic conditions.[4] But four decades later, almost none of his provocative leads for historical research have been explored. The health hazards
of twentieth-century workplaces are the subject of a growing body of
scholarship.[5] Nonetheless, the preceding century of industrial transformation remains virtually the prehistoric age with regard to the impact of
work on health.

Occupational disease among U.S. coal workers arose in a burgeoning industry essential to the developing economy. Commercial coal extraction
began inauspiciously in Virginia in the eighteenth century. But by the second half of the nineteenth century, large-scale production for regional,

national, and export markets took place in fields scattered across more than twenty states, with major centers in the Midwest and central Appalachia. Demand for fuel for rail transportation, home heating, and industrial manufacturing soared in the decades after the Civil War. In 1870, U.S. firms dug forty million tons of anthracite and bituminous coal. By 1900, production had multiplied more than sixfold. The industry's work force grew from just under 100,000 in 1870 to almost 500,000 in 1900. These producers made the United States by far the foremost coal-producing nation at the turn of the century, with roughly one-third of world output.[6]

Coal-mining technology in the late nineteenth and early twentieth centuries remained essentially preindustrial. To be sure, methods of extraction changed over the period and varied widely among mines at any given time. Nonetheless, before 1900 most mines depended primarily on animate sources of power and hand tools to extract coal. As Keith Dix and others have demonstrated, the most distinctive characteristic of the labor process in this era was the time-consuming, worker-paced loading of coal cars by hand shoveling.[7]

Coal diggers in the Gilded Age all too often toiled in an environment that presented a serious respiratory hazard. Many routine tasks raised dust. Preparing for the explosion of charges involved undercutting the coal face with a hand pick. Lying on his side at arm's length from the point of dust generation, the miner could not avoid breathing mineral particles. In the late 1870s, the journalist Henry Sheafer reported that "every stroke of the pick dislodges a fresh shower of dust, to be inhaled by the miner." The strenuous exercise of undercutting raised the miner's rate of respiration, increasing the dose of dust. The shift to undercutting machines at the end of the century dramatically exacerbated this hazard. Using an auger drill to bore the holes into which blasting powder was placed further exposed coal workers to dust. Blasting itself produced immense quantities of mineral particles. The common practice of returning to the working face soon after the detonation of charges meant entering an area filled with particulate matter. The laborious chore of loading broken coal into cars stirred large amounts of dust into the air. Transporting, unloading, and cleaning the extracted material gave a dose of dust to laborers far from the mine face. "The wonder is not that men die of clogged-up lungs," Sheafer concluded, "but that they manage to exist so long in an atmosphere which seems to contain at least fifty per cent of solid matter."[8]

Almost everywhere in the years before 1900, and for long thereafter in small operations, ventilation systems did too little to abate air contamination. Primitive workings, particularly drift mines that reached a coal seam by tunneling into a hillside, often relied on natural ventilation. Many mines went only one step beyond natural airflow by setting up furnaces at the bottom of the mine shaft to create an updraft to move air. John Brophy worked under such an arrangement in the bituminous fields of central Pennsylania in the 1890s. "An elaborate system of fans and blowers was 'too costly,'" Brophy sardonically explained, "so the miner had to pay for bad ventilation by 'miners' asthma' and other ailments caused by bad air, stagnant at best." Even where fans operated, they sometimes did not deliver fresh air to the far reaches of the underground labyrinths where many employees were stationed. When air flow did not remove mineral particles, layers of dust accumulated on the floor of the mine and on other surfaces. Inevitably, the movements of workers and mules recirculated this dust.[9]

By the second half of the nineteenth century, an extensive medical literature linked coal mine dust with workers' ill health. European science shaped North American understanding of miners' respiratory distress in important ways. Of particular significance, the French school of pathological anatomy, though past its heyday, exerted both direct influence on American developments and indirect influence via Britain. The work of several British anatomical investigators paved the way for what became the dominant paradigm. Andrew Meiklejohn astutely concluded that British physicians of the mid-nineteenth century "were dependent almost entirely on the correlation of clinical observations with morbid anatomical changes observed at post-mortem inspections." Tying unmistakable, readily perceived signs and symptoms to anatomical discoveries offered strong substantiation of the existence of miners' pneumoconiosis. More important for the diffusion of knowledge across society, pathological anatomy demystified coal workers' disease by extracting and revealing the physical damage done by dust accumulation and by connecting this damage to lay observations of illness. Accessible to both the general public and clinical practitioners, who generally lacked a strong foundation in the biological sciences, this form of scientific inquiry yielded especially convincing evidence of the miners' condition.[10]

The long-established coal industry of Britain gave rise to a stream of case studies. James Gregory at the Royal Infirmary of Edinburgh took a major step toward clarification of the respiratory ailments of coal workers in 1831 with the publication of a "Case of Peculiar Black Infiltration of the Whole Lungs, Resembling Melanosis." Gregory began by sounding an alarm for "those practitioners who reside in the vicinity of the great coal mines, and who may have charge of the health of the miners, to the existence of a disease, to which that numerous class of the community would appear to be peculiarly exposed." He then presented the case of John Hogg, a fifty-nine-year-old miner, who had died under his care earlier that year. He enumerated Hogg's main symptoms—dyspnea, chest pain, palpitations, expectoration, and cough—and his sinking trajectory. Gregory reported in detail on his postmortem examination:

> When cut into, both lungs presented one uniform black carbonaceous colour, pervading every part of their substance. The right lung was much disorganized, and exhibited in its upper and middle lobes several large irregular cavities, communicating with one another and traversed by numerous bands of pulmonary substance and vessels. The cavities contained a good deal of fluid, which, as well as the walls of the cavities, partook of the same black colour.

The Scottish physician explained this condition by the patient's inhalation of coal dust on the job. He backed this inference by recounting that Hogg "himself attributed the complaint of which he died to the air of the coal mines in which he had been working for so many years."[11] Gregory, like most other nineteenth-century investigators, took as valid his patient's self-report.

Seven years later, the *Edinburgh Medical and Surgical Journal* printed a case study by Thomas Stratton that advanced a novel term for the disease: "What has been called the black lung of coal-miners . . . may more shortly be defined anthracosis." Widely, if not universally, adopted by biomedical professionals on both sides of the Atlantic, Stratton's label stuck for a century. Other British journals in the mid-nineteenth century published pathological studies that found blackened, damaged lung tissue and attributed this damage to coal dust and other underground air contaminants.[12]

By the late 1860s, a sizable literature identified a discrete clinical entity.

Without question, the symptoms of anthracosis were indistinct. Shortness of breath, chest pain, and cough could accompany any number of disorders. Similarly, the gradual deterioration over many years that typified the natural history of anthracosis hardly stood out as unique. But anatomical explorers seized upon one crucial connection and held out its importance. They had traced to its source in necrotic cavities within the lungs the extraordinary black sputum often seen in the clinical setting and often remarked upon by the miners themselves. Indeed, as James Merchant and his colleagues recently observed, "Melanoptysis, the often dramatic production of several ounces of black inky sputum from a ruptured lesion, can be considered the only specific, although somewhat unusual, clinical sign of CWP [coal workers' pneumoconiosis]." Melanoptysis made anthracosis.[13]

In the mid-nineteenth century, the pathognomonic sign of coal workers' dust disease elicited considerable commentary. The title of William Thomson's 1837 article—"On Black Expectoration and the Deposition of Black Matter in the Lungs, Particularly as Occurring in Coal Miners, Etc."—fixed attention on melanoptysis, while relating this overt manifestation to internal damage. Investigators took pains to indicate that this dense black substance differed markedly from ordinary sputum speckled with dark mineral particles. Edward Greenhow described a former miner who spat up a fluid "closely resembling black paint." Comparison to ink also recurred well before H. A. Lemen's presentation. Moreover, British scientists commented on another sensational attribute of melanoptysis, its copious quantity. J. W. Begbie found that with one of his hospital patients, "for a period of several months, the spit-box was daily filled with a dark, heavy mass." William Thomson dissected the lungs of a miner who for months before his death spat "a large quantity of a dark-coloured sputum." Despite the ambiguities surrounding miners' respiratory maladies, the pathognomonic quality of melanoptysis cast the affliction in stark terms that were neither easily dismissed nor easily confused.[14]

John Carpenter, a physician in Pottsville, Pennsylvania, drew on the British literature when he gave a paper at the annual meeting of the Schuylkill County Medical Society in 1869. Reviewing fifteen years' clinical experience, Carpenter portrayed local hard-coal workers as men beset by manifold risks. Although some threats were obvious, the practitioner asserted that "it remains for the skilled professional man to trace out the predisposing and exciting causes of disease that encompass the miner in his daily surroundings—to note the effects of the altered temperature, the deprivation of sunlight, the inhalation of gases, as well as of insoluble, solid, carbonaceous material into the lungs, and the results of severe labor, for hours, in constrained and unnatural positions of the body." He asserted that inhalation of gases and dust "must be estimated the most serious of the many causes which assail life and health in our mines." Rather than specifying coal dust or rock dust as the sole agent of disease, Carpenter assumed that stagnant, contaminated environments harboring decaying or otherwise noxious substances gave rise to miasmas, which caused disorders of many kinds. This long-standing etiologic notion found a receptive audience, given that coal is formed from decomposed, compressed vegetable matter. The doctrine of specific etiology lay beyond the horizon of the medical profession in the North American coalfields in 1869.[15]

Working within the investigative mode of pathological anatomy, Carpenter linked the carbonaceous state of autopsy specimens to "the characteristic black sputa which accompany every case of bronchial or lung disease among miners." He went on to delineate a composite clinical picture of his patients: "A peculiar asthmatic character of cough is generally noticed; emphysema is detected on physical exploration, and the sputa are black, often streaked with blood. Miner's asthma is chronic bronchitis, with thickening of the air-passages, emphysema and nervous distress in breathing. . . . The black expectoration is observed for years after ceasing work in mines." Carpenter also emphasized the "very remarkable" persistence of symptoms by citing the case of a man suffering "chronic bronchitis, with coal-dirt sputa, who has not entered a mine for nineteen years."[16]

The Pottsville physician plotted the trajectory of this relentless malady. He maintained that miners' asthma "becomes often a constitutional affection attended by great debility." He qualified this assessment by assuring that "these chronic troubles may last a lifetime, without being rapidly fatal, or necessarily so." Nonetheless, he had found that few anthracite workers lived past fifty-five years of age. Similarly, the "great excess of old women over old men" in mining villages struck him as remarkable. Carpenter closed his paper with a bit of underwriting advice: "I could not conscientiously advise any life insurance company to do business among miners, except on short periods of risk, and at large increase of percentage." No such solicitude extended to the men and boys working in or planning to go to work in this industry. Insurance carriers apparently needed more protection from risk than did either the hardy individuals who labored in the mines or their prospective widows.[17]

Carpenter relied primarily on the designation "miner's asthma," but used other terms as well. In the case of McKeever, the former miner whom Lemen described in Colorado twelve years later, the diagnosis was "phthisis pulmonalis nigra." Reflective of the uncertainty surrounding this condition, Lemen hastened to append a string of synonyms: "anthracosis, black phthisis, carbonaceous bronchitis, coal heavers' consumption." These terms indicate more than the imprecision of medical knowledge in the late nineteenth century; anything with five names has gained wide recognition. Lemen remarked that "coal heavers' consumption, anthracosis pulmonum, is referred to by a number of writers on pulmonary diseases, by pathologists and microscopists." In the late 1870s, union leader John Siney was diagnosed by his family physician as suffering from "miner's consumption," yet another name for this condition. (Siney succumbed to this disorder in 1880.)[18]

Some in the biomedical community tried to impose better order on this unsettled situation. Gottfried Merkel's overview of dust diseases in 1874 reflected the confusing proliferation of terms. In discussing the effects of the deposition of coal dust on the respiratory system, Merkel listed a series of names, including false melanosis, coal-miner's lung, and anthracosis pulmonum. But over this loose terminology, he cast the blanketing concept of pneumokoniosis (more commonly in the U.S. spelled "pneumoconiosis," but also occasionally "pneumonoconiosis" or "pneumonokoniosis"), a unifying term for the respiratory dust diseases, which had been coined seven years earlier by the German investigator Friedrich Zenker. Merkel considered coal miners' disease "the most thoroughly studied of all the pneumokonioses." His discussion encompassed pathological anatomy and the startling black fluid in the lungs. An 1885 overview of dust diseases that embraced this conceptual framework described miners' lungs as "miniature coal mines."[19] Medical comprehension thus advanced by including anthracosis in a classificatory scheme that related coal miners' ailments to those of other dust-exposed workers.

Some critical commentators promoted preventive measures. In 1896, J. W. Exline's summary of underground air contaminants in Colorado warned of "the clouds of dust contributed to the air in the processes of mining." Exline recommended a stringent state law requiring improved ventilation. Such breadth of vision by a clinician, quite extraordinary by late-twentieth-century standards, epitomized the untrammeled analysis of a time before the division of professional labor in this field.[20]

North American medical textbooks helped to legitimate and to distribute the expanding corpus of knowledge. H. A. Lemen quoted a passage from Austin Flint's *Treatise on the Principles and Practice of Medicine* to convey anatomical features of anthracosis. Beginning with its 1873 edition, this widely used tome carried an entry on anthracosis. In addition to his enumeration of symptoms and signs, Flint declared that the disorder was "caused by the inhalation of coal dust." The text even specified a pathogenic mechanism: large doses of dust induced disease by simple mechanical irritation of lung tissue.[21]

Flint's discussion reinforced the privileged place of pathological data in explaining coal workers' disease. The author had to discard the erroneous contention of the eminent German pathologist Rudolf Virchow that blood, not dust, caused dark pigmentation in lung tissue. "By their microscopical character the carbon-pigment is readily distinguished from that derived from the blood," Flint argued, "and sometimes the particles of coal are sufficiently large to be recognized by the naked eye." Such reports of unassisted observation of deposited dust undoubtedly encouraged general practitioners without microscopes to make their own postmortem examinations.[22]

The consensus supported the exogenous origin of the disorder in excessive dust exposure. In a departure from previous contributions to North American texts, Edward Bruen in 1885 located anthracosis within the family of pneumoconioses. Bruen maintained that "the injurious action of dust upon the lungs is in proportion to the quantity deposited in them." Adolf Strumpell differentiated the pathological condition miners' anthracosis from the darkening of the lungs found in urban residents exposed only to the polluted air of the ambient environment. Although these texts extended and codified growing recognition of anthracosis, they did so in a somewhat disjointed way. Compartmentalized summaries of signs and symptoms now increasingly stood apart from and made no reference to findings on postmortem dissection. This style of presentation severed physical damage from human distress.[23]

The schematic approach had its compensatory virtues, however. Textbook authors were locked into a format that left them no way to evade difficult questions for which clinicians needed practical answers. Primary-care physicians wanted to be able to address their patients' fears about how this illness would change their lives. No alarmist, Austin Flint held that "if the quantity [of dust deposited] be not large, there is no appreciable diminution of respiratory function." The question of treatment was another inescapable clinical concern. Flint recommended palliative therapy, including inhalation of turpentine vapor. Bruen offered no efficacious treatment. Instead, like Exline, he emphasized prophylaxis: "The most practical plans consist in thoroughly ventilating the atmosphere, and thus preventing the dust from reaching the artisan." Moreover, Bruen preferred engineering controls over "the use of masks or respirators, which possess the obvious disadvantages of clumsiness and inteference with respiration." With no chance to effect a cure and no power to order prevention, clinicians had to confront the unpleasant topic of prognosis. Flint warned that the prospects for victims of anthracosis were grim. In contrast, Bruen held that "the prognosis depends very largely upon the withdrawal of the sufferer from the unhealthy environment."[24]

In 1892, an authoritative new textbook took up the miners' distinctive ailment. The inaugural edition of William Osler's *Principles and Practice of Medicine* included a section on "pneumonokoniosis." The short list of dust diseases consisted of siderosis, caused by inhalation of metallic particles, chalicosis (soon to be supplanted by silicosis), caused by inhalation of rock dust, and anthracosis. These distinctions further underscore the point that the chronic disease resulting from coal mine dust was not always conflated with silicosis before the mid-twentieth century. Beyond his command of the scientific literature, Osler brought to the topic his own experience of performing postmortem studies on miners. On the pathogenesis of coal disease, Osler argued that the natural dust-clearing devices of the respiratory system sometimes proved inadequate under the onslaught of sustained, intense particulate exposure. With phagocytic and muco-ciliar defenses overwhelmed, deposits of dust particles accumulated and fibrosis ensued. On a more practical plane, Osler considered diagnosis of anthracosis "rarely difficult," given the characteristic expectoration. The Johns Hopkins professor also delineated the course of the disorder: "The symptoms do not come on until the patient has worked for a variable number of years in a dusty atmosphere. As a rule there are cough and failing health for a prolonged period of time before complete disability." Subsequent editions of this singularly influential work advised medical students and practitioners on the hazard of coal dust and pointed to the notorious black spit.[25]

Despite Osler's guidance, one formidable obstacle continued to curtail diffusion of knowledge among clinicians and, in turn, its transmission from physicians to the lay population. Like their patients, medical practitioners wanted a rigorous scientific description and explanation of this condition much less than they wanted an effective cure for it. Like his predecessors, Osler could not promise any efficacious therapy. The first edition of *The Principles and Practice of Medicine* spent one unencouraging sentence on the topic. In the absence of an outright cure, miners turned to patent medicines and home remedies for symptomatic relief. Miners' reliance on self-medication probably kept many cases of chronic dust disease from the observation of medical practitioners.[26]

Biomedical professionals oriented toward the nuances of pathological anatomy were ill prepared to ascertain the extent of dust disease across the nation's coalfields. Case reports fixed analysis at the individual level. Persistent controversy over the propriety of autopsies ensured that these procedures remained relatively rare, limiting the quantity of data available to begin to assess pneumoconiosis prevalence. Preoccupied with uncovering and precisely describing the internal damage within the lungs of individuals, through increasing emphasis on microscopic findings, late-nineteenth-century textbooks generally avoided any consideration of the distribution of this disorder in the mining workforce. Although conveying a sense of the frequency of occurrence of this condition would have helped to alert clinicians to its likelihood among their patients, these guides to practice prudently refused to hazard any guess as to the prevalence of dust disease in the coalfields. A few comments suggested the magnitude of the phenomenon. Roberts Bartholow's textbook remarked that "miners' lung" was "very common in the coal regions of Pennsylvania, and other mining localities." J. W. Exline's paper alluded to the extent of the ailment in Colorado: "Most of us have treated patients of this class, and know something of the pathology of this form of phthisis so prevalent among men who handle coal." However, no private practitioner of medicine was expected to carry out the epidemiological tasks necessary to deliver an informed answer to this question.[27]

Private organizations did not take on the challenge of measuring the magnitude of this affliction either. Besides the various state and national medical societies, voluntary groups for the advancement of knowledge, such as the American Social Science Association and the American Public Health Association, provided the institutional base from which civil society might have considered the health cost of industrialization, but none sponsored such studies. Biological and social scientists at the universities in coal-mining states did not inquire into the extent of pneumoconiosis nearby. Philanthropists and charity leaders were preoccupied with other matters; there were no middle- and upper-class activists operating settlement houses in the mine-patch villages. The formidable and often aggressively intrusive organizational forces of elite civil society did virtually nothing to help expose the scale of this social problem.[28]

The state had the potential to generate much knowledge on the extent of miners' disease. To be sure, federal administrative capacity was quite minimal in the late nineteenth century. But at the state level, public officials carved out a mandate to produce and distribute information on diverse manifestations of the impact of industrialization on social welfare. Both temporary exploratory bodies and permanent data-gathering agencies looked toward building a knowledge base for public understanding and remedial policy on miners' health. To this end, the state set out to buttress and amplify private findings regarding miners' asthma. Of particular relevance to political discourse on this subject, the state increasingly took responsibility for marshalling quantitive evidence. William Brock saw a faith in statistics driving governmental investigation in this period: "A method which divested itself of preconceived theory, concentrated upon the collection of data, and presented the results objectively was conceived as the essential instrument of material and moral progress in nineteenth-century civilization. With the help of figures one could trace long-term movements in social evolution . . . and the influence of unhealthy environment or occupations." An adventuresome inquisitiveness about the effects of the enormous industrial experiment under way set the stage for advances in the recognition of occupational diseases.[29]

Despite its broad mandate and wholistic perspective, governmental pursuit of knowledge was crippled by numerous serious limitations in the late nineteenth century. Constraints imposed by meager resources often prevented information-gathering initiatives. In an era of Darwinistic individualism, modest ambitions regarding state intervention to protect the weaker elements in society served to dampen inquiry. With capital opposed to general awareness of the deleterious effects of its operations, governmental agents came under pressure to mediate social relations by obfuscation or neglect. The fragmentation of state power further vitiated efforts to clarify the extent of the damage wrought by unhealthful conditions in coal mining. In particular, devolution of power to local government prevented the production and distribution of knowledge on occupational disease across the society as a whole.[30]

Historians have recently disinterred several forms of social investigation into the plight of the working class in the industrializing era. With a few notable exceptions, these historical studies have given little more than passing notice to the assessments of health status that were integral to these inquiries into lower-class life.[31] However, wide-ranging public investigations commonly did consider the health status of coal workers. Moreover, even relatively narrowly focused surveys explored the social and environmental determinants of disease.

Under the weak state of courts and parties, ad hoc institutions filled some administrative gaps in the late nineteenth century. A succession of commissions took up questions of miners' health. However short-lived and understaffed, these bodies publicized various facets of anthracosis.

In 1871, Ohio governor Rutherford B. Hayes appointed a Mining Commission to look into conditions in the state's coal industry, with a view to formulating protective legislation. On September 16, 1871, Daniel Rathben appeared before the commission to give testimony drawn from his extensive background as a medical practitioner in Middleport. Like John Carpenter, Rathben could not restrict himself to one name for the respiratory condition he had repeatedly encountered among his coal-digging patients. Besides referring to work-induced asthma, Rathben stated that "Scotch people call it spurious melanosis, really a coal miner's consumption." He informed the commission that this disorder arose "from the peculiar atmosphere charged with carbonaceous particles." Besides coal dust, the physician indicted carbon monoxide gas and the airborne residue from the incomplete combustion of explosives as contributing factors. He had conducted anatomical examinations: "I examined them after death because before their decease they spit a black substance, whose real character I wished to ascertain." On the epidemiological front, Rathben pointed out that dust exposure brought on "a good many cases of Asthma." The commissioners did not pursue this passing reference.[32]

The Ohio commission called attention to "the dust and fine coal held so injurious, by English physicians, to the miners' lungs." One of its members, Andrew Roy, toured the state's coalfields and made a long list of underground risks that included "breathing coal-dust." Rank-and-file miner William John advised the panel that inadequate ventilation had damaged his health. John joined Roy in encouraging the appointment of professional public inspectors, who "would give more reliable information as to the status of ventilation in a mine than any miner or other person sent down by a court." The commission recommended legislation providing for workplace ventilation.[33]

The Board of Commissioners for Pennsylvania's Second Geological Survey sent a geologist, Henry Chance, into the anthracite fields to study extractive technology in the early 1880s. His sweeping findings struck a fatalistic tone: "Miners working in dry dusty workings, and breaker hands working in breakers where the coal is prepared dry, undoubtedly become the victims, sooner or later, of the disease known as 'miners' consumption,' 'miners' asthma,' 'miners' anemia,' and by various other names." "There is little doubt," Chance concluded, "but that these terms have all been applied to cases of one and the same disease, having as a common origin the presence of large quantities of dust in the lungs." Combining an eyewitness account with a diligent review of the medical literature, this report painted a nuanced clinical picture. In addition to paying attention to the distinctive expectoration, Chance pointed out that "this disease is not asthma" but merely shared with it the symptom of extreme dyspnea. He also illuminated the insidious clinical course of miners' asthma, from a slight shortness of breath through total disability to death.[34]

The U.S. Industrial Commission, created by Congress in 1898 to conduct an encyclopedic study of employee-employer relations, caught a glimpse of the health consequences of digging coal. Thomas Davis, vice president of the United Mine Workers of America and himself a victim of miners' asthma, testified before the commission on April 14, 1899. From his own work experience and his observations as a union official, Davis presented salient aspects of the pneumoconiosis threat confronting his members. He publicized the characteristic shortness of breath that he and others suffered. This survivor of twenty-eight years underground—sixteen years in anthracite, twelve in bituminous—distinguished variations in trajectory: "Some men endure it for a number of years; others pass away very rapidly with it." Davis considered miners' asthma to be "very prevalent" in the anthracite fields. "Hundreds of miners become afflicted with it at a very early age, some of them as young as thirty years, and possibly younger than that," he contended. Davis believed that miners' asthma also plagued soft-coal districts, but not so extensively. When asked for statistical corroboration for his statements, he admitted that he had none. Nonetheless, perhaps because none of the coal operators appearing before the panel disputed his assertions, the commission's summary of Davis's presentation emphasized its epidemiological dimensions: "In the anthracite regions, and in a less degree in the bituminous mines, miner's asthma is common and frequently proves fatal." Federal investigators did not go on, however, to advocate more systematic surveillance of miners' health.[35]

With the exception of the Industrial Commission, the federal government disregarded miners' diseases during the late nineteenth century. The national decennial censuses, which became important instruments for examining societal problems, did not probe industrial diseases. The Census Office began to gather mortality data in 1880. However, this data base had no discrete category for pneumoconiosis, much less the pneumoconiosis peculiar to the coal industry. The 1890 census reported how many sheep were killed per year by dogs in every county in the United States but not how many miners were killed by dust inhalation. Moreover, at the close of the century only ten states participated in the death registration system. No cabinet-level agencies for health or labor existed to initiate inquiries. Neither the Marine Hospital Service, predecessor of the Public Health Service, nor the short-lived National Health Board ventured to investigate this noninfectious condition. The Department of the Interior concerned itself with promoting exploitation of the nation's mineral resources, not publicizing exploitation of the nation's human resources.[36]

Responsibility for investigating miners' respiratory disease fell primarily to state governments. In several coal-producing states, bureaucratic institutions arose whose jurisdiction extended to the well-being of mine workers. Permanent specialized agencies charged with understanding and protecting public health, labor, and mining proliferated after 1870. Direct surveillance, statistical analysis, and recordkeeping activities expanded markedly, especially in Pennsylvania, where most of the nation's coal was mined.

State boards of health were the primary candidates to ascertain the extent of anthracosis. Illinois, Pennsylvania, Ohio, and other mining states created health agencies after 1870. These bodies took on diverse data-gathering functions in the areas of vital statistics and community health surveillance. Their officers often entered the field of public health with an optimistic, expansive view of the role of the state as an instrument for disclosing, if not preventing, illness.[37]

The Pennsylvania State Board of Health and Vital Statistics set out on a lofty mission upon its founding in 1885. Its manifesto to the people of the commonwealth declared that the human rights set forth in Pennsylvania's constitution "necessarily include the inherent right to the enjoyment of pure air, pure water, and pure soil, since without them life can neither be enjoyed nor successfully defended and the pursuit of happiness becomes a cruel mockery." To this high purpose, it asserted that "no man or combination of men, however rich or powerful, shall be allowed to trespass on these rights of the humblest citizen, whether from negligence, from greed or gain, or simply from ignorance. It is no mere empty figure of speech by which we call disease a public enemy." In its pursuit of this enemy, the board explicitly placed the unhealthful workplace within its purview. The stage was seemingly set for an attack on an eradicable disease like anthracosis.[38]

At the same moment, however, the agency hastened to express its solicitude of business interests. The board admitted that where economic and health concerns clashed, it would proceed with "the least possible interference." Consistent with this policy, it sought only to "diffuse information which shall develop an enlightened public sentiment in regard to both rights and duties from a sanitation standpoint." In fact, its enabling legislation had unequivocally granted the board the right to investigate occupational diseases and disseminate its findings but had not granted it comparably strong powers to abate hazards. The board had to rely on moral suasion, not police action, to ameliorate working conditions.[39]

Before its inaugural year was out, the Pennsylvania board undertook "a careful investigation into the sanitary condition of the mining populations" of the state, including the "character and effects of labor, and sanitary condition of mines." Despite this explicit charge, medical inspector

Spencer Free neglected the working environment. Free concentrated instead on the unhygienic personal habits of mine employees, especially the most recent immigrants from southern and eastern Europe, and on the manifest deficiencies of community sanitation, especially the absence of modern sewerage arrangements. Understandably preoccupied with infectious conditions such as typhoid fever, Free failed to focus on pneumoconiosis. Similar priorities for elemental measures to control epidemics led to similar lack of awareness among public health officials in other mining states.[40]

Free described at length the model community health program developed by the Rochester and Pittsburgh Coal and Iron Company at its operations in western Pennsylvania. In these company towns, the health boards consisted of Rochester and Pittsburgh's managers and company physicians. In Pennsylvania, as in other mining regions, state officials in the late nineteenth century had to depend on local agencies for information on the existence of problems as well as for leadership in remedying them. Community boards in company-controlled towns and villages were disinclined to blame disease on working conditions, which created a formidable impediment to the recognition of pneumoconiosis in a sizable share of coal communities. This structural impediment would remain in place in hundreds of localities for decades to come.[41]

Yet management did not monolithically deny the problem. Mine foreman W. B. Owens served on the health board in the anthracite community of Taylor. In a paper presented at the 1901 Pennsylvania sanitary convention, Owens alleged that one in two coal workers had miners' asthma and would eventually die of the disorder. This claim prompted an angry riposte from engineer John Fulton, representative of a bituminous enterprise. From his forty years in coal, Fulton countered that "not five per cent of the miners are affected with miner's asthma." "There is nothing in mining that makes it insanitary," he maintained, "and any insanitary conditions which may exist are doubtless closely related to the rum shop." However, even Fulton's far lower rate would yield a statewide prevalence of dust disease exceeding 10,000 cases.[42]

When Pennsylvania surveyed physicians regarding consumption in the mid-1880s, the responses showed some awareness of pneumoconiosis. One respondent from a mining community observed that coal dust "induces a form of consumption in which asthma is a prominent symptom."

This practitioner also drew the distinction between silicosis and anthracosis: "The miners who cut the rock tunnels suffer from a disease known among them as rock-miners' consumption; of this the prominent symptom is a shortness of breath, not generally asthmatic." Another respondent, situated in the soft-coal village of Arnot, commented on the frequency of miners' asthma among his patients.[43]

State officials looked to ongoing collection of vital statistics, not one-time surveys, to disclose major disorders. It was assumed that disease recognition depended heavily on systematic aggregation of morbidity and mortality data. In theory, this axiom applied to occupational disorders. In 1889, Pemberton Dudley, a member of the Pennsylvania health board, described the hazards, including respirable dust, to workers in the metal trades in a paper at the Third State Sanitary Convention. Dudley's study led him to criticize the inadequacies of current methods of collecting data: "So long as we are deprived of the facilities for accumulating and preserving statistics relating to these subjects, so long shall we make but indifferent progress in our investigations, and we shall go on in our present course, sacrificing the lives of our people, through an ignorance born to a false economy." The stage was seemingly being set for a more careful oversight of the deleterious impact of industrialization on workers' health.[44]

Despite Dudley's forceful encouragement, statistical evidence of occupational diseases was not forthcoming. Benjamin Lee, secretary of the Pennsylvania health board, bluntly characterized the state's vital statistics program as "simply upon paper" in 1889. Official sources in Pennsylvania's coal-mining areas did attribute a few deaths to dust diseases. For example, Luzerne County, where extant records go back to 1893, reported that thirty-one men succumbed to miners' asthma, one to miners' consumption, and one to miners' croup before 1900. In its tabulations, however, the Pennsylvania health board lumped mortality from respiratory disorders into broad classifications that buried not just miners' asthma but pneumoconiosis in general. Other mining states performed even more poorly. Kentucky officials damned the vital statistics statute under which they functioned as "wholly inoperative." "Until the law is amended and vitalized," advised the Kentucky State Board of Health, "any compilation and publication of the returns would be worse than useless." This lack of state capacity posed a major barrier to any decisive policy initiatives regarding dust disease.[45]

In Ohio, the state mine inspector tried to promote awareness of the dust threat. Daniel Rathben's testimony before the Mining Commission in 1871 had alerted Andrew Roy, who shortly thereafter became the state's first mine safety officer. In his report for 1876, Roy asserted that over time bituminous workers' lungs "become clogged up from inhaling coal dust, and from breathing noxious air." He used the common vernacular term for the mixture of vapors, gases, and dusts that miners inhaled on the job: "bad air." The inspector, whose repertoire did not include dissection, turned to Rathben to convey the deterioration of coal workers' lungs: "After twelve years they are black, and after twenty years they are densely black, not a vestige of natural color remaining, and are little better than carbon itself." The gross anatomy of this disorder again proved disturbingly persuasive.[46]

Roy's long tenure as mine inspector, in ongoing, close contact with working miners, led him to believe that pneumoconiosis pervaded the coalfields. In 1889, after he had left office, he argued that a state hospital should be established to accommodate victims of dust disease. His case for this institution rested on the controversial claim that disease took as great a toll among coal workers as did trauma:

> In war there are fully as many soldiers who fall victims to the diseases resulting from exposure, hard marching, and imperfect food and clothing as fall in battle. In mining also, a similar condition of facts are [sic] true. The carbonaceous solidification of the air cells of the lungs, the contracted chest and the prostrated energies perform the work of death as surely as the ponderous masses of coal and shale.

Roy's comparison of deaths from illness to the number of fatal injuries, however crude and unsubstantiated, represented an attempt to develop an equivalence that would stand as a rough estimate of cumulative mortality. Public policy in Ohio did not proceed from analogies, however colorful: the state did not build a special hospital for coal workers.[47]

Roy's counterparts in Pennsylvania were most suspicious of the above-ground breakers where coal was sorted and cleaned. In 1881, inspector Samuel Gay condemned conditions in the breakers: "Often while groping my way through those concerns, I have felt as though I would suffocate before reaching the outside. Such an atmosphere, loaded with dust, as it is, certainly must be injurious to those who are obliged to breathe it." Four years later, perhaps in response to Gay's indictment and concomitant plea for corrective legislation, Pennsylvania amended its mining law to require managers of anthracite coal-processing plants to abate air contamination "where the coal dust is so dense as to be injurious to the health of persons employed therein." Enforcement of this measure was lax. In 1892, for example, inspector G. M. Williams did not seek to impose sanctions after discovering extremely dusty breakers in his district. Williams's inaction suggests that he looked on airborne coal particles as a mere nuisance, despite the fact that the law held otherwise.[48]

The same official disregard predominated with regard to conditions underground. Pennsylvania inspectors, like those in other coal states, largely ignored the threat of respirable dust as they strove to minimize the concentration of methane and other gases, blasting-powder residue, and lamp smoke. Apprehension accompanied the arrival of undercutting machines in the nineties, however. Joseph Knapper's report from the bituminous fields in 1899 expressed concern that the new coal-cutting equipment threw off more dust, which in his view was "unhealthy to breathe." But most inspectors' commentary on dust focused on its explosivity. This obliviousness stands out as all the more remarkable because the 1885 law had put inspectors on notice that coal mine dust represented a respiratory risk.[49]

Whereas mining bureaus passed over a hazard that lay unquestionably within their purview, specialized labor agencies could ignore mine dust because their jurisdiction generally excluded the mining industries. Protective legislation covering industrial workers commonly excluded coal diggers. Hence, the investigatory efforts of the first cohort of labor inspectors, who often delved into the wide-ranging adverse effects of work, centered on sweatshops and factories in urban areas and gave no notice to comparable hazards in rural coal mines. Under this disjointed arrangement, dawning cognizance of the hazards of industrial dust did not carry over to the mining industry.[50]

Overall, the state stopped at the threshold of recognition of pneumoconiosis in coal mining in the late nineteenth century. Governmental officials caught glimpses of some facets of the disease and communicated bits of factual information to the public. But no substantial findings emerged that could help provide a foundation for a thoroughgoing commitment to disease prevention.[51]

Medical investigators were quite aware of this occupational illness. By 1900, miners' asthma or anthracosis had gained wide recognition in biomedical circles as a clinical entity. Its natural history as a slowly disabling chronic condition was understood. Clinicians had identified many of its signs and symptoms. The pathognomonic melanoptysis particularly captivated medical observers. Individual signs and symptoms were commonly combined into a characteristic syndrome. The professional construction of a chronic illness was largely completed by the turn of the century.

At the same time, wide recognition coexisted with somewat shallow understanding. Persistence of the nebulous notion of bad air indicated that, by today's standards, chronic dust-induced respiratory disease did not yet constitute a clear-cut disease entity. To be sure, for William Osler and the fraction of the medical community that held anthracosis to be the type of pneumoconiosis caused specifically by coal mine dust, a disease entity did exist. Such awareness appears to have been outweighed, however, by lingering confusion over the etiology of the condition.[52]

As an epidemiological entity, whose distribution across the at-risk population was known with any certitude, miners' pneumoconiosis did not exist. Private agencies made no pretense of pursuing this daunting task systematically. The state served as little more than a platform for soliciting informal impressions and recapitulating doctors' determinations regarding individual cases. Governmental agents lacked not the mandate but rather the administrative capacity and, more important, the will to generate knowledge on the prevalence of coal miners' breathlessness. In the absence of a strong movement demanding such inquiry, the state would not take on such an inevitably controversial assignment.

CHAPTER TWO

TWICE A BOY

Coal workers had an acute sense of the perils of their industry. They came to the dilemma of dust disease with a pragmatism driven by concerns very different from those of the biomedical community. Explication of pathogenesis meant far less to them than estimation of future chances for subsistence. Above all, miners tried to fend off and to accommodate growing respiratory impairment. Translation of impairment into disability and lost wages dominated rank-and-file thinking. Some miners tried to warn their sons to avoid the industry. William Keating sang this ballad at the turn of the century:

> When I was a boy says my daddy to me:
> "Stay out of Oak Hill, take my warning," says he,
> "Or with dust you'll be choked and a pauper you'll be,
> Broken down, down, down."
>
> But I went to Oak Hill and I asked for a job,
> A mule for to drive or a gangway to rob.
> The boss said, "Come out, Bill, and follow the mob
> That goes down, down, down."[1]

Other fathers felt they had no choice but to ask their sons to take a mining job in order to help the family survive.

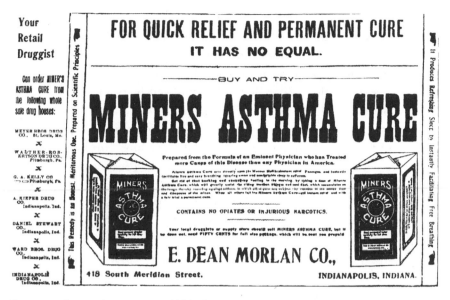

Patent medicine advertisement, 1901. (Reprinted from *United Mine Workers Journal*)

Coal workers' families could not absorb the costs of pneumoconiosis. At the turn of the century, miners built a mass movement to press for better terms and conditions of employment. From its founding, the United Mine Workers of America (UMW) fought to protect its membership against work-induced disease. The titanic anthracite strike of 1902 gave the union an unparalleled opportunity to publicize the predicament of those members who were no longer able to toil because of work-related illness.

Coal miners embraced a collective response to occupational disease only after realizing the inefficacy of individual coping. Miners learned that the ministrations of medical practitioners against the ravages of pneumoconiosis were fruitless. The only helpful, although naive, pieces of advice doctors offered were to leave the mines or to improve the circulation of air underground. Coal workers experimented with all kinds of self-medication. The traditional ritual of drinking a shot of whiskey with a beer chaser after the day's work supposedly brought up dust. Nineteenth-century coal miners took curative measures at the beginning as well as at the end of the day. According to George Korson, "morning bitters," a popular home remedy that stimulated the coughing up of dust, consisted of "whiskey with a mixture of snakeroot, gold seal, and/or calamus root, sweetened with rock candy." Merchants in mining communities promoted

the medicinal use of bourbon, gin, brandy, and other potent liquors. Whatever symptomatic relief these alcoholic formulations offered, however,
came at the price of the opprobrium their consumption engendered.[2]

From the volume of advertising for patent medicines in mining-town
newspapers, it would appear that individual self-help relied heavily on
commercial concoctions. Innumerable nostrums were aggressively mar-
keted. By the 1840s, Pottsville, Pennsylvania, not far from Philadelphia, already had local agents hawking such putative asthma cures as Wright's
Indian Vegetable Pills and Dr. Bechter's Pulmonary Preservative. In more
remote localities, mail-order products predominated. In western Maryland, the *Frostburg Mining Journal* carried instructions for sending away for
various panaceas. At the turn of the century, the *United Mine Workers Journal* regularly published advertisements for patent medicines, including a
special cure for the coal workers' peculiar ailment:

> Get rid of that hacking and choked-up feeling in the morning, by taking a
> dose of Miners Asthma Cure, which will greatly assist the rising mucous
> [sic], phlegm and coal dust, which accumulates on the lungs, thereby in-
> suring against asthma, to which all miners are subject—by reasons of the
> smoke, dust and dampness of the mines. When all others fail try Miners
> Asthma Cure—get instant relief, and with a fair trial a permanent cure.

The campaign of chemical warfare against occupational disease continued
for decades, but to no avail.[3]

The self-help approach underscored personal responsibility for health.
Hard-selling patent medicine manufacturers were not above blaming the
victim. One advertisement for a respiratory cure-all declared that there
was "No Excuse for Being Sick." In the same vein, another drug company
proposed a regimen that combined doses of Doctor Pierce's Golden Medical Discovery with regular breathing exercises to expand the lungs. In an
individualistic culture, such injunctions undoubtedly struck a responsive
chord.[4]

Lay cognizance of respiratory disease in the nineteenth century developed
most rapidly in the anthracite region of eastern Pennsylvania. The extant
evidence suggests that, in fact, work-induced lung disorders were more
prevalent in the nation's hard-coal center than in soft-coal regions. Several

factors contributed to this difference. Large-scale anthracite mining commenced during the first quarter of the nineteenth century. Here, in contrast to more recently opened fields in West Virginia or Alabama, by the closing decades of the century thousands of men had pursued mining long enough to pass through the latency period between the initial exposure to mine dust and the manifestation of symptoms. As extractive enterprise progressed, mining operations extended deeper underground, making effective ventilation more difficult. The irregular, often extreme, inclination of the hard-coal seams further complicated the task of maintaining sufficient air flow.[5]

Perhaps most important, the social relations of anthracite production fostered chronic respiratory disease. With the maturation of this segment of the industry came a tendency toward long-term employment. Although hardly inescapable, the mines held large cohorts of career employees. Reviewing trends in anthracite since the 1860s, George Virtue reported in 1897 that "miners rarely leave the calling to which they have been brought up." The decisions of these men, made and remade as part of their families' strategies for subsistence, guaranteed substantial cumulative exposure to mine dust.[6]

In the first half of the nineteenth century, extraction of hard coal grew into a major industry in Pennsylvania. Anthracite output rose from an annual total of 235,000 tons in 1830 to 20,000,000 tons in 1870, at which time it roughly equaled bituminous output. Donald Miller and Richard Sharpless did not exaggerate in asserting that, given its importance as a fuel during the formative period of iron-making and rail transportation, anthracite ignited the Industrial Revolution in the United States. In the decades after 1870, the hard-coal side of the industry continued to grow dramatically, albeit less dramatically than soft coal. In 1900, 150,000 employees produced 57,000,000 tons of anthracite.[7]

Industrialization in anthracite was a contradictory and incomplete process. The stumbling advance of technology not only left much arduous hand labor but at the same time created new manual tasks in and around the mines. One of these gaps in mechanization involved processing anthracite immediately after extraction. Coal hoisted up out of the mine was not ready for market, especially not for the increasingly demanding home consumer. Chunks of raw material had to be broken into smaller pieces, these pieces had to be sorted by size, and bits of slate and other rock had to be removed. In the initial phase of anthracite mining, men working in the open air outside the mine placed large chunks of coal on iron plat-forms, smashed them with sledge hammers, and threw out the bits of slate that invariably mixed with the coal.[8]

By mid-century the collieries had built elaborate breaker facilities near the top of the mine shaft. Inside these towers of 100 feet or more in height, the main factors of production were gravity, steam-driven mechanisms, and unskilled laborers. Loads of coal dumped into the top of the breaker tumbled down through one or more sets of revolving cylinders that crushed large lumps and then through a series of sorting screens. Beneath the screens the anthracite flowed down a number of chutes. Three or four workers sat on planks a few inches above each chute. Their job was simply to catch and discard pieces of slate and other impurities.[9]

Soon after the introduction of this technology, at least by 1866, boys were picking slate in breakers. Contemporary data on the number and age distribution of breaker boys were invariably rough. By the early 1880s, al-most 20,000 boys under the age of sixteen reportedly toiled in hard coal. In 1885, Pennsylvania prohibited the employment in breakers of children below age twelve, but failed to enforce the law with any rigor. Persistent, widespread illegal practices necessarily led to systematic misrepresenta-tion of the ages and numbers of very young workers. State statistics that put the total number of breaker boys at 13,133 in 1902 no doubt under-stated the extent of child labor in anthracite.[10]

Many children began their careers in hard coal at a very young age. In 1877, journalist Phoebe Gibbons found six-year-olds picking slate in the coal mills around Scranton. A quarter-century later, little had changed. In 1902, James Moore, a Methodist minister in the mine patch of Avoca, claimed, "I have seen boys going to the breaker that did not seem really able to carry their dinner pail." Although some parents evidently put their sons to work as early as the age of six, more often the juvenile laborers commenced at eight, nine, or ten. Thomas D. Nicholls, who went on to become president of District 1 of the United Mine Workers, started clean-ing coal in the late 1870s at age nine. Because the only skill needed to pick slate was manual dexterity, management counted as an asset the nimble little fingers of laborers under ten. (For the same reason, their sisters were deemed ideally suited to piecing up ends in the silk mills of the region.)[11]

No immigrant group withheld its children from the breakers. All shared essentially the same economic plight. In his 1889 survey of the industry, Homer Greene noted, "The miner is fond of his family; his children are dear to him, and, whenever the grim necessities of life permit, he sends them to the schools instead of to the mines or breakers." Greene explained that "the scant wages that they earn may serve to keep bread in the mouths of the younger children of their households and clothing on their own backs." Against allegations that parental intemperance explained most child labor, miners and their supporters steadfastly maintained that the employment of boys resulted from the low rates of pay and the high rates of disability and death of their fathers.[12]

Breaker boys labored in a highly contaminated environment. In fact, virtually every operation performed in a breaker created dust. The coal-milling began with the indelicate dumping of a loaded coal car into the maw of the crusher located at the top of the facility. The early crushers were crude, slowly revolving cast-iron cylinders. As their name indicates, they did not cleave the coal so much as pulverize it, releasing many small particles into the air. As the anthracite lumps fell through a series of screens, they gave off dust. The friction caused by coal traveling down the chutes generated more air contamination, as did the activities of the laborers themselves as they burrowed through the piles. In addition, the large and ever-increasing scale of operations entailed correspondingly heavier and heavier doses of mineral dust for colliery workers. In 1872, a new plant broke 1,000 tons of coal per day. By the turn of the twentieth century, many breakers in eastern Pennsylvania had an even larger daily capacity.[13]

We have no quantitative data on the anthracite dust hazard in the nineteenth century. Neither colliery operators nor state inspectors possessed the technology to monitor workplace air pollution. Yet numerous eyewitnesses concurred about the severity of air contamination. In fact, the appearance of the atmosphere outside breakers disturbed some observers. Henry Sheafer expressed alarm in 1879: "Any one who has . . . watched the thick clouds of dust which sometimes envelop the huge coal-breakers of the anthracite region so completely as almost to hide them from sight can form an idea of the injurious effect upon health of constantly working in such an atmosphere."[14]

Inside, of course, it was much worse. Homer Greene claimed that the boys "must breathe an atmosphere thick with the dust of coal, so thick that one can barely see across the screen room." The dismal darkness shocked novelist Stephen Crane, who visited a breaker in 1894. "The dust lay inches deep on every motionless thing," reported Crane, "and clouds of it made the air dark as from a violent tempest." When at the age of eight Robert Reid took a job at the Continental Breaker in Scranton around 1880, the place had no ventilation. "You breathed an atmosphere thick with coal dust," recalled Reid, "so thick that you could hardly see across the room where the boys picked out the slate."[15]

To be sure, an enlightened minority among the operators took steps to limit the hazard. Various types of ventilation systems carried a share of particulate matter out of some breakers. Systems that relied primarily on exhaust fans were most effective. Greene exclaimed that such engineering controls "pass beyond the domain of science and progress into that of humanitarianism." It was, however, more common simply to design breaker buildings with a large number of windows. Under this plan, no dust control existed on calm days and during the winter months when the windows were closed. Another effective, but infrequently implemented, way to abate dust was to wet down the coal. The want of employer-initiated engineering measures shifted responsibility to the employees at risk. Some breaker boys wore handkerchieves over their mouths; others used a wad of chewing tobacco to catch mineral particles.[16]

Although childhood exposure to coal mine dust had minimal immediate adverse effects, it was nonetheless not innocuous. Coal workers' pneumoconiosis is a dose-related disorder, and boys usually incurred a substantial dose of particulate matter during their tenure in the coal-processing plants. Breathing high levels of this deleterious substance nine or ten hours a day for a period of two to five years contributed significantly to the pathological process that eventuated in debilitating respiratory disease years later. In 1881, one of Pennsylvania's mine inspectors wondered about the health of anthracite miners "after serving an apprenticeship in one of those dust mills." Perhaps more important, however, were the indirect consequences of picking slate. Boys quit school to work in the breaker. The large proportion who ended their formal education before the age of twelve had few, if any, alternatives to continued employment in the mines. Many were functionally illiterate. Young anthracite laborers were thus set on a career path that predisposed them to protracted exposure to mine dust.[17]

The prospect of upward mobility within the industry lured many to persevere. The job ladder extended even to the worker in his first menial position: the youngest breaker boy aspired to move down the coal chute. The most experienced slate picker customarily sat at the bottom of the chute and took responsibility for removing the last bits of rock. For this he received slightly higher pay than the two or three laborers who sat above him.[18]

Beyond this modest promotion, boys planned to escape the breaker altogether. Phoebe Gibbons plotted the normal route to a skilled position in the 1870s: "As soon as the boy earns fifty cents at the mine, his sole ambition is to earn seventy-five, and then to be a driver. From driving one mule his desire is to drive a team, then to become a laborer, and then a full miner." The probability of advancement surely induced some employees to endure the extremely hazardous conditions in the breaker.[19]

After cleaning coal for a few years, boys went into the mine itself to open and close the doors that regulated ventilation. Despite the fact that the state child labor law of 1885 barred anyone under the age of fourteen from working inside an anthracite mine, ten- and eleven-year-olds held many doortending jobs. Far removed from both the breaker and the working face of the mine, door boys gained a respite from intense exposure to mineral dust. Adolescents soon graduated to a series of haulage jobs. First, they "spragged" cars, i.e., stopped coal cars at the top of inclines on haulage ways by inserting pieces of wood called sprags between the spokes of the cars' wheels. Then they drove mules. In general, workers on the transportation crew also managed to avoid the worst air contamination, except when they entered miners' chambers to deliver or retrieve cars.[20]

By the age of twenty, a typical employee had climbed to the next rung on the ladder. As a miners' laborer, a young man took part in the actual extraction of coal. Often working under his father, the laborer cleaved masses of blasted coal into smaller chunks with a pick, culled some of the rock and other refuse from the freshly hewn material, shoveled the anthracite into cars, and assisted the skilled miner. After a few years in this informal apprenticeship, the laborer became a full-fledged miner, responsible for directing the excavation process. Within their underground chambers, often out of range of the mine's ventilation system, miners and their assistants shared a dust-filled work space. Miners' helpers incurred the greater exposure to mine dust. Whereas many miners set up a round of charges, ignited them, and went home for the day, their helpers returned to the breast of the mine shortly after the explosion to pick, sort, and load coal.[21]

For all but a small minority of miners, attainment of craftsman status marked the apex of one's career. Opportunities to move into the ranks of management were scarce. In 1890, only 1,301 of the 123,676 individuals employed in hard coal were foremen or overseers. Union leader John Mitchell guessed that "only one in five hundred can even be given place as a foreman or superintendent." The vast majority of miners could not curtail their dust exposure by further upward mobility. In addition, their independence on the job, skills specific to the industry, and relatively good earnings ensured that few men left anthracite in their prime.[22]

After practicing their trade for a decade or two, many miners found themselves in declining health. Mitchell illuminated the crucial turning point: "If he is fortunate enough to escape the falls of rock and coal, he may retain this position as a miner for a number of years; but as age creeps on and he is attacked by some of the many diseases incident to work in the mines, he makes way for those younger and more vigorous following him up the ladder whose summit he has reached." Unquestionably, there were "many diseases incident to work in the mines" during this period, including arthritis and a number of cumulative trauma disorders. But the most feared of the degenerative conditions afflicting hard-coal workers remained miners' asthma.[23]

Under the working conditions that prevailed in late-nineteenth-century anthracite, pneumoconiosis followed an insidious course. The latency period before the first clinical evidence of disease appears to have been at least fifteen years, with considerable variation among individuals, depending upon the dose of dust and other factors. An initially unremarkable cough and slight shortness of breath were the first manifestations of the malady. Some mine workers experienced a degree of dyspnea by the age of thirty. As respiratory function slowly deteriorated, miners found it increasingly difficult to continue at their strenuous work. The anthracite craftsman had to carry out numerous arduous tasks beyond the capability of anyone with significant respiratory impairment.[24]

Prevailing personnel policy contradictorily accommodated and exacerbated disability. Victims of miners' asthma tried to retrace their steps on the job ladder. As their strength faded, anthracite workers took less arduous assignments. Mitchell observed that the aging miner went "back to become a miner's helper, then a mine laborer, now a door-boy; and when old and decrepit, he finally returns to the breaker where he started as a child." Some individuals descended the job ladder more precipitously. At age fifty-one, John Devenney plunged from miner directly to slate picker. In the early 1880s, Henry Chance watched "old men too feeble to perform hard labor" at the picking chute. Two decades later, Frank Warne judged that "no more heartrending scene can be depicted than the sight of this type of an old man—a class appearing old even when in middle life— seated alongside the breaker boys just entering their teens and picking slate for 75 to 90 cents a day." In all probability, during the nineteenth century the final phase of most hard-coal careers was one of abject downward mobility.[25] Ironically, this accommodation to debility increased ailing workers' exposure to coal dust.

During the period before the miners' union won seniority provisions governing transfer rights, management had sole discretion over job reassignments. Although the principles and mechanics of managerial decision-making in this realm remain obscure, fragmentary evidence suggests that well-intended, informal paternalism guided practice. In 1892, for example, the wife of an employee debilitated by miners' asthma asked Benjamin Hughes, a superintendent of coal operations for the Delaware, Lackawanna, and Western Railroad, to give her husband a less arduous job. Hughes, in turn, urged one of his foremen to try to place this man and others like him: "We must sympathize with them[;] you will get old yourself if you live long enough."[26] In all likelihood, however, the power of foremen in the prebureaucratic era to hire, fire, and move workers at will limited the extent of systematic reassignment to lighter tasks outside an individual foreman's jurisdiction. Indeed, just as Mrs. Hughes approached the mine superintendent, not her husband's foreman, John Devenney obtained his seat over the coal chute by repeatedly imploring the superintendent at J. C. Wentz & Company. Gratitude for the chance to keep working mixed with bitterness. In 1884, Jack Johnson expressed in song the humiliation of downward mobility:

> Little I thought when I grew old and mining could do no more,
> I'd go back to the breaker where I spent my days before.
> This world is full of trouble, hardship, care and strife,
> It's twice a boy and once a man, is a poor miner's life.

Back in the breaker, aging employees breathed the same air as their young co-workers, of course.[27]

Men like Devenney and Johnson had little choice but to work in spite of respiratory impairment. Disabled miners commonly had sizable families to support. Like other male industrial workers in their fading years, aging anthracite workers relied upon multiple wage earners to support their families. Even the low pay of old slate pickers, when combined with the earnings of other family members, could be critical to subsistence. Accordingly, retirement meant not a benign freedom from work but rather a distressing loss of an income. The desperate scramble for family income ensured that aging workers would grasp at any remaining employment option.[28]

Perversely, although their condition resulted in part from boyhood dust exposure, the decline of men in their middle years served to perpetuate, not to eradicate, the child labor system. Henry George saw the vicious cycle emerging in the 1880s. First, he quoted a broken ex-miner:

> I will be thirty-eight next September, and am, as you know, gray and old. . . . My mind goes back to the hundreds of boys who with me were little slate-pickers. I recall lots of them who are in the grave-yards, and those yet among the living whom I occasionally meet are gray-headed, old young men, worn out before their time. Asthma, consumption, weak back, gravel and rheumatism follow the breaker and mine work.

George went on to attribute much of the child labor in anthracite to this phenomenon: "Where the natural bread-winner can with difficulty support his family, any pittance that the children can earn becomes important. Still more is this the case where the natural bread-winner is disabled or taken away, and many of the little fellows employed in the mines are the sons of such men." Thirteen years later, Charles Spahr encountered a mule driver, the son of a fifty-two-year-old victim of miners' asthma, who had become such a breadwinner: "Outside work his father could still do, but there was none to be had. His sisters were only ten years old and four, so they couldn't earn anything yet. Therefore, he, a boy of only sixteen, was the only support of his family." Under these pressing circumstances, colliery management generally did not have to coerce employees to bring their children to work. The destruction of labor power generated fresh supplies.[29]

The lack of alternative sources of income in the late nineteenth century made it imperative to overcome this difficulty within the family. A miner disabled by occupational disease had no hope of winning a lawsuit for damages against his employer. Those operators who administered disability benefit programs paid indemnities only to accident victims who might otherwise bring legal action. Employer-financed pensions for old or permanently disabled employees were virtually unknown in the anthracite industry prior to the 1930s.[30]

Public assistance meant not monetary allowances but confinement in state or county institutions. The state miners' hospitals erected in the anthracite region after 1880 refused to admit individuals with incurable chronic diseases. The absence of state services left only the county poorhouses. Although dread of the primitive conditions in these institutions and of the stigma of such confinement kept the disabled at their jobs as long as possible, many former miners ultimately could not avoid this degradation. "The Old Miner's Refrain" expressed the resignation that characterized the end of many careers:

> I started in the breaker and went back to it again,
> But now my work is finished for all time;
> The only place that's left me is the almshouse for a home,
> That's where I'll lay this weary head of mine.[31]

Such a sorry conclusion to a lifetime of honest labor stood in sharp contrast to the comfortable old age of mine employers.

An unrelenting, incurable condition, pneumoconiosis hastened the demise of many anthracite veterans. For the deaths officially attributed to pneumoconiosis in the decade 1893–1902, the mean age at death was fifty-five. Stephen Crane contended that for the miner lucky enough to avoid a fatal injury "there usually comes . . . an attack of 'miner's asthma' that slowly racks and shakes him into the grave." Condy Brislin of Hazleton, who succumbed to the disease in 1880, considered death a relief. His epitaph, composed by his son, expressed not only that feeling but also immortal bitterness:

> Fourty [sic] years I worked with pick and drill
> Down in the mines against my will
> The Coal Kings slave but now it's passed
> Thanks be to God I am free at last.[32]

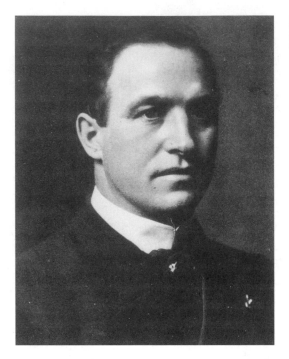

John Mitchell, ca. 1902.
(Courtesy of the United Mine
Workers of America)

The growing disparity between the operators' fortunes and the miners' misfortunes led to a dramatic confrontation at the turn of the century. Beginning in the late 1890s, hard-coal workers attempted to improve their chances for a better life by joining the United Mine Workers of America. Throughout the union organizing campaign, deepening consciousness of the human cost of industrialization helped to confer legitimacy on increasingly forceful collective action. Shocked by the unhealthful working conditions and other miseries of the breaker boys, John Mitchell applauded their youthful militance. "In their parades they carry banners saying 'Give our fathers justice and we can go to school,'" Mitchell sympathetically observed during the strike of 1900. If the union could increase pay sufficiently, it could make the system of family employment unnecessary, and children would be liberated from the breakers. The compromise settlement in the 1900 dispute fell short of this grand objective, however.[33]

The climactic encounter in this struggle came two years later. The strike that broke out in May 1902 was, among many other things, an attempt to curtail child labor by raising adults' compensation. Pursuing demands for better pay, shorter hours, and union recognition, the organized workforce of 150,000 shut down the anthracite mines for five months. In terms of worker-days lost, this was by far the largest strike in the nation's history up to that time. As winter approached, the dispute threatened to create a shortage of home-heating fuel across the eastern United States.[34]

The mounting crisis precipitated federal intervention. Whereas Eugene Debs went to jail on federal charges for his role in the Pullman strike only eight years earlier, the UMW's John Mitchell went to the White House on October 3, 1902, to confer with Theodore Roosevelt. The operators' arrogance at the White House conference, together with the indispensability of hard coal to the national economy, forced innovative action. After refusing the mine owners' request for U.S. troops, Roosevelt prevailed upon them to accede to the union's proposal to submit the dispute to a presidential arbitration commission, whose decision would bind the parties. On October 23, the miners went back to work.[35]

The UMW welcomed the opportunity to present its grievances in an unprecedented open forum. The moderate Mitchell sought not only to gain a favorable settlement but to demonstrate to the general public that unions were respectable institutions with just aims. These aims included not merely the immediate objectives of higher wages and shorter hours. They also encompassed a more thorough reckoning of the human cost of the development of the hard-coal industry. In its appeals for public support, the union underscored its sacrifices in enhancing the welfare of the nation as a whole: "When we look upon the enormous fortunes that our labor has made possible, with the innumerable comforts and luxuries that it brings to the people at large, and then examine the paltry pittance we undergo [sic], the dampness we must endure, the foul air we must breathe, and the peculiar rheumatic and lung troubles superinduced by these conditions which we must bear, we naturally feel that we are being unjustly dealt with." The proceedings of the Anthracite Coal Strike Commission gave the UMW a unique chance to win popular sympathy for its cause.[36]

Observers outside the union also cast the dispute in terms of human progress. The inveterate radical Mother Jones portrayed the battle as an accounting for many years of suffering under the "most intolerable and inhuman conditions." At the other end of the ideological spectrum, at least one highly conservative member of the business community treated this as a matter of national importance. "Most of the arguments against child labor are based on the highest considerations of good citizenship and the future of the race," maintained Frederick Hoffman, an executive at Prudential Life Insurance much involved with health policy. "Children deprived of light and air, exposed to dust, and at work underground, must needs suffer bodily injury if such work is carried to excess." Whether viewed in terms of prospective developments or past injustices, the work stoppage in eastern Pennsylvania took on a larger significance.[37]

The UMW hurriedly put together a comprehensive case for the strike commission. In the midst of these preparations, union leaders received a long, apparently unsolicited letter. After twenty-nine years of medical practice in the region, John Jones wrote to advise Mitchell and his colleagues that "[p]erhaps there are no 'trade' diseases better known or more constantly occurring than those to which coal miners are addicted, and notably that very common one—Miner's Consumption." Jones attested to the decline of the typical victim: "It will not be many years before he becomes a confirmed and incurable Asthmatic, which will incapacitate him from following the work of an active miner and eventually compel him to take a subordinate position, which does not require much exertion, such as that of door keeper." He also shed light on the miners' tenacity against deepening impairment: "I have in the course of my experience seen many evidences where patients would continue working at the mines when scarcely able to crawl and when they knew that it meant sure death to them in a few years." This experienced practitioner offered a graphic description of the final state of pneumoconiotics: "I have often seen them, post mortem, in such a carbonaceous condition that I could write with the fluid that could be expressed from the lungs."[38] Jones articulated themes and images that the Mine Workers could readily elaborate in portraying miners as hard-working martyrs to industrialism. The union would stand for men who crawled to work.

In the hearings that commenced in Scranton on November 14, 1902, the UMW case, coordinated by attorney Clarence Darrow, dwelt at length on the dire consequences of underground work. To be sure, at no time did the miners' organization demand eradication of the dust hazard in the hard-coal mines. Instead, the UMW reasoned that the heavy toll taken by chronic respiratory ailments helped to justify higher wages and shorter hours. In his opening statement, John Mitchell contended that health risks warranted a wage increase: "If he [the miner] escapes death or injury by falls of rock or coal, he cannot escape attacks of miners' asthma." In his summation, Darrow decried a system that sentenced young children to labor in an "everlasting cloud" of dust because of the inadequate wages paid their fathers. Mitchell maintained that part of the rationale for the eight-hour workday was the unhealthful nature of anthracite extraction.[39]

The union brought in a number of physicians and disabled miners to corroborate its claims. These witnesses described miners' asthma in stark detail, from beginning to end. Dr. John O'Malley of Scranton considered this a disorder brought about by "the inhalation of great quantities of coal dust and powder smoke and vitiated air." O'Malley held that the lungs became "saturated with this coal dust, . . . [which] acts as an irritant." He noted that on postmortem examination, the veteran miner's lung "looks like a chunk of anthracite coal." Dr. Eugene Butler testified that sections of miners' lung tissue removed at autopsy sank when placed in water, whereas normal lung tissue floated. He explained the difference in tissue density by the retention of mineral particles. The union's medical consultants maintained that many workers' difficulties stemmed from the heavy doses of dust incurred while picking slate as boys.[40]

The UMW physicians identified several clinical facets of pneumoconiosis. The disorder was called miners' asthma mainly because of the extreme, often paroxysmal, dyspnea that its victims exhibited. Dr. James Lenahan informed the commission that some individuals could not lie down to sleep and had to "sit up at night gasping for breath." In Lenahan's assessment, "Many times they are unable to walk." Dr. Richard Gibbons focused on those who were somewhat less disabled. Gibbons characterized the typical advanced patient as "the marked picture of distress that is commonly seen, an individual walking along and being overtaken by air starvation, so to speak." Men with miners' asthma who testified also confirmed their difficulty in breathing. Melanoptysis particularly impressed Dr. Butler. When asked to describe the sputum of one of his patients, he replied, "You could use it for ink."[41]

The pro-union physicians traced their patients' decline. When dust exposure began in boyhood, symptoms emerged at a relatively early age. Lenehan claimed to have seen asthmatic miners only thirty years old. O'Malley held that the typical victim was "really as old at the age of 40 as another man in another vocation at the age of 70. He has a decrepid [sic], dull, haggard, emaciated appearance, and he looks prematurely old; in fact, is prematurely old." O'Malley also noted that some individuals with miners' asthma eventually developed emphysema. He and his colleagues concurred that the disease ultimately became quite crippling. The overriding practical question remained the capacity to perform work. Lenehan reported that pneumoconiotics lost earnings due to their respiratory impairment and that many were not even able to walk. Patrick Welsh testified that miners' asthma significantly limited his ability to labor underground. John Devenney told the commission that at age fifty-one the disorder had driven him down into a job cleaning coal along with children, for $0.90 per ten-hour day. Butler pointed out that "these old men that pick slate in the breakers, they do not last long." Some of those who dropped out of the work force sought Civil War veterans' pensions when they reached sixty-five. A former federal pension examiner, O'Malley averred that almost 90 percent of the former coal workers who applied for these entitlements had miners' asthma.[42]

Not every search for respectable relief ended well. The hearings shed harsh light on the plight of disabled elders who fell into the poorhouse. From four years' experience as medical director of the Wilkes-Barre almshouse, Eugene Butler estimated that about 70 percent of its inhabitants were former anthracite workers, "a great many" of whom suffered from miners' asthma. Lenahan likewise believed that 70 percent of the inmates of another nearby poorhouse came from the mines. He estimated that 60 percent of these ex-miners had lung trouble. Given their disability and their humiliation, it is not surprising that no pneumoconiotic inmates of these institutions appeared to testify.[43]

The UMW case lacked corroborating vital statistics. It offered no quantitative evidence on the average longevity for victims of occupational disease. In fact, the miners' organization attempted to gather such data from the insurance industry, only to learn that life insurance carriers refused to cover anthracite miners. Because the union had based its wage and hour demands in part on claims of diminished life expectancy and, more specifically, claims of shortened careers, the absence of statistical data weakened its case. In the same vein, labor witnesses made only the most informal estimates of the prevalence of miners' asthma. In O'Malley's view, there were "very few . . . who can escape at least moderate attacks of this, whose occupation or environment is such that they they inhale this dust." Under cross-examination, however, he conceded that he possessed "no statistics about it whatever." Butler called miners' asthma "quite a com-

mon occurrence among the miners, after a number of years in the mines."
In defense of this assertion, he offered to bring one hundred patients to the
next day's hearings. Without giving a reason, the arbitrators chose not
to pursue this opportunity to venture into makeshift clinical epidemiology. (Nor did the UMW take advantage of a chance to dramatize the issue
by summoning a crowd of pneumoconiotics to the Lackawanna County
Courthouse.) Veteran miner John Stannix boldly estimated that half the
anthracite work force had miners' asthma. John Mitchell went even further, asserting that "there is scarcely a mine-worker who has not contracted this malady to some degree." A strong, if vague, sense of the sizable magnitude of the dust-disease problem had diffused throughout the
hard-coal territory.[44]

Obviously, the revelations of these witnesses helped physicians, operators, miners, and the general public within the anthracite region to comprehend industrial disease. The press carried the story to a national audience. The *New York Times* recounted O'Malley's observation of lungs
black as coal and quoted Mitchell's contention that older miners could
not escape occupational disease. The *Chicago Tribune* also seized on O'Malley's vivid description of autopsies in an article subtitled "Few Escape the
Asthma." The *Pittsburgh Press* ran a front-page story, which declared that
"the avocation of miner usually brings on miners' asthma" and that "com-
plications resulting from miners' asthma were usually fatal." Unsurpris-
ingly, the media stressed the most sensational statements on the matter.[45]

As expected, the mine owners counterattacked. In his opening statement, S. P. Wolverton of the Philadelphia and Reading Coal and Iron Company promised to show that "mining is not an unhealthy occupation."
James H. Torrey of the Delaware and Hudson Railroad advised the commission that digging anthracite was "more than ordinarily healthful." To
this end, the operators leaned heavily on British mortality data that appeared to show that overall death rates for coal mining were relatively low.
Clarence Darrow and commissioner John Spalding replied that such occupational data were distorted by the departure of a substantial share of the
disabled from mining before they died, so that their deaths were charged
against some other occupation (like watchman) or against no occupation
at all.[46]

The attorneys and witnesses for the operators attempted not to deny the
existence of dust-induced disease but rather to minimize the issue. Com-

pany doctors held that they seldom encountered miners' asthma. After acknowledging that miners' asthma was the vernacular term for the pneumoconiosis anthracosis, Dr. W. G. Fulton discounted the disorder as "not very prevalent." William Dolan testified that his survey of poorhouse residents turned up only thirty-three cases of miners' asthma, most of whom he dismissed as disabled primarily by alcohol, not by mine dust. The mine owners brought in several foremen and superintendents to swear that they had a minimal number of asthma victims and a large complement of robust elderly employees. Seward Button had many healthy old men working underground and only one case of miners' asthma among the 200 employees he supervised for the Hillside Coal and Iron Company. Medical representatives of management explained the infrequency of pneumoconiosis in anthracite workers by arguing that coal particles posed less risk than other types of industrial dust. But when asked whether inhalation of coal dust would tend to prolong or shorten one's life, company doctor Fulton stated that "probably it would shorten it." The union had set the terms of this debate, placing management in a defensive posture. Yet at the same time, the coal operators were beginning to shift the battleground to more favorable terrain by their questioning of the magnitude of the dust-disease phenomenon.[47]

Pressed for an immediate decision and buried by an avalanche of contradictory and often unverifiable testimony (amounting to more than 10,000 pages) and accompanying exhibits on a long list of complex issues, the Anthracite Coal Strike Commission faced an impossible task. Hence, it is understandable that in crafting a compromise settlement the commissioners devoted very little attention to industrial disease, which it regarded as a difficult question of secondary importance. In its report to President Roosevelt on March 18, 1903 (i.e., less than five weeks after adjournment of its hearings), the commission granted, without delving into the respiratory-disease controversy per se, that some increase in wages should be made in part because of "the hazardous nature of the employment."[48]

The 1903 arbitration commission settled nothing with regard to the nature and magnitude of the respiratory diseases besetting hard-coal miners. Federal intervention did not extend to initiatives to gather new information that would bear the imprimatur of national authority. In its circum-

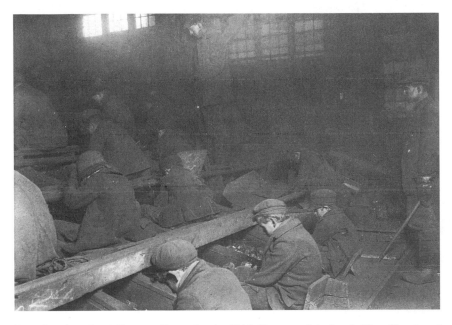

Ewen breaker, South Pittston, Pennsylvania, 1911. Photograph by Lewis Hine. (Reprinted from *Child Labor Bulletin*)

scribed role as the ad hoc adjudicator of exceptional labor disputes, the federal government lacked the time and resources to uncover the full extent of the miners' afflictions. Nonetheless, the strike inquiry raised considerably the visibility of pneumoconiosis. Even in a forum that only recorded and attempted to resolve conflicting private claims, the relatively passive state served to illuminate the human cost of industrialization.

This struggle also brought the United Mine Workers to the forefront of the effort to create public understanding of pneumoconiosis. The union established itself as the champion of aging laborers who struggled to work to help support their families. Despite lacking its own scientific expertise, organized labor managed to frame the debate. Even the coal operators grudgingly conceded that miners' asthma existed. Management fell back to a defensive insistence that not very many men crawled to work. Thus, the union effectively used the deliberations of the Anthracite Coal Strike Commission as a platform to promote understanding of miners' respiratory disease.

In the short term, however, expanded knowledge did not transform the social relations of producing coal. The federal commission did not grant a pay increase sufficient to allow anthracite miners to keep their sons in school. In the aftermath of the strike, the number of children employed in the breakers and in other unhealthful worksites in and around the mines continued to grow. In 1906, the National Child Labor Committee estimated that approximately ten thousand boys under the age of fourteen worked illegally in the hard-coal fields.[49]

CHAPTER THREE

THE ATMOSPHERE OF THE MINE IS NOW VINDICATED

An amazing reversal occurred after the 1902 anthracite strike. The working environment in both hard coal and soft coal came to be widely regarded as relatively harmless. In the assessment of leading representatives of medicine and industry, the ailment known as miners' asthma became a small problem or no problem at all. The voices of a few dissenters went virtually unheard outside the ranks of the miners. The production of misunderstanding took considerable exertion and even some contortions. Nonetheless, by 1930 denial of coal workers' respiratory difficulties had triumphed in the United States.

Physicians and other professionals led the campaign to exonerate coal mine dust. Confronting the Progressive reformers who disentangled the intricacies of many working-class problems during this period, conservatives in the professions moved decisively to dominate the discussion of miners' lung disorders. In a time of socialist and other mass working-class radical movements, class polarization turned many middle-class doctors, engineers, and journalists into loyal partners of the mine operators. The underdeveloped middle class in small mining communities often lacked the autonomy to promote an independent perspective on matters such as industrial disease. In particular, physicians aligned with coal management aggressively proclaimed the innocence of underground conditions. The expansion of trade and professional associations and other voluntary organizations helped to spread the message that mining did little or no damage to miners' lungs.[1]

Defenders of the working conditions in coal challenged their opponents' scientific claims. They launched a frontal assault on the anatomists' sensational accounts of the state of deceased miners' lungs. In the aftermath of the anthracite settlement, the coal industry heralded British assertions that anthracosis constituted neither a disease nor a cause of disease. Instead, in R. S. Trotter's formulation, black lung tissue merely coincided with some cases of respiratory illness.[2] A number of investigators went further, denying that anthracosis provided even a reliable marker for disease. To Samuel Haythorn, among others, blackened tissue represented only a harmless discoloration. Haythorn, a pathologist at the University of Pittsburgh, conducted inhalation experiments of ten days' duration on one guinea pig and of eighty-seven days' duration on one rabbit. On this basis, he decided that "moderate anthracosis in an otherwise normal lung is not detrimental to health." The fact that residents of polluted urban areas who had not died from any lung condition commonly had darkened lungs on necropsy permitted the inference that similar pigmentation in miners by itself might well indicate little or nothing regarding respiratory impairment.[3]

Even the melanoptysis that had so cogently confirmed the connection between the clinical condition of the living and the findings of postmortem examination took on a positive meaning in the early twentieth century. Contributing an entry on dust diseases to an American textbook in occupational medicine, the prominent British authority Thomas Oliver in 1924 pronounced this sign a blessing: "Miners keep bringing up large quantities of black spit for years after they have ceased working in coal—a circumstance which shows not only that considerable deposits of carbon had taken place in the lungs but that the lungs tend to rid themselves of the deposited carbon largely by means of the action of pulmonary phagocytes." The body's natural defenses were amply capable of defeating potential lung disorders.[4]

The revanchists pushed furthest with the contention that inhaled coal dust guarded miners against tuberculosis. This claim won considerable support in the early twentieth century. At a time when tuberculosis still loomed as the scourge of the working class, this was no small matter.[5] The protective hypothesis turned attention away from any deleterious effects of inhalation of microscopic coal particles. Moreover, it accentuated the contrast between coal dust and the increasingly well known hazard posed by silicious dusts, which fostered a predisposition to tubercular infection.

Dusts generally were regarded with suspicion in relation to tuberculosis at the turn of the century. Prevailing hygienic doctrine deemed dust particles natural vehicles for the airborne transmission of the tubercle bacillus. Biomedical science held these inanimate vectors responsible for carrying germs into the breathing zone of individuals at home, in the workplace, and on the street. In addition, mineral and metallic dusts were seen as irritants that increased the lung's vulnerability to infection. In the Progressive Era, public health analysts began to comment on the high rates of consumption among employees in the dusty trades.[6]

In this context it was extraordinary to consider dust not an accomplice in the induction of tuberculosis but rather an impediment to that process. But just such a line of reasoning came into prominence. Once again, British work guided thinking in the United States. In 1885, three years after Robert Koch's discovery of the tubercle bacillus, Andrew Smart, in a presentation before the British Medical Association, explained the rarity of consumption among coal workers by postulating that "there must be some special protective feature in coal-mining operations not shared in by the rest of the dusty trades." Reflecting the influence of germ theory, Smart cited the "antiseptic properties of carbon" as the beneficial factor at work. Pennsylvania coal operators made this argument before the anthracite strike commission, but had difficulty sustaining it.[7]

In the years after the hard-coal dispute, advocates of the anti-tubercular qualities of coal dust regrouped for a forceful counterattack. Jonathan Wainwright, a Scranton physician who had testified on the operators' behalf before the ACSC, and Harry Nichols, a Washington, D.C., physician, assessed the relationship between anthracosis and tuberculosis in a seminal article in the *American Journal of the Medical Sciences* in 1905. "We have all heard," Wainwright and Nichols began, "that miners have a tendency to immunity from tuberculosis, that coal dust prevents tuberculosis, and that it even has a curative effect when tuberculosis is once developed." They reinforced these points by a review of the extensive European literature, including reports that doctors treated pulmonary tuberculosis with doses of coal particles.[8]

Wainwright and Nichols tested and rejected the hypothesis that coal dust (or, more specifically, the sulphur or some other chemical substance in coal) acted directly to kill bacteria. Their laboratory experiments found that "the dust has no germicidal action whatever." Having dispatched the most widespread explanation for the apparent infrequency of tuberculosis in coal workers, they proposed an alternative. Their research suggested that coal particles in the lung helped to protect against the tubercle bacillus by stimulating the growth of fibrotic connective tissue. Fibrosis, in this analysis, functioned both in "preventing the bacilli from getting a foothold and in overcoming them when once established."[9]

Wainwright and Nichols also maintained that coal mines presented an environment inhospitable to infection. Bacteria had difficulty traveling to the main worksites underground: "The air supplied to chambers passes slowly through damp gangways sometimes a half mile. During this passage many bacteria fall to the ground so that the air when supplied to the chambers has undergone a purification by sedimentation just as takes place in rivers." In addition, such sprawling, uncrowded working spaces gave little opportunity for contagion. Coal mines compared favorably to cramped sweatshops and other disease-ridden places of employment.[10]

Many in medicine embraced and built upon this assessment. When, for example, Wainwright and Nichols presented their analysis in the heart of the hard-coal region, one member of the Luzerne County Medical Society hailed it as "a treat for the members of the Society." Another physician at the meeting speculated that the mechanical action of inhaled coal particles in the lung conferred invulnerability to infection. By 1911, Osler's textbook used Wainwright and Nichols to explain the low rates of tuberculosis among anthracite workers. Recurrent citation of this study long after 1905 both further established and reflected its authoritative status.[11]

At least one physician agnostically endorsed extractive labor without delving into the question of the sources of immunity from tuberculosis. After twenty-five years treating bituminous miners in Illinois, Dr. M. C. Carr considered them "practically immune from tubercular infection" but gave no scientific rationale for this position. Instead, Carr demonstrated consensus by conducting a survey of practitioners in mining communities in Illinois, Indiana, Ohio, Pennsylvania, and West Virginia. Among more than 200 colleagues who responded to his questionnaire, approximately three quarters agreed that mine workers were not susceptible to tuberculosis.[12]

The coal industry itself often proclaimed the salubrity of its working conditions with respect to the "white plague." In 1904, the *Coal Trade Journal* announced that the disinfective power of coal dust had prompted a proposal in Silesia to erect a sanitarium at the mines. *Coal Age* continually asserted that the sulphur in coal acted as a germicide, despite mounting medical skepticism of this hypothesis. In 1912, this preeminent trade journal reacted angrily to plans by the U.S. Public Health Service (PHS) and the U.S. Bureau of Mines (BOM) to study tuberculosis in the mining workforce. Contrasting coal miners and metal miners, an editorial averred the "comparative immunity among men working at the coal face." Shortly thereafter, the weekly underscored that message with a series of articles by Wainwright and Nichols.[13]

With the seemingly overwhelming accumulation of evidence that anthracite and bituminous workplaces harbored no bacteria, all that remained was to declare victory. In 1915, the editor of *Coal Age* announced that "the atmosphere of the mine is now vindicated even though its healthfulness has not yet been extolled." The following year, the journal pronounced the coal mine "always a healthful place for men and a baleful place for microbes." In 1924, a participant in the annual meeting of the Coal Mining Institute of America reported the case of a man who cured his tuberculosis by taking a highly dusty job. The coal mine had acquired the image of a sort of underground sanitarium. Civil society not only solved this problem without state interference but educated the public on the accomplishment.[14]

The view that inhaling coal dust was harmless also derived in large measure from repeated comparison with the threat posed by another type of particulate frequently encountered in bituminous and anthracite workplaces. Unquestionably, exposure to the silicious dusts associated with sandstone, slate, and other minerals that occurred with coal deposits posed a serious threat to some mine workers. In the early twentieth century, however, for many observers this undeniable threat overshadowed the coal dust hazard to the point that the latter virtually disappeared. Indeed, by the 1920s the study of pneumoconiosis faced the seductive hazard of reductionism.

Contrasts between carbonaceous and silicious dusts predated the twentieth century. From the mid-nineteenth century on, British, German, and French clinicians and scientists differentiated among dust hazards of the workplace. North Americans took cognizance of numerous European studies of silicosis among extractive workers. Moreover, those in this country concerned with chronic respiratory disorders could hardly avoid the comparisons repeatedly drawn between the plainly deleterious effects of inhaling microscopic rock particles and the less dramatic effects of in-haling coal particles. By 1905 it was uncontroversial for Wainwright and Nichols to note in passing that "all agree that stone-dust is much more in-jurious than coal-dust."[15]

Before the 1920s, the predominant theory of the pathogenesis of pneu-moconiosis emphasized the physical characteristics of dust particles. The hard, sharp, angular nature of silica particles was thought to induce dis-ease by a mechanical process of irritation. Conversely, the softer, less an-gular nature of the smallest coal fragments explained their relatively lower propensity to produce respiratory disease. To Henry Landis of the Univer-sity of Pennsylvania, lower risk expressed itself not by the simple absence of pathology but instead by its delayed onset: "Owing to the fact that coal dust is relatively the least dangerous of the inorganic dusts, years may elapse before symptoms arise which are indicative of serious pulmonary damage." Initially, coal particles were still believed to be a risk to respira-tory health, but a lesser one than silica.[16]

This contrast opened the way to the view that coal dust posed no hazard at all. British science again played a key role in reorienting North Ameri-can thinking. In the Milroy Lectures of 1915, Edgar Collis virtually col-lapsed pneumoconiosis into silicosis. Collis made the analogy that "just as all germs are not pathogenic, so all kinds of non-viable particles do not give rise to pneumoconioses." Appropriating the principle of specificity from the hegemonic germ theory, Collis carefully linked the specific etio-logic agent silica to specific pathological processes. He related these, in turn, to the characteristic clinical picture of silicosis. Collis illustrated his interpretation with numerous cases of illness among potters, tool and cut-lery grinders, and gold and tin miners—a collective portrait that gave only scant mention to coal workers. If coal miners incurred pneumoconio-sis, they must have inhaled rock dust. To leave no doubt on this question, Collis flatly declared coal dust "not injurious." Against this lucid, elegant formulation, the relatively unclear pathogenesis and generally amorphous adverse effects of coal dust and of the mixed dusts of coal mines receded into inauthenticity. Collis thus in one stroke attacked both anthracosis and the generic conceptualization of pneumoconiosis.[17]

Collis also underscored the exceptional capacity of silica to foster tuber-culosis. His study of national mortality data determined that excess deaths from tuberculosis in dusty occupations were "always found associated with exposure to dust containing crystalline silica." He contrasted this predisposition to infection with the favored status of those who breathed coal dust. Indeed, in the finale to his last lecture, Collis made a point of repeating that "some dusts, such as coal . . . not only appear to have no power of producing pneumonoconioses, but even may possess some inhibitory influence on phthisis." Together with his other findings, this assessment forged a single-minded preoccupation with silicious dust.[18]

Collis used a set of radiographs of silicosis to illustrate his final Milroy Lecture. Though hardly the centerpiece of his presentation, these images were helpful in making differential diagnoses in chronic lung disease cases, he maintained. None of the X-rays showed the lungs of a coal miner. None referred to the characteristic radiographic appearance presented by large deposits of coal mine dust. The reductionism implicit in this particular facet of his handling of pneumoconiosis would prove to be crucial for decades to come.[19]

Collis's lectures found a substantial and receptive audience in the United States. Many accepted without hesitation his equation of dust disease with silicosis. No participant in the 1927 meeting of the American Institute of Mining and Metallurgical Engineers took exception to Collis's statement that "coal dust does not in itself appear to exert any particularly harmful effect on the lungs." In 1923, the hygiene publication of the American Medical Association declared that "exact and particular observation has shown that the inhalation of coal dust unmixed with sand does not lead to diseases of the lungs, even though it may lead to anthracosis." Anthracosis had become a benign, if ugly, discoloration of the lungs. The same year, Henry Pancoast defended fixation on silicosis in a paper at the American Congress of Internal Medicine. The University of Pennsylvania investigator presumed scientific consensus:

> It has been generally conceded that the important injurious constituent of dust is silica, and it is the constituent that is active in the production of fibrosis in any dusty occupation in which individuals acquire pneumoconiosis. This condition is in reality the effect produced by silica, and it might just as well be termed silicosis. It is true that among coal miners, coal dust is taken up into the pulmonary lymphatics in rather large amounts, . . . but it probably plays a very minor part in the production of fibrosis.

Whereas in the scientific study of infectious disease after 1880 the discovery of one germ gave impetus to searches for a host of others, in the study of the pneumoconioses after 1915 there arose a systematic attempt to explain every illness by one cause. In a sense, biomedical science imploded.[20]

In partnership with protégé Eugene Pendergrass, Pancoast took advantage of the growing legitimacy and importance of silicosis to establish industrial radiology as a medical subspecialty. The first professor of roentgenology appointed at any U.S. medical school and a former president of the American Roentgen Ray Society, Pancoast possessed by the mid-twenties the personal authority and institutional resources to sponsor a new branch of applied science. Moreover, armed with expertise in a technology that appeared objective and efficient, the University of Pennsylvania radiologist set out to contribute to the rationalization as well as the specialization of medicine. Dismissal of anthracosis demonstrated a rigor deemed imperative in this discipline-building project. In 1925, Pancoast and Pendergrass issued a reductionist manifesto in the *American Journal of Roentgenology and Radium Therapy*: "Anthracosis, siderosis and chalicosis imply occupation only, as the active agent in all of them is silica." Coal dust, on the other hand, was classified as inert. In a foray beyond their sphere of expertise, the radiologists interpreted even melanoptysis as a sign of silicosis, and a positive one at that: "A coal miner who stops work may have black sputum for two to four years afterwards. Certainly these and many other observations would seem to indicate that silicosis may be arrested or even regress." Under this ambitious revisionism, out-of-work miners spewing black spit would soon virtually disappear, abstracted into little more than nebulous X-ray shadows.[21]

To accomplish the central task of elucidating the radiologic indications of dust disease, Pancoast and Pendergrass turned their article into a monograph. The title of this volume, *Pneumoconiosis [Silicosis]*, perfectly conveyed its fundamental theme. The authors reiterated the need to differentiate among the hazards posed by various dusts, including their opinion that coal dust was "relatively harmless." They then gave a detailed, extensively illustrated overview of silicosis. Throughout, the partners endeavored to synthesize other recent advances with their own radiological studies. Silica dust retained in the lungs gave rise to fibrotic nodules and other lesions that the imaging technology of the 1920s captured quite vividly. Hence, Pancoast and Pendergrass could guide their colleagues through the progression of fibrosis, culminating in the dramatic coalescence of masses of scar tissue, often with the complication of tuberculosis. By offering a

three-stage classification system to order this progression and by expli-
cating the pathological process that drove cases through it, they neatly
packaged the chronic illness caused by silicious dusts. Needless to say, the
now-obsolete condition of anthracosis did not receive similar attention in
this book.[22]

Even as they narrowed the horizons of occupational respiratory disease,
Pancoast and Pendergrass allowed for the small possibility that silicosis
might not constitute the whole domain. Yet this judicious concession itself
came with a measure of skepticism: "We have assumed that silica is not the
sole etiological factor in pneumoconiosis, but in this we may be wrong."
Although Pancoast and Pendergrass nominally rejected reductionism,
they never seriously explored the hypothesis that coal dust caused any
significant disease. Most amazingly, they took passing notice of but failed
to attach any importance to the occurrence of pneumoconiosis among lo-
comotive firemen, a group of coal shovelers who experienced negligible, if
any, exposure to silicious dust. In light of such obliviousness to this potentially provocative fact, their profession of open-mindedness on the haz-
ardousness of nonsilicious dusts rang hollow.[23]

Pancoast and Pendergrass strained to install their own subspecialty as
the best way to comprehend dust disease. "The roentgen-ray examination
is really the most important means of studying the condition in the living
individual," they declaimed, "and this aspect of the subject should be fostered in every possible way." To be sure, they acknowledged that full
understanding of pneumoconiosis depended upon a firm grasp of the underlying morbid anatomy. But whereas pathological anatomists had correlated clinical features of illness with injured lung tissue seen on postmortem dissection, the industrial radiologists endeavored to visualize
internal damage in their patients and to identify certain X-ray images as lesions. Implicitly set aside in this approach were the sick person's symptoms and signs. Accordingly, this volume gave cursory lists of clinical observations of patients without integrating these to any significant extent
into the interpretation of the case at hand. Even the melanoptysis that had
stirred the imagination of nineteenth-century students of dust disease
merited no comment. Thus, the authors' assertion that they possessed the
"most important means of studying the condition in the living individual"
was vitiated by treating the living individual as if he were already dead
and incapable of helping to describe and explain his situation. Special-

ization caused a fragmentation of knowledge, and some fragments got misplaced.[24]

Pancoast and Pendergrass drew out another key difference. Deposits of coal dust tended to make fuzzy radiographic images, in contrast to the more well-defined markings associated with silica retention. In this regard, *Pneumoconiosis [Silicosis]* continued a line of interpretation that Pancoast and others had pursued as early as 1918. In 1919, for instance, Henry Landis, Pancoast's colleague at the University of Pennsylvania, had noticed that "in the case of the less irritating form of dust the spots are not so sharply defined." The less distinct quality of the shadows found in many aging coal miners made it easier to dismiss uncertain self-reports of difficult breathing and to return to the relative simplicity of classical silicosis.[25]

A third line of reasoning helped exonerate coal dust. This was the contention that even if sustained exposure to very high doses of microscopic bits of coal might lead to respiratory impairment, no such exposure occurred in U.S. mines in the early twentieth century.

The argument depended upon a sort of retrospective recognition. The coal industry admitted that air quality had been unhealthful in years past. But, it contended, the underground dust hazard no longer existed. The British again created the template for North American apologists. In 1908, for instance, Thomas Oliver's text in occupational medicine announced great progress: "Fifty years ago coal-miners' phthisis, or anthracosis, was a well-known disease; today, thanks to the well-ventilated condition of our coal-mines, the malady has remarkably diminished in Great Britain." In a subsequent article in the *Journal of Industrial Hygiene*, Oliver put this idea directly before occupational health specialists in this country.[26] In 1916, *Coal Age* happily reported similar advances in the United States: "In the olden days, many of the miners had miners' asthma, and it was thought to be owing to coal dust inhalation. In recent years, however, asthma among miners is rare, and this improvement is due in a measure to better ventilation in the mines." A large-scale survey by Metropolitan Life Insurance Company in 1917 put the prevalence of miners' asthma at less than one per thousand for bituminous employees and at less than three per thousand for anthracite employees. But historical data on changes in underground dust concentrations were entirely absent from these reports.[27]

Coal miners' overall health purportedly reflected all these blessings. Employed in well-ventilated workplaces where they inhaled little silica and some harmless coal dust, bituminous and anthracite workers enjoyed above-average longevity, according to some analysts. After subtracting fatal injuries, Wainwright and Nichols found that hard-coal miners in Scranton outlived males in other occupations. Dr. Samuel Mengel of the Lehigh Valley Coal Company boasted that mortality rates for miners were below those of farmers, whose work in the open air remained the benchmark for healthful employment.[28]

Industry representatives broadcast this optimistic message. The paucity of relevant statistics for the United States permitted continued citation of British data. When, for instance, Edgar Collis discussed the low mortality from lung ailments in Nottinghamshire and Derbyshire in a 1927 presentation in this country, *Coal Age* quoted excerpts from his paper.[29] Rather than confine itself to tedious comparative analysis of occupational mortality statistics, the trade journal offered up numerous flesh-and-blood cases of hearty elderly miners. An article in 1915 titled "The Long Life of Coal Miners" featured a photograph of five active employees of the Susquehanna Coal Company. This stalwart group, whose tenure with the firm ranged from thirty-two to forty-four years, averaged seventy-three years of age. "That the life of the miner is laborious but is not unhealthy," this article reasoned, "is proved by the large number of old men in and around the mines, many of whom started work long before what is now the legal age." Thus, even child labor became a source of pride (as, apparently, did the absence of a pension plan for employees over the age of seventy who had given their employer more than thirty years of service). Later the same year, *Coal Age* celebrated the ninety-eighth birthday of James Farrar, who had worked in the mines of Alabama past age seventy-five. The occasion provided another opportunity to proclaim the longevity of the coal workforce and to dismiss anthracosis as an inconsequential discoloration of the lungs. "There are no healthier men anywhere," the editorial on Farrar's birthday stated, "than in the mining industry."[30]

In 1916, the industry journal invited scientific investigation into the "phenomenally long life" of miners. At the same time, with the mine laborers' difficulties swept aside, other occupational ailments rose in priority. In 1919, *Coal Age* warned of the threats facing some aboveground employees:

The chief executive himself is . . . apt to think that because he has the distinction of control conferred on him, he is bound to exhibit a greater persistence in labors and a more ardent devotion to his duties than any of his subordinates. As a result he breaks down in a few years. He loses his poise and develops executivitis—an occupational disease in which the stomach ceases to function, sleep is denied and the nerves give way.

Plainly, by the 1920, the coal industry had shifted to an offensive stance regarding its occupational health hazards.[31]

Exoneration of coal dust exercised less than hegemonic influence, however. A number of observers contested the glowing assessment of working conditions and their human consequences. Certainly, accounts of the situation in hard coal in the years after the big strike gave no indication of any substantial abatement of the dust hazard. Coal breakers, for example, remained exceedingly dusty. In 1905, Owen Lovejoy of the National Child Labor Committee (NCLC) lamented that young slate pickers still had to wear miner's lamps in order to see the coal at their feet. Lovejoy did note one sign of progress: in one anthracite mill, an exhaust fan cleared the air so that he had enough light to obtain "a dim picture" with his camera. Photographer Lewis Hine, whom the NCLC sent to the anthracite region in 1911, gained access to a breaker but found that "the dust was so thick, most of the time I was there, as to obscure the view of the boys." In addition to the many journalists and reformers who elaborated on the sorry air quality in the anthracite-processing plants, Progressives found at least one representative of management to confirm their appraisal. "No boy of mine will ever go in that hell," foreman Thomas Walker told an NCLC investigator in 1912. "About twenty boys working in [my] breaker, and I bet that you could shovel fifty pounds of coal dust out of their systems." Walker made no mention of the prophylactic value of dust exposure against tuberculosis.[32]

A modicum of quantitative data supported this negative view. In their often-cited 1905 article, Wainwright and Nichols published the results of dust monitoring conducted in an unspecified number of anthracite breakers. They found a mean concentration of 396 milligrams of particulate matter per cubic meter of air, that is, almost two hundred times the current federal limit on permissible exposure to coal mine dust. Technical concerns yielded a rough measure of the severity of the hazard. One mining engineer estimated in 1910 that, on average, the 320 breakers in eastern Pennsylvania reduced to dust about 2 percent of the raw coal they handled. This meant that the typical breaker generated at least twenty tons of dust per working day.[33]

For the industry as a whole, the acclaimed advances in ventilation were, in all probability, offset by other forms of mechanization that exacerbated respiratory hazards. Use of mechanical undercutting devices gradually spread across the coalfields. By the 1910s, cutting machines were engaged in producing more than half of all U.S. coal. By 1930, machines cut over 80 percent of the nation's coal, ending the era of pick mining. Power drills came into use by World War I. Like cutting machinery, these power tools greatly elevated dust concentrations. Throughout this period, hoisting operations and horizontal transport also were increasingly harnessed to motors driven by steam, gasoline, or electricity. More rapid movement of coal and equipment contributed to keeping microscopic mineral particles suspended in the air.[34]

Quantitative analysis of air contaminants in the bituminous mines revealed conditions comparable to those found in anthracite. In 1925, one engineer recalled encountering numerous situations in which shovelers toiled in an environment containing between one billion and eight billion particles of coal dust per cubic meter of air. In a mine deploying undercutting machinery, he found respirable dust, i.e., dust particles less than ten microns in diameter, concentrated at more than four billion particles per cubic meter. Other industrial-hygiene studies done during the twenties detected high dust levels for both mechanized and unmechanized tasks. In an assessment of mines in six states, federal officials determined that hand-auger drilling resulted in an average dust contamination of sixteen milligrams per cubic meter of air, a level eight times the current Mine Safety and Health Administration standard. This exercise also found that hand loading took place in an environment that averaged twenty-eight milligrams of coal mine dust per cubic meter of air and that pick mining generated six milligrams. Even haulage work away from the coal face exposed laborers to a hazard that was almost double today's limit on permissible exposure.[35]

With so many points of dust generation throughout the typical mine and with deficient ventilation that recirculated particulate matter without removing it from the mine, the dust hazard was widely shared across the mining workforce. In 1916, Frederick Crum of Prudential Life Insurance

Company estimated that at least 650,000 of 800,000 U.S. coal employees faced "an exceptional amount of coal dust in the course of their respective specific employments." Crum estimated that only 50,000 of Pennsylvania's 300,000 mine workers escaped dust exposure. Thus it appears that the early twentieth century was hardly the golden age of improved working conditions that some imagined.[36]

Union officials objected to the dismissal of their members' sufferings. In 1906, UMW Secretary-Treasurer William B. Wilson, who seven years later would become the first U.S. secretary of labor, commented on both the extent and the severity of the problem. "A great percentage of miners have miners' asthma," Wilson, a former bituminous worker, maintained. "The miners' asthma is caused by the miners inhaling the dust. I was laid up last week with the asthma, . . . though I have not worked in the mines since 1898." The *United Mine Workers Journal* refused to let pass the assertion that union members enjoyed long and healthy lives. A 1911 editorial held that more long-term coal employees prematurely fell prey to dust disease than attained old age. The journal rejected as exceptions the operators' reports of superannuated miners: "We must take the craft as a whole, and it will be found that very few of them are bothered with old age, because they have passed in their checks before they reach it." On the concomitant question of disability, the union editor maintained that few mining veterans possessed normal respiratory capacity. In 1924, an anthracite workers' leader reiterated that "impure air tends toward a slow but sure decline in health and ultimately results in lung and asthmatic troubles that bring on premature old age and death." Unionists were unswayed by scientific authorities exonerating underground conditions.[37]

Coal workers themselves vehemently disputed the notion that their peculiar respiratory ailments were either trivial or a thing of the past. Joseph Pico, a rank-and-file miner in Missouri, saw occupational disease as both serious and widespread. In a letter to the Mine Workers' newspaper in 1911, Pico reeled off a list of coworkers weakened by pneumoconiosis. Against the argument that continued employment indicated good health, he indignantly countered that sick men clung to their jobs because their options were to "dig coal or the poorhouse." To Pico, the predicament of these aging men demonstrated not the healthfulness of mining but rather that low earnings kept miners from saving for retirement. Accordingly, he considered it "a disgrace to this country to see them go to work." Pico suggested that anyone who took up mining to cure his lung disease "will soon be where he doesn't need any cure." Taking aim at two of the industry's best-known investors, he added that he would like J. P. Morgan and John D. Rockefeller to try this remedy. Dismissal of self-evident maladies seemed absurd to underground workers.[38]

Some within the biomedical community either doubted or rejected the hypothesis that inhalation of coal dust prevented tuberculosis. Oskar Klotz, writing in the *American Journal of Public Health* in 1914, only conceded that it was possible that coal particles set up protection against this bacterial infection. Henry Landis considered the proposition "still debatable" in 1925, based on the fact that "a large proportion of the workers suffering from anthracosis do develop tuberculosis." Some U.S. physicians may well have been swayed by Edgar Collis's critique of the immunity thesis in the *Journal of Industrial Hygiene* in 1922. Collis showed that although coal miners as a whole had a relatively low incidence of this disease, the rate of incidence of particular mining jobs correlated positively with coal dust exposure. Along the same lines, Henry Willis specified irritation as the mechanism by which coal dust promoted infection.[39]

Miners' leaders seem to have generally shared this view. William Wilson believed that coal diggers enjoyed no immunity from the tubercle bacillus. Some in the union accepted the premise of lower rates of infection among the membership but offered alternative explanations. Vice President T. L. Lewis contended that individuals with incipient consumption did not choose this arduous occupation. The *UMW Journal* argued that unionism prevented tuberculosis. An editorial in 1915 pointed out that long hours of labor, unsanitary working conditions, and a low standard of living fostered vulnerability to this disorder. Hence, the union's achievements in lowering hours, improving conditions, and raising wages built resistance to tuberculosis.[40]

But miners and their union did not confront squarely the shifting paradigm of pneumoconiosis. They generally failed to engage the crucial question of etiology, so that the growing preoccupation with silicious rock dust largely escaped rejoinder. On at least one occasion the UMW newspaper went so far as to pass along without criticism a central tenet of the reductionist formulation; in 1911, the journal advised its readers that particles of coal dust, softer and rounder than those of stone dust, were relatively harmless.[41]

Many health professionals held to the traditional view that long-term exposure to coal dust induced chronic respiratory ailments. Even for Wainwright and Nichols, the most advanced cases of anthracosis involved a loss of lung elasticity that accounted for "the condition inaccurately termed 'miners' asthma.'" These researchers did not label this impairment as a pneumoconiosis per se, but did identify it as "clinically a chronic bronchitis and emphysema." Other early-twentieth-century investigators continued to discuss anthracosis as a major type of pneumoconiosis. Some, like Henry Landis, considered coal dust less a threat than silica dust but still quite dangerous. In a textbook chapter published in 1917, Landis identified anthracosis as "by far the commonest form of dust disease and the one about which the most has been written."[42]

Against the rising pressure for specification, a few dissenters upheld a more wholistic perspective. Use of the generic concept of pneumoconiosis persisted, based on the recognition that coal workers were not laboratory animals who inhaled only one type of dust. Exposure to mixed dusts—coal, silicious rock, and other mineral particles—invalidated strict, often speciously precise, categorization of respiratory ailments. In such a mixed situation, the broader conceptualization still seemed more appropriate to some. Robert Legge of the University of California, for one, defended the more encompassing term as "the proper nomenclature in occupational medicine for all inorganic and organic dusts that produce lung disease among workers" in the *Journal of the American Medical Association* in 1923. Yet even Legge devoted the bulk of his article to defining the three stages of silicosis.[43]

After the turn of the century, anthracosis, previously a relatively well-understood, prominent form of industrial disease, virtually disappeared from the view of those outside the working class. Coal operators promoted the healthful nature of extractive work, with the intention of refuting the claims of the United Mine Workers. Biomedical investigators appear to have had a variety of motives, partisan and nonpartisan. Whereas some, like Wainwright and Nichols, had close ties with the mine owners and shared their interests, others were interested not in the ongoing debate between labor and capital but rather in refining understanding of disease entities by use of prevailing scientific theories and emerging diagnostic technology. Irrespective of their divergent intentions, biomedical rethinking and industrial public relations effectively combined to marginalize miners' grievances regarding their lung ailments. By 1930, few looking down on the coal workforce considered miners' asthma a significant industrial disorder.

CHAPTER FOUR

SHEEP-LIKE ACCEPTANCE OF HALF-BAKED STATEMENTS

Governmental scientific expertise failed to reverse the exoneration of coal mine dust in the early twentieth century. Instead, public health authorities helped whitewash black lung. It could well have been otherwise. After 1900, both new and old public agencies generated much more knowledge of social ills. The Progressive Era seemed to offer a propitious time to examine such matters as occupational disease in the coalfields.[1]

Governmental experts pursued several avenues of inquiry regarding respiratory disorders among anthracite and bituminous workers in the first three decades of the twentieth century. Most importantly, the U.S. Public Health Service and the U.S. Bureau of Mines made extensive epidemiological studies during the 1920s. However, because the facts uncovered in the field contradicted the prevailing interpretation, they were disregarded or made to conform to it. Indeed, given the procrustean confines of the reigning conceptualization of miners' respiratory disease, it was remarkable that a few observers refused to ratify this misunderstanding.

In early-twentieth-century federalism, state officials continued to hold primary responsibility for the welfare of miners. But coal workers were subject to much obfuscation, little edification, and minimal protection from this quarter. Mounting economic rivalry among mining states created pressure to minimize disease investigation and concomitant regulatory activity. Too many states were anxious to attract investments and to preserve jobs in the ferociously competitive coal industry. The structural constraints imposed by what David Moss aptly termed "degenerative competition" all but forbade state-level intrusions.[2]

State health departments nominally remained the primary institutional site for producing knowledge of miners' diseases. Surveying the domain of the "new public health" in 1917, Alice Hamilton and Gertrude Seymour noted that "responsibility for occupational disease . . . has been specially recognized" by state health units. A chasm separated formal assumption of responsibility and actual oversight, however. Ossifying agencies continued to commit their limited resources almost entirely to the control of infectious conditions. Regarding dust disease, they largely confined themselves to passing comments, taken from the medical literature, that reinforced conventional wisdom. In 1906, the Iowa State Board of Health passed on the idea that the rounded edges of coal particles made them "far less dangerous" than particles of stone or metal. In a survey of mortality from industrial diseases in 1909, another state health official referred to coal dust as "apparently harmless." Despite a supposedly thorough investigation of the state's main work-related disorders in 1913–14, the Ohio State Board of Health gave only fleeting attention to anthracosis. In subsequent publications, Emery Hayhurst, director of the Ohio board's Division of Occupational Diseases, placed coal at the bottom of the list of harmful dusts to which miners might be exposed. Hayhurst refused to go so far as to declare coal dust beneficial. In 1920, he used the lack of conclusive quantitative research to retain some skepticism: "Nowhere do statisticians find that the inhalation of dust of any type is virtuous."[3]

State health expertise came to bear on this question by a roundabout route. During the 1910s, Ohio, Illinois, and Pennsylvania tried to take into account the effects of occupational diseases in the course of assessing the need for and potential costs of compulsory health insurance plans. The Pennsylvania Health Insurance Commission speculated about the magnitude of disabling anthracosis in the commonwealth. The commission underscored the insignificance of miners' asthma by placing the disability rate at roughly four per thousand anthracite miners and roughly two per thousand bituminous miners. In the Ohio social insurance report, Emery Hayhurst cautioned that "the health of coal miners in the United States remains a matter of considerable doubt and uncertainty" and lamented that "practically no statistics are available concerning sickness among Ohio coal miners." But he nonetheless proceeded to label miners' asthma a diminishing phenomenon, affecting only 1 or 2 percent of the state's coal workers. In his capacity as an expert consultant to the Illinois commissioners, Hayhurst reached an identical conclusion.[4]

Intensified federal investigative work filled the void left by the states. The shifting and sometimes porous boundaries of Progressive federalism allowed more thorough engagement by the national government with a wide range of health-related issues. Showing unprecedented initiative, Washington ventured to take on such problems as impure meat, dangerous drugs, pellagra, leprosy, child and maternal welfare, and (of most direct relevance here) workplace exposure to phosphorus. Perhaps most indicative of the fluidity and expansiveness that characterized this period were plans for a cabinet-level health department; one proposal even placed the U.S. Bureau of Mines within this department. Although that quest failed, the founding of the Bureau of Mines in 1910 and the reconstitution of the Marine Hospital Service as the Public Health and Marine Hospital Service in 1902 and then as the Public Health Service in 1912 laid the institutional foundation for more systematic investigation of the causes, effects, and extent of miners' dust disease. By the 1920s, federal officials moved beyond mere crisis management to a central, authoritative role in generating fresh information on pneumoconiosis and related conditions in coal workers.[5]

No part of the federal government could claim exclusive jurisdiction over miners' diseases in the Progressive Era. In 1913, establishment of the Department of Labor gave U.S. workers an information-gathering institution closely attuned to many of their vital interests, including working conditions. Shortly after its founding, the agency undertook an exhaustive field study of industrial lead poisoning. But no comparable investigation of miners' respiratory disease followed, even though the first secretary of labor, William B. Wilson, was himself a victim of miners' asthma. Wilson's new department lacked sufficient funds and autonomy to proceed rapidly with research into such a controversial issue.[6]

A paucity of internal expertise also kept the Department of Labor from launching more than an exceptional inquiry. (A consultant, Alice Hamilton, performed the lead studies.) In 1918, the department's Bureau of Labor Statistics (BLS) published a lengthy review of the biomedical literature on the dust diseases by Frederick Hoffman, a vice president at the Prudential Life Insurance Company. That the Department of Labor had to enlist an insurance executive for this task tells a great deal about the underdevelopment of federal administrative capacity regarding matters of workers' wellbeing. Hoffman remained unconvinced that tuberculosis rarely struck coal workers. He found the evidence on U.S. miners inconclusive and questioned the ailment's purported infrequency among British coal diggers, arguing that the high rate of mortality from trauma concealed respiratory maladies. The Prudential executive also refused to acquit coal particles of causing dust disease. Hoffman held to the older view that "health-injurious consequences must in course of time result from an extensive coal-dust infiltration." He took anthracosis to be a debilitating condition, not a meaningless discoloration. Wainwright and Nichols's assurances that large deposits of coal in the lungs posed no danger left him incredulous.[7]

Hoffman found much to criticize in the quantitative aspects of Wainwright and Nichols's work. Scornful of their analysis of occupational mortality data, he asserted that the widespread failure of North American clinicians to identify nontuberculous lung disorders as a cause of death had misled the two physicians. He contended that Wainwright and Nichols, despite reliance on flawed data, could have detected a problem. "The authors," Hoffman maintained, "do not draw sufficient attention to the fact that the proportion of deaths from asthma in their own figures was 7.07 per cent for anthracite coal miners against 1.58 per cent for all other occupied males." Moreover, he reasserted the importance of distortions caused by mobility: "To anyone thoroughly familiar with the conditions in the mining districts of the United States there can be no question of doubt that labor changes are quite common and that in a measure they are directly attributable to a desire to replace an apparently unhealthful employment underground by an occupation with a lesser liability to diseases resulting from continuous and considerable coal-dust exposure."[8]

Hoffman discarded the trade journals' sanguine assertions. Citing one of the *Coal Age* editorials, he protested that "an occasional obituary notice of an aged miner is erroneously construed into an argument in favor of the noninjuriousness of coal dust, or underground work." Against what he took to be a patently fallacious approach, Hoffman offered sobering statistics on differential occupational longevity. From the 1910 census, he noted that whereas 29 percent of employees in agriculture were over the age of forty-five, only 17 percent of coal workers exceeded that age. All in all, the corporate actuary made a spirited defense of the legitimacy of the miners' ailments.[9]

Such advocacy might have stimulated a research program by "labor's voice in the cabinet" to resurrect the issue, rather than allowing it to be set aside in the preoccupation with silicosis and tuberculosis. Continued dependence on the insurance industry's expertise sharply limited the ability of the Department of Labor to follow up on Hoffman's insights. To be sure, a BLS compilation of mortality data from Metropolitan Life Insurance appearing in 1930 identified more than a hundred fatal cases of miners' asthma. But reprinting Metropolitan's influential guidelines for the diagnosis of occupational disease contributed to the trend to trivialization. The 1922 edition of *Occupation Hazards and Diagnostic Signs* advised that coal dust might produce "slight changes [in miners' lungs] and then only after long exposure," in the context of an exonerative comparison with free silica. The subsequent edition of this guide, also published as a BLS bulletin, made no reference to coal dust, while devoting much attention to silica and asbestos dust. The silence only deepened with the reminder that "many inorganic dusts found in industry have been inhaled for long periods without noticeable injury." For the most part, the Bureau of Labor Statistics and its parent department kept away from this subject.[10]

In November 1919, the United Mine Workers led a strike in most of the nation's far-flung bituminous mines for higher wages, shorter hours, and other demands. The miners' organization reiterated the charge that its members suffered a frightful toll from occupational disease. At the convention at which it wrote its bargaining agenda, the UMW invoked miners' asthma as part of the rationale for the six-hour day and the five-day week. The soft-coal workers struck for more than a month in defiance of a federal injunction. The deadlock broke when acting union president John L. Lewis accepted the Wilson administration's proposal to submit unresolved issues to a federal arbitration panel. Both its experience in hard coal seventeen years earlier and the presence of a Democratic administration led the union to expect a sympathetic hearing from this panel.[11]

In January 1920, representatives of the soft-coal workers pleaded their case before the U.S. Bituminous Coal Commission in Washington. John L. Lewis grounded the demand for the thirty-hour week in fears over his members' wellbeing. "If a man works in a mine for twenty years steadily, he acquires an occupational disease that unfits him for any service practi-

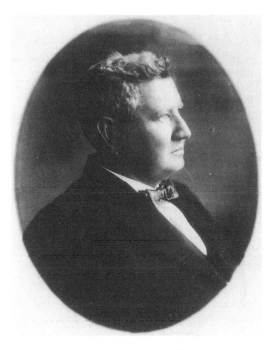

William B. Wilson, ca. 1920. The first secretary of labor suffered from miners' asthma. (Courtesy of the United Mine Workers of America)

cally during the remainder of his life," Lewis declared in his opening statement. "From a humane, health standpoint, the miner is entitled to a shorter work-day." But with the callousness that would typify his long involvement with this issue, the UMW leader neglected to mention either miners' asthma per se or the dust hazard as its cause.[12]

The mine owners pounced on this vague assertion. Ralph Crews, counsel for the operators of the Central Competitive Field, properly characterized it as "not very strongly urged." Taking the offensive, Crews retorted, "We are not informed of any occupational diseases in the mining industry." Quite to the contrary, he upheld coal mining as beneficial to health. Crews praised the robust appearance of the union delegation, all survivors of many years underground, as "exhibits, if the Commission please, as to the general healthful character of the industry." Operator T. W. Guthrie showed less restraint in his appraisal of Secretary of Labor William B. Wilson, a participant in the hearings. "I heard Secretary Wilson say that he had swung a pick in the coal mine for twenty-three years," Guthrie taunted, "and I am surprised they did not make use of him as being an illustration of the serious effect which it has on the physical condition of a man, because I have never seen a more rugged, intellectual, vigorous, virile man than Secretary Wilson is after his twenty-three years work." The operators thus shrewdly attempted to maneuver the unionists into a choice between asserting their masculinity and improving their members' terms and conditions of employment.[13]

Unmoved by this flattery, a number of miners' officers tried to improve upon Lewis's performance. Van Bittner, president of the UMW district surrounding Pittsburgh, cited insurance carriers' data to demonstrate that coal workers' mortality rate exceeded the average for all industrial workers by 32 percent. Bittner identified respiratory diseases, along with occupational injuries, as the leading causes of death among his members. International Secretary-Treasurer William Green noted that an operators' survey of doctors in western Pennsylvania, introduced to confirm the absence of any occupational diseases, did just the opposite. Indeed, in contradiction to the exculpatory interpretation contrived by the mine owners, this study had found that more than one-third of the medical practitioners surveyed (who, Green pointed out, were company doctors) had encountered industrial respiratory disorders among their coal-digging patients. In the process, however, Green confusedly expressed the view that rock dust caused miners' asthma. Moreover, somewhat surprisingly, neither Green nor any of William Wilson's other long-time comrades nor even Wilson himself explained to the commission that, like his father before him, the Secretary of Labor suffered partial disability from pneumoconiosis, his hearty, manly appearance notwithstanding. On balance, the flawed case put forward by the union did little to advance understanding of pneumoconiosis.[14]

In its decision, rendered in March 1920, the Bituminous Coal Commission found a way to treat the hours issue in strictly economic terms. The majority report denied the request for the six-hour day, noting the inconsistency between the union's demand for shorter daily exposure to health hazards and its professed desire for more regular employment (and concomitant elevated exposure to hazards). The majority held to this position in the face of the dissent of commissioner John White, who leaned on the precedent of Britain, where shorter hours had brought improvements in miners' health status. The commission managed to dodge the tough question of the existence and severity of work-related diseases among the soft-coal workers.[15]

The UMW fared even worse a few months later when federal arbitrators settled a similar impasse in the anthracite mines. Union leaders in eastern Pennsylvania looked forward to an opportunity to condemn the exorbitant profiteering that had occurred during World War I in this oligopolized segment of the industry. As in the soft-coal negotiations, the Mine Workers defended their demands for the six-hour day not only by reference to the enormous profits they produced but also by the argument that reduced hours would curtail the risk of work-induced disease. At the joint convention of the three anthracite districts in August 1919, William Green gave this rationale for the six-hour proposal: "The dampness, the dust, the dangers of the mine require that men should not be called upon to work more than a reasonable number of hours per day. From a health standpoint, from a humane standpoint, from the highest considerations that move men sentimentally, we have a right to demand and press for favorable consideration that demand for a shorter work-day." In his presentation of the union's contract proposals to the operators in March 1920, District 7 president Thomas Kennedy argued, "We are not doing justice to our men who must go into the mines eight, nine or more hours per day, depending upon their occupation and their work, in artificial light and air, and as a result contract what is known in the local medical parlance in the region as 'Miners' Asthma.' We believe that from this standpoint alone the mine workers are justified in demanding a shorter workday." The anthracite miners opened this round of negotiations by emphasizing that deleterious environmental conditions justified decreased hours.[16]

The UMW addressed its arguments to the public at large as well as to the Anthracite Coal Commission. For the hearings that opened in June 1920, it prepared numerous news releases and distributed thousands of copies of its exhibits of evidence to the press, universities, and libraries across the nation. One of these exhibits, *Occupation Hazard of Anthracite Miners*, drew on Frederick Hoffman's analysis of mortality data for the Bureau of Labor Statistics. The union used this and other material, as it had two decades earlier, to contend that elevated rates of miners' asthma and other chronic lung disorders warranted both higher pay and shorter hours. However, the miners' negotiators shifted position in the midst of the negotiations in a way that made it more difficult to hold the high ground. In the wake of the disappointing bituminous settlement, the UMW replaced its six-hour demand with a more modest eight-hour standard and proposed a 50 percent premium in pay for all time worked beyond eight hours per day. Such an economistic approach, tacitly accepting respiratory risk in exchange for extra remuneration, vitiated the humanitarian argument, which had stressed shorter hours of dust exposure. By selecting Jett Lauck of the Bureau of Applied Economics to prepare its case, the Lewis administration reinforced its dollars-and-cents orientation.[17]

Moreover, the UMW decision to rely on Frederick Hoffman proved to be unfortunate. Troubled by the miners' use of his publications in a class confrontation, Hoffman worked behind the scenes to refute the conclusions that the union had drawn from his evidence. Indeed, the insurance man armed the operators with a detailed rebuttal of the union case. In introducing his brief as an exhibit for the commission's consideration, operator S. D. Warriner took pains to identify the Prudential executive as "an authority who was partially quoted" by the Mine Workers. Taking the prudent stance of the professional statistician with very high standards of proof, Hoffman denied that any worthwhile data existed on the rates of respiratory diseases in the anthracite workforce. But then the management consultant dropped his cautious skepticism and made a series of quantitative judgments. He advised the commission that few hard-coal workers suffered from either silicosis or anthracosis. Pirouetting away from his previous concern over Wainwright and Nichols's finding of elevated asthma mortality in anthracite, Hoffman now belittled that issue as "numerically not of the importance generally assumed." Two years earlier, he had expressed doubt as to whether coal workers really had a lower rate of tuberculosis. For the edification of the federal arbitrators, however, he uncritically affirmed the miners' lower vulnerability to that disorder and explained it by the protective action of coal dust. Moreover, he questioned the seriousness of anthracosis, contending that its victims often were hardly disabled. Regarding the contentions about miners' longevity that he had derided in 1918, Hoffman announced, without giving any corroborating data, that research by the Mellon Institute of Industrial Research had "show[n] conclusively that . . . many miners live to an advanced age regardless of exposure to coal dust." In his overall appraisal, the Mine Workers' case was "not a contribution to the facts in the matters at issue, but a contribution to further controversy, and as such is unworthy of the confidence of this Commission." An eminent actuarial authority and former president of the American Statistical Association, Hoffman dealt a serious blow to the credibility of the union's claims.[18]

The federal commissioners made no explicit comment on this facet of the controversy in rendering their decision in August 1920. The commission construed its charge narrowly and refused to consider many issues raised by the union. It awarded the miners a minimal raise and no reduction in working hours. Instrumental use of the occupational disease issue yielded no gains for the hard-coal workers.[19]

The union's disillusionment hardened further after its next experience with intercession by Washington. In 1922, Congress set up the U.S. Coal Commission after unprecedented simultaneous work stoppages in both anthracite and bituminous, involving more than 500,000 miners.[20] Unlike the previous strike commissions, this body did more than merely receive claims and counterclaims from the interested parties. Instead, it took advantage of a permissive statutory license to send its own investigators into the field to find facts relevant to the perennial disputes in the industry. A team of public health workers retained by the commission systematically evaluated conditions in mining towns and villages across the nation. However, these health officers focused on sewage disposal, insect eradication, water purification, and other means of infectious-disease control. Certainly, this orientation was understandable in light of the investigators' professional training and the rudimentary infrastructure of most mining communities. Yet because the investigators inspected seemingly every aspect of the coal-mining environment except the workplace, the dust hazard went unnoticed. Over the protests of the UMW, the commission announced that it had found "no positive evidence" that either hard- or soft-coal workers suffered from any "special occupational disease." The institution of the federal commission, which at the turn of the century seemed such a promising forum for bringing broad public enlightenment on miners' suffering, had come to a dead end two decades later.[21]

Throughout the half century prior to the enactment of the Coal Mine Health and Safety Act of 1969, the U.S. Bureau of Mines (BOM) and the U.S. Public Health Service (PHS) shared primary ongoing responsibility within the federal government for studying and publicizing the health hazards of coal mining. In the legislation establishing the mining bureau in 1910, Congress unmistakably assigned it the task of protecting the lives of miners. However, the bureau possessed neither police powers nor medical expertise to meet that enormous challenge. Not long after the bureau's founding, BOM director Joseph Holmes entered into a partnership with the public health agency, which had a large corps of physicians and long experience in investigating epidemics. For decades, the PHS loaned members of its medical staff to the mining bureau for temporary assignments. At the same time, the PHS occasionally carried out field investigations of mine dust under its own auspices.[22] This makeshift arrangement virtually ensured an indecisive, fractured approach to producing and disseminating information.

During the 1910s, these bureaucratic partners embraced the priority of silicosis. In their first foray into the field, the agencies passed over an opportunity to explore the hazards of respirable coal mine dust. Based on his 1911 visit to the hardrock and coal districts of Colorado as a special investigator for the BOM, Samuel Hotchkiss of the Public Health and Marine Hospital Service made this distinction: "Hard, insoluble dust particles, having sharp edges and corners, are believed to be more injurious to the lung tissue than are particles which are comparatively free from these sharp points. Coal dust is of this latter type, while the dust of many metalliferous mines conforms to the former type." Accordingly, the agencies spent the rest of the decade discovering silicosis in the hardrock mines. Washington joined the chorus of reassurances on the relationship between dust exposure and tuberculosis. At the 1915 meeting of the National Safety Council, W. A. Lynott of the BOM attributed the infrequency of tuberculosis among coal workers to their inhalation of coal dust. In its promotional campaign to acquit working conditions of charges that they harmed miners' health, the coal industry had nothing to fear from federal officials during the heyday of Progressivism.[23]

The Office of Industrial Hygiene and Sanitation at the PHS conducted a series of field investigations of particulate hazards throughout the twenties. Along with explorations of the effects of metal dust, granite dust, cotton dust, and street dust, the PHS studied the dust danger in anthracite and bituminous mines. At its inception, the anthracite project examined hard-coal dust as a threat in its own right. The Public Health Service in Februrary 1923 sent two medical officers to eastern Pennsylvania to investigate anthracosis. From the outset, the investigators sought to work closely with both the mine owners and the miners, locating their first office in the Lehigh Valley Coal Company in Wilkes-Barre but then soon relocating to Luzerne to be closer to the miners' residences.[24]

Like the other studies in this series, the Luzerne inquiry involved three activities. First, the PHS monitored environmental contamination. Sanitary engineer J. J. Bloomfield took eighty air samples at work sites in and around two mines in 1926. Bloomfield found that employees directly involved in coal extraction were exposed to an average dust concentration of 232 million respirable particles per cubic foot of air; laborers employed away from the coal face incurred an average exposure of 31 million particles per cubic foot of air. Chemical analysis determined that free silica constituted less than 2 percent of the anthracite dust. The hard-coal workers inhaled very high levels of dust, but the dust was virtually free of the dreaded silica.[25]

Second, the Public Health Service examined approximately half of the 700 employees of the two mines. It conducted a physical examination and took a medical history of all participants. In addition, the PHS ran pulmonary function tests on ninety-two subjects. Using a spirometer to measure vital capacity, the researchers learned that the "air capacity of the lungs" of men over the age of forty who had spent ten or more years in the hard-coal mines averaged 16 percent less than that of men in the same age bracket who were employed in other manual occupations. A strike thwarted plans for an X-ray screening component of the project. Nonetheless, the data indicated significant, widespread respiratory impairment.[26]

The third facet of the Luzerne study took the Public Health Service beyond its accustomed focus on health status. Employers' concerns prompted the investigators to evaluate miners in terms of their inability to work: the coal operators cared about absenteeism, always a drag on efficiency. Nurses followed up on medical examinations with home visits to ascertain lost work days per episode of illness. This investigation discovered that respiratory conditions accounted for almost half of the miners' absences that were due to sickness. The PHS found disabling respiratory disorders in general, and bronchitis in particular, far more common in this industry than in others. Each year 9 percent of anthracite workers experienced an episode of lung disease that caused the loss of eight or more days from work, compared with only 4 percent of manufacturing laborers.[27]

The Public Health Service wrestled with the meaning of its findings. The agency had to explain an obvious pattern of elevated respiratory disease in workers exposed to high levels of mineral dust. Reducing the subject to silicosis was not a viable alternative for a group of employees practically free from silica exposure. The PHS conceded the existence of what it termed "evidences of anthracosis and other type [sic] of pneumoconiosis" in 8 percent of the anthracite workers, including 21 percent of those over age forty-five who had more than fifteen years' service in the industry. But then federal agents crucially qualified their acknowledgment of anthracosis. Regarding the question of disease severity, the PHS held that "serious physical impairment was noted only where the workers were exposed for long periods to large amounts of dust containing a high percentage of quartz." This accommodation to the preeminence of silicosis made no sense in view of the evidence of diminished respiratory capacity in longtime mine workers. Especially given miners' need to continue to work despite impairment, which misleadingly reduced their rates of absenteeism, this interpretation also did not square with the finding that almost one in ten hard-coal employees missed eight or more days per year due to respiratory ailments. Nonetheless, determined to follow the tendency to treat pneumoconiosis as silicosis, the PHS gave no explanation for the condition of most ailing anthracite workers.[28]

The Public Health Service proved even less helpful in clarifying pneumoconiosis among bituminous workers. The dust study series included an investigation of the effects of inhaling particles of soft coal, conducted in Wyco, West Virginia, between 1923 and 1927. The Wyco operations of the Gulf Smokeless Coal Company employed roughly 200 men at that time. In this instance, the approach departed from the uniform plan specified by the Office of Industrial Hygiene and Sanitation for its pneumoconiosis field research program. Rather than send its own physician to conduct medical examinations, the PHS allowed the local company doctor, George Fordham, to evaluate the research subjects. Fordham followed no standardized examination protocol. No visiting nurses confirmed the reason for absences from work. Instead, an informal system of data collection received the approval of the Public Health Service: "Inasmuch as the number of employees was small and the mine physician acquainted with them all, it was possible to check the foreman's record of absences with the physician's record of visits and calls." A PHS technician took X-rays of a group of Wyco miners. By this time employment in bituminous mines greatly exceeded that in anthracite and the bituminous segment of the industry was growing while anthracite was stagnating, so the disparity between the resources allocated for this project and the one in hard coal seems questionable.[29]

Irregularities in research protocol set the stage for dubious analysis of results. PHS engineer J. J. Bloomfield calculated that dust exposure for coal cutters and loaders in Wyco averaged an astronomical 112 million particles per cubic foot of air. Yet "dyspnea, emphysema, and miners' asthma were not encountered" by Fordham, who diagnosed none of his charges as pneumoconiotic. The physician could not see "any evidence of physical impairment" among this group, which consisted largely of workers who labored in close proximity to mechanical coal-cutting devices. Given the absence of positive clinical findings, federal authorities chose to disregard the fact that forty of ninety-five chest X-rays from the Wyco miners displayed "generalized fibrosis." Similarly, the finding that 6 percent of the Gulf Smokeless workers missed eight or more days of work per year due to respiratory disease was discounted because this rate of disability fell below that of hard-coal labor, even though the bituminous respiratory disability was 50 percent higher than that for manufacturing workers. The federal government thus uncritically accepted and disseminated the judgment of a company doctor that no disabling dust disease existed among bituminous miners. The Public Health Service was apparently untroubled by Fordham's manifest conflict of interest and oblivious to the strong incentives for employees being examined by a manager to conceal illness in order to keep their jobs.[30]

The PHS used its harmonious relations with Gulf Smokeless to facilitate a second federally financed study at Wyco. The service arranged for one of its consultants, Leroy Gardner, director of the Saranac Laboratory for the Study of Tuberculosis, to test experimentally the hypothesis that coal dust prevented tuberculosis. While Gardner for the most part stayed at his laboratory in upstate New York, Fordham oversaw two groups of guinea pigs housed in his firm's dusty coal-cleaning plant. A control group of animals breathed only the dust-filled air of the cleaning plant. The experimental group inhaled this atmosphere after inoculation with the tubercle bacillus. Gardner found that infections healed rapidly in the dust-exposed guinea pigs. In an article in the *Journal of Industrial Hygiene* in 1933, he concluded that "there may be some protective action by inhaled bituminous coal dust against the development of a tuberculous infection."[31]

In the southern coalfields, the Public Health Service acted as the junior partner in a major study mounted by the Bureau of Mines. In late 1922, J. J. Forbes, a BOM engineer, and F. V. Meriwether, a PHS physician, began to analyze conditions in the iron mines surrounding Birmingham, Alabama. Not unexpectedly, they identified both a significant hazard from silicious dust and a substantial rate of silicosis among metal miners. In August 1923, one of the local firms, Gulf States Steel Company, asked Meriwether to extend the study to its coal operations. The federal team eagerly accepted the chance to broaden its inquiry into a nonunion bituminous field.[32]

In autumn 1923, the BOM-PHS team studied the Gulf States Virginia Mine near Birmingham. Under the format it would use in subsequent investigations in the district, Meriwether and Forbes delved deeply into the nature of the underground dust hazard and its effects. Forbes conducted comprehensive environmental monitoring. Meriwether screened a sizable sample, roughly one-quarter, of the Virginia workers. His examinations included an occupational and medical history, a thorough physical examination, and a chest X-ray. In addition to interpreting the radiographs himself, the PHS physician received guidance on the meaning of the X-ray opacities from Henry Pancoast. From the outset, Meriwether took this as an opportunity not merely to determine whether soft-coal workers incurred classic silicosis (from exposure to particles of rock around the coal seam) but also to ascertain whether coal dust posed a risk. That the Virginia Mine employed predominantly miners of long tenure improved the prospects for discovering coal workers' dust disease.[33]

The findings from the examinations at this mine were disturbing. A third of those examined had pneumoconiosis of some form. Against the tendency to collapse everything into silicosis, Meriwether drew on his recent experience in the iron mines to tease out a key distinction. He began with the fact that the X-ray images from the lungs of bituminous workers lacked the reassuringly distinctive density of those obtained from metal miners. Paradoxically, such indistinctiveness made the condition distinctive to Meriwether. Soon after finishing the Virginia investigation, he leaned toward the view that a coal workers' dust disease other than silicosis did exist. In February 1924, Meriwether told a colleague, "After considering for some time, I have about made up my mind that the two diseases are separate and distinct." Further study would confirm this tentative decision.[34]

The BOM initially attempted to communicate news of this discrete hazard. In June 1924, the bureau's acting director, D. A. Lyon, sent Meriwether and Forbes's report on the Virginia Mine to Gulf States Steel. Lyon directed the firm's attention to its conclusions regarding "the apparent effect upon the miners of breathing coal dust," which he considered "of particular interest to the Bureau, since most of its efforts hitherto have been directed to the effects of breathing rock dust." On the other hand, senior mining engineer George Rice hastened to mute the warning by invoking racial stereotypes of biological and social inferiority. Thirty of the thirty-one Gulf States employees examined were African American, "a poor lot as regards diseased condition," in Rice's view. "I feel doubtful," he cautioned, "if one should, from this evidence alone, conclude that the dustiness in the Virginia mine is responsible." Although Rice's hesitation to generalize from a small group seemed prudent, his dismissive attitude also served to undermine the cumulative process by which small findings contribute to the gradual building up of a body of evidence. Indeed, white supremacist notions had served to discount reports of miners' respiratory disorders in Alabama for at least thirty years. In 1893, Russell Cunningham elucidated for the Medical Association of Alabama the lung ailments found among black convicts put to work in the Pratt mines. Cunningham advised his medical colleagues that disease followed not merely from dusty working conditions but also, more importantly, from the degrading effects of incarceration. Whereas free white miners (who often had less dusty jobs) did not appear to Cunningham to suffer from "miners' consumption," black prisoners did, because their "personal manhood, energy, industry, pride [and] self-esteem are things of the past." Rice thus perpetuated a line of racist reasoning to which medical practitioners and mine operators—in the North as well as in the South—were, in all likelihood, quite receptive.[35]

The mining bureau gathered more evidence in order to test the validity of the Virginia findings. Meriwether and Forbes studied four more Alabama coal camps by mid-1924. In addition, BOM officials authorized investigations outside Alabama, making preliminary plans for work in Tennessee, Kentucky, and Virginia. In the fall of 1924, Meriwether and Forbes continued their work in Coal Valley, Corona, Sipsey, and Sayre and began a sixth coal-dust investigation at Carbon Hill, Alabama. After failing to secure access to groups of miners in southwestern Virginia, the BOM received permission to screen employees of the West Kentucky Coal Company. The bureau's mining engineer for Kentucky guided the investigators to this nonunion firm in part because "they have very good control over their men and could arrange for the physical examinations." With the administration of one hundred examinations in Sturgis, Kentucky, in early 1925, the bureau reached its objective of studying 500 men.[36]

The Bureau of Mines' commitment to promote understanding of the dust hazard operated within tight constraints. These limitations became painfully clear at the end of the investigation at Corona Mine No. 12 of the DeBardeleben Coal Corporation. Transmitting Forbes and Meriwether's analysis to DeBardeleben management on July 24, 1924, BOM director H. Foster Bain assured the corporation of his organization's policy of confidentiality: "This report is not intended for publication but is a private report between the Bureau and your company. If the Bureau should desire later to use any of the data or conclusions contained in the present report for publication purposes, your permission will first be sought." Similar promises were made to other operators. Accordingly, neither in Corona nor in the other research sites did federal authorities inform workers at risk of their scientific findings. No one told any miner his diagnosis, and no one advised miners as a group of the discovery of a pattern of work-related disease.[37]

To be sure, governmental consultants did encourage coal operators to take preventive measures. Forbes pressed for improvements in ventilation and for wet methods of dust suppression. Where extremely hazardous mechanical undercutting prevailed, he advocated killing dust at the point of its generation by spraying the cutting bar.[38]

Despite his superiors' promises to the businesses involved, Meriwether sought a wider distribution of his findings. After all, he had done a large-scale, potentially path-breaking study and had come to provocative conclusions. Meriwether repeatedly raised the possibility of issuing a comprehensive report that drew on the wealth of data collected. The presumption of eventual dissemination extended to the top of the PHS. In his 1924 annual report, Surgeon General Hugh Cumming summed up the progress of this cooperative venture with the BOM and stated his expectation that "a general report on this work will be prepared for publication." Meriwether spent a considerable amount of time during 1926 writing a final report on this project.[39]

But such a publication would have to come from the mining bureau, which controlled the study, not from the PHS. Certainly, the bureau had several outlets for such a work. It regularly put out brief reports of investigations and information circulars. It also published series of longer technical papers and bulletins, which were more appropriate venues for discussing an inquiry of this scale. Indeed, when Forbes's supervisor wrote to commend him on his field work in July 1925, he made the case for publication of his expected report in either of these series.[40]

As Meriwether analyzed his data, he found in the observations of a colleague strong support for his growing conviction as to the danger of coal dust. Daniel Harrington, a veteran BOM engineer, mounted a withering attack on the general failure to confront all the respiratory hazards in coal. In a paper presented before the American Institute of Mining and Metallurgical Engineers in February 1924, Harrington asserted that "any dust insoluble in the fluids of the respiratory passages, and in sufficiently finely divided form to float in the air and be breathed by underground workers, will ultimately be harmful to health if the dust is in the air in large quantities and is breathed by workers for long periods of time. This applies to . . . coal dust or mixtures of coal and other dusts." In an especially inflammatory statement for this period, he conjectured that "it is entirely probable that a much greater number of men who have worked in our coal mines die annually of bronchitis, pneumonia, miners' asthma or other diseases caused directly or indirectly from coal dust, than die from mine explosions." Recognizing that some parameters of this phenomenon defied quantification, he acknowledged that the misery caused by dust disease was inestimable. The engineer went on to propose practical means of dust abatement.[41]

Harrington continued his lonely crusade through the mid-twenties. He sought to shatter what he took to be the complacent misunderstanding surrounding this subject. To this end, he pressed further his comparison with the much-publicized explosions. In an article in *Coal Age* in November 1924, shortly after leaving the federal service, he extended the comparison beyond mortality, arguing that lung disease caused "more deaths and far more misery, lost time and other humanitarian and economic losses among our coal miners than do mine explosions, and it appears that dust inhalation—chiefly of coal dust—is mainly responsible."[42] Without divulging details, he borrowed data from Forbes and Meriwether to support the assertion that pneumoconiosis was no rarity among coal workers.

He offered this evidence as an antidote to the "sheep-like acceptance of half-baked statements and misinterpreted statistics, largely of English origin, that . . . [had fostered] a positive belief that coal mining is one of the most healthful of occupations." Harrington attributed some nonrecognition of dust disease to the shift of partly disabled miners into farming and storekeeping. He also pointed to a less innocuous cause of ignorance:

> Seldom does a coal-mine doctor write his views for publication, generally because he is too busy, frequently because he doesn't know how to do it and often because he is afraid that his standing with the company will be injured if he gives undue publicity to health danger from dust or from other cause. The mine doctor knows that the coal operator in most parts of this country would much dislike to be compelled to spend the money necessary to preserve the health of his employees, though he ought to do it for the benefit of his own purse.[43]

In an article published in the *Journal of Industrial Hygiene*, Harrington repeated his appeal to company doctors to confess openly what they knew. He also urged public health officials to share their findings with those at risk: "State and federal authorities should cooperate in making studies and publishing results as to the health situation of workers in dusty places in coal mines." Ever protective of the industry (but not so protective as to refuse to print Harrington's critique), *Coal Age* responded with a skeptical editorial. The trade journal suggested that Harrington may have been misled by conditions peculiar to the western locales in which he had done much of his work. It also questioned the sources for his assertions.[44]

Amid this simmering controversy, Meriwether offered the main lessons of his extensive research to the mining section of the National Safety Council on September 29, 1927. He commenced by noting that preoccupation with silica dust and with the depressed rate of tuberculosis in active coal miners had "led many investigators to believe that coal dust was harmless." He then described collecting medical data on more than 500 miners. On this basis, he advanced the thesis that "coal dust when inhaled in large quantities over a long period of time will produce pneumonoconiosis."[45]

Meriwether explained chronic respiratory disease among coal workers primarily in terms of cumulative dust exposure. Hence, he stressed the susceptibility of men occupied at the working face itself, where cutting and loading machinery raised "dense clouds of dust" that enveloped workers. Although the PHS physician characterized those exposed to dust-generating machines as a relatively small segment of the extractive workforce, this characterization could hardly have relieved the mine operators, who were embarking on a major expansion of mechanization into coal loading. In the same discomforting vein, Meriwether left the operators little opportunity to blame disease victims themselves for their fate. His analysis of family histories and miners' lifestyles led him to reject genetics and personal behavior as important factors in respiratory illness. Instead, under his interpretation, the major determinants of disease lay in the working environment. It ineluctably followed that eliminating pneumoconiosis would require transforming that environment.[46]

Meriwether sketched for the assembled mine managers the clinical picture of dust disease among southern coal miners. He assured his audience that "symptoms of pneumonoconiosis can be detected by an ordinary layman." To clarify this point, he asked the operators present to recall a familiar scene: "You men who have slope mines will notice that the older men will walk out of the slope and rest at frequent intervals. . . . If you will question the old man, you will find that he claims he has asthma, or as he says, miner's asthma. It is pneumonoconiosis." Notwithstanding this attempt to demystify the recognition of the disease, Meriwether insisted that medical expertise was crucial to solving this problem. He encouraged operators to take company doctors into the mine and advised that every employee receive a physical examination at least annually. Moreover, though no engineer, he repeated the well-known prescription for dust controls.[47]

The discussant of this paper was none other than Daniel Harrington, who had returned to the staff of the BOM. Harrington welcomed Meriwether to "the ranks of the bolshevists on coal dust" and offered corroborative observations from his own long experience underground. He demonstrated that his recent spate of articles had exhausted neither his fund of anecdotes nor his capacity for sarcasm:

> Very often you find the coal mining man, the coal superintendent or general manager, will practically tell you that you are an anarchist if you say that coal dust will harm persons who breath [sic] it. . . . I have gone underground with those same men and have tried to get them to stay with me while I was observing the effects of dust while men were overcutting or

undercutting the coal. But they would not stay in a working place during the period when the place was being cut. It was harmless, all right enough, but they wouldn't stay in there and allow their precious lungs to breathe it. That's the attitude of a large number of our coal mining men toward the dust.

Another discussant, R. Dawson Hall, the engineering editor of *Coal Age*, admitted that Meriwether had "proved a very good case" and hoped that these revelations would prompt remedial measures. Hall also apologized to Harrington for previous criticism of his allegations.[48]

This campaign for enlightenment was aborted. To be sure, Harrington continued to hammer away. Reassigned to Oklahoma to study silicosis among zinc-lead miners, Meriwether fell silent.[49] No further publications from the Alabama-Kentucky research project appeared in the literature of medicine, public health, or engineering. Most surprisingly, given the resources expended on this inquiry and given the agency's tendency toward profuse publication of its own work, the Bureau of Mines never issued a technical paper or bulletin devoted to the discoveries in Alabama and Kentucky. At the very minimum, the agency might have released (in its reports of investigations) the manuscript Meriwether had prepared for the National Safety Council, which he straightforwardly titled "Pneumonoconiosis Due to Coal Dust." Such a publication would have been especially valuable in light of the fact that the published proceedings of the council's meeting carried only Meriwether's brief remarks summarizing that lengthy manuscript. Neglected in his oral presentation, for example, were the critical epidemiological findings that 20 percent of the miners examined had pneumoconiosis and that another 41 displayed abnormally high amounts of fibrosis in their lungs. Also buried from public view were laboriously collected data on dust contamination in the mines. For example, twenty-seven air samples taken at a range of jobs at the Sipsey Mine averaged an unhealthful twenty milligrams of respirable dust per cubic meter of air. These and many other findings remained impounded, the secret possession of the mine owner and a handful of bureaucrats. The federal government thus squandered a unique opportunity to educate the coal industry and the biomedical professions on the extent and severity of the nonsilicious dust hazard.[50]

Top officials of the mining bureau simply suppressed publication of these unpleasant facts, according to Harrington. However cynical, this assessment certainly accords well with the BOM's general policy of subservience to employers' interests, narrowly defined as the pursuit of productivity, with minimal interference for nonproductive activities like spraying and ventilating mines. For example, when in 1931 a steel-making firm inquired as to the nature of the dust risk in its coke and coal handling operations, the bureau's acting director replied that silica was the only hazard worthy of attention. The insights of Meriwether and Forbes apparently had no real impact on those in charge of the agency.[51]

Harrington's view also undoubtedly reflected his awareness of the beliefs of his nemesis, R. R. Sayers. Sayers, a member of the PHS staff who served as the chief medical officer of the BOM throughout the 1920s, considered silica dust the only important respiratory threat in the coalfields. His presentation before the Coal Mining Institute of America in 1924 contrasted the pathogenic properties of free silica particles with the harmlessness of coal particles. While allowing the possibility that enormous doses of coal dust might induce disease, Sayers emphasized the way that improved ventilation had reduced this hazard to the point that miners' asthma was disappearing.[52]

Beset by a plethora of problems stemming from productive overcapacity in general and the growth of nonunion centers of production in the South in particular, the United Mine Workers of America did not seize on the observations of Meriwether and Harrington. Indeed, the UMW was fighting for its life. In the early twenties, with roughly half a million members, it was by far the largest labor union in the nation. A decade later, after a series of lost strikes and other setbacks, the organization had fewer than 100,000 members. Lacking any professional staff of its own in occupational health, the miners' union was ill-equipped to enter the sophisticated scientific and professional debates on the dust issue.[53] Moreover, widespread permanent debility among its aging members forced the union to concentrate on the welfare side of the occupational disease issue.

Throughout the early twentieth century, the UMW looked to the state for relief for its pneumoconiotic members, not for better understanding of the causes and prevention of future cases of dust disease. Initially, the union continued to pursue the traditional institutional approach to welfare. Capitalizing on heightened public awareness of industrial disease in the immediate aftermath of the great anthracite strike, it sought to make the state the custodian of those who were incapacitated. In April 1903, the Pennsylvania legislature created a Miners' Home. The lawmakers waived the age requirement of sixty years for admission when "an employe has become a victim of what is commonly called 'miner's asthma.'" The Pennsylvania law called for bilateral private financing of this project. Employees were to contribute to the construction and operation of the home by payroll deductions; employers were to incur an assessment on each ton of coal produced. Such a financing mechanism aimed to set apart miners as the respectable poor, who took not charity but merely services for which they had paid. Elevating support for this experiment to a formal policy, the UMW international convention of 1904 voted to pursue legislation to establish such facilities in all coal-producing states.[54]

Pennsylvania never built the Miners' Home. While specific plans for self-assessment were being devised, union president John Mitchell toured Europe during 1904. In the course of his travels, Mitchell was impressed with the redistributive political demands of labor in general and of miners' unions in particular. He also took note of European reliance on social insurance to deal with such common misfortunes as disability. From this vantage point, he came to oppose the proposition that Pennsylvania coal workers pay five cents per month and operators pay one mill per ton to support a long-term care center. "I am not willing that the miners shall build their own poorhouses," Mitchell told the joint convention of the three anthracite districts upon his return in 1905. He offered a progressive alternative: "What we ought to do is to ask the Legislature of Pennsylvania to make provision as is done in the countries of Europe to pay pensions, not only to aged and crippled miners, but to wornout veterans of industry, no matter where they are employed." The anthracite convention agreed to withhold support from the home. The union as a whole soon embraced this objective. The international convention of 1909 resolved to fight for old-age pension legislation. Shortly thereafter, UMW leader William B. Wilson, serving as a member of the U.S. House of Representatives, sponsored the first federal old-age pension bill. This proposal went down to defeat, as did many other union-supported initiatives at the state level during the next two decades.[55]

The UMW also mounted a campaign specifically to aid victims of work-induced chronic respiratory disease. For Progressives of all classes in the United States, workers' compensation for occupational injuries stood as the prototype of social insurance. Middle-class reformers such as John Andrews of the American Association for Labor Legislation (AALL) looked to this form of insurance as a panacea for the amelioration of working conditions. In theory, the financial burden of experience-based compensation insurance premiums would ineluctably drive employers to eliminate hazards from the workplace. The *United Mine Workers Journal* reported in 1913 that Andrews had pressed the American Public Health Association to support workers' compensation, citing miners' asthma as one object of his concern. Beginning with the first version of its model bill, published in 1914, the AALL stood for blanket coverage of all diseases contracted in the course of employment, a position it held for three decades.[56]

Pragmatic unionists approached this subject with trepidation. No UMW representative appears to have espoused the view that workers' compensation would automatically prevent occupational disease. Union officials worried that the enactment of compensation might instead prevent the continued employment of thousands of rank-and-file members. At the AALL annual meeting in 1914, both Mitchell and District 5 president Van Bittner voiced fears that enactment of compensation would provoke mass firings. Bittner sketched one plausible scenario for the assemblage of middle- and upper-class reformers: "I say that 65 per cent or 67 per cent of the men who work in the mines of this state over ten years have miners' asthma, and under existing conditions it would be a crime to compel these men to undergo a physical examination and then discharge them, simply because they could not stand the test, in order that the employers may not have to pay them compensation." If management were indeed to terminate all older employees who had signs of respiratory impairment, tens of thousands of coal workers might be jettisoned in states like Pennsylvania. This standing threat long tempered the union's enthusiasm for workers' compensation.[57]

Nonetheless, district affiliates of the UMW soon became the champions of social insurance for miners' asthma. Indignation at the patent injustice of excluding from compensation illnesses that were induced by work apparently overcame apprehension over the possibility of discriminatory discharge. Serious agitation for change began in the anthracite fields. Within a month of the passage of the Pennsylvania Workmen's Compensation Act of 1915, which failed to provide for victims of work-related illness, UMW District 7 President Thomas Kennedy, who had started his career at the age of nine picking slate out of hard coal, took up the issue. In an address to leaders of neighboring District 1, Kennedy set forth an ambitious social-democratic agenda, including mothers' pensions, old-age pensions, unemployment insurance, and workers' compensation reform. The vision of a "perfect Compensation law" that he offered convention delegates included coverage of occupational diseases. The following year Kennedy's own district resolved to win compensation for workers totally disabled by occupational disease, including "persons who were forced to quit work on account of miners' asthma." A similar resolution passed in District 9, the third anthracite organization, at the same time.[58]

Throughout the twenties, anthracite unionists continued to push for compensation reform. Although they never completely abandoned the comprehensive demand for protection for all those afflicted by work-related maladies, the miners increasingly confined their advocacy to the peculiar interests of their own industry. Influenced by the British system of compensating only specified conditions, hard-coal activists drifted away from universalistic proposals for blanket coverage of all occupational illnesses. But even this circumscribed proposition did not open the way to a compromise with employers, who easily defeated labor's reform measures. In 1923, already frustrated by repeated failures, Kennedy cynically explained the tactics of the opposition: "They used barrels and barrels of money along with barrels of whiskey." Despite implacable resistance, the Pennsylvania miners persisted in their demand.[59]

A compensation campaign also emerged in the twenties in Illinois, where the miners' organization had long been active politically. The president of the state labor federation, former miner John Walker, lobbied for an occupational disease amendment drafted by UMW District 12. Walker brought a keen personal interest to this issue. He had watched his father's deterioration over the course of thirty years, ending in his death in 1926. He carried a vivid impression of the autopsy findings: "His heart, stomach, liver and all his organs were in good condition, no sign of aterial [sic] hardening, but his lungs were caked with coal dust, baked as hard as a board and black as a shoe." Such intimate knowledge of the problem did not, however, enable Walker to secure expanded compensation coverage in the legislative sessions of 1927 and 1929.[60]

Although district organizations naturally took the lead in state-level political work, the international union did address the issue during this phase of agitation. At its 1924 convention the UMW committed itself to social insurance for victims of miners' asthma. Despite sympathy for the progressive principle of insuring all types of occupational disorders, the UMW tended to limit its demands to miners' pneumoconiosis, along with a few other conditions common to the coal industry, such as rheumatism and bursitis. Compensation reform thus became increasingly a struggle to add miners' respiratory disease to a preexisting list of compensable disorders or to begin such a schedule in states where none existed. As was the case in Pennsylvania anthracite, the union as a whole departed from the more elegant universalistic approach perennially advocated by the AALL because of the fierce opposition to it by mine operators and other employers. However, with the rising tide of denial surrounding miners' dust disease, even a circumscribed proposition was doomed.[61]

Efforts to secure preventive measures shared the same fate. No mining state enacted strong ventilation requirements during this period. In the absence of compelling evidence of a widely prevalent, disabling, preventable condition, economic considerations prevailed over public health or social welfare. In 1909, unionist Patrick Gilday fought in vain for stronger ventilation standards: "We have hundreds of people in the State of Pennsylvania who have miner's asthma. If there were purer air put into the mines, there would be no miner's asthma. But they are refused that because it keeps the fans going all night; the employer says it is not necessary. They tell you it is going to put the mines out of business." In a vacuum of manufactured ignorance, the exigencies of the market ruled in an industry already plagued by overcapacity. Increasingly, weak ventilation provisions in mining codes and niggardly social provision became sources of degenerative competitive advantage for the southern fields. The federal government, by producing and disseminating knowledge of a nationwide dust threat, might have shifted the terms of discussion.[62]

For coal miners facing the threat or the reality of dust disease, the Progressive Era brought no progress. Although government capacity to address the consequences of industrialization expanded greatly after 1900, the state stopped short of aiding some of those who were most victimized by that process. Certainly, as a wealth of recent scholarship on the development of social policy has demonstrated, the deeply gendered nature of the incipient welfare state in large measure determined access to societal provision for those in need of help. The miners were all men; they could either fend for themselves in the labor market or press for social insurance.[63] But entitlement under a "workmen's" compensation system that was not designed for chronic diseases hinged on clarification of the workplace origins, disabling nature, and wide extent of the miners' respiratory ailments. Such clarification was not forthcoming from public investigation during this regressive era. Instead, at a time when liberal reformers both inside and outside government innovatively refined and applied methods of social empiricism to lay bare many facets of diverse societal maladies, the preponderant weight of scientistic public authority promoted the fallacy that coal miners' diseases did not exist. Most paradoxically, increased state scrutiny mainly brought not liberating revelations but a sequestration of knowledge that helped stifle reform.[64]

Moreover, in the context of rampant reductionism, even production of a substantial body of quantitative data did not bring enlightenment. Because they could be misconstrued to exonerate coal dust, the epidemiological results from Pennsylvania and West Virginia took their place in the biomedical literature. Conversely, because they proved insusceptible to any such manipulation, findings from a more elaborate study in Alabama and Kentucky were deliberately buried. By 1930, only a small cohort of unreconstructed advocates within the United Mine Workers persevered in pursuit of legislation to protect pneumoconiotics in the coal fields.

CHAPTER FIVE

TO BITS

After 1930, redefinition of coal workers' respiratory disease became more openly political. Throughout the depression years, battles over workers' compensation legislation raged in coal-producing states. Economic hardships on both sides intensified this conflict: displaced miners waged a desperate struggle for subsistence amid the Great Depression; mine owners felt it imperative to avoid taking on an onerous competitive disadvantage in an ever more ruthless market. The contest over redistribution shaped not just the application of biomedical knowledge but its generation as well.

An altered balance of forces made possible a renewed drive for social insurance for industrial disease. The resurgence of the United Mine Workers brought stronger demands for state intervention. Alarmed at the prospect of internalizing even a fraction of the health costs of production, operators responded to the growth of union power by attempting to limit the disorders deemed compensable. Amid the contentious legislative politics that unfolded in the thirties, the state played the role of broker as well as that of producer of biomedical information. Public officials exerted a decisive influence in promoting the minimalistic conception of miners' disease as anthraco-silicosis. This compromise, negotiated by labor and capital with state mediation, yielded only a small bit of entitlement to societal provision. The turbulent years wrought no transformative recognition of the miners' predicament, but only rearrangements that institutionalized its underrecognition.

For the coal industry, the collapse of the late twenties and early thirties was not merely a downward swing in the business cycle but the close of a long era of expansion. After World War I, stiffer competition from petroleum cut into the market for coal. Bituminous output dropped from 573 million tons in 1926 to 310 million in 1932; anthracite output sank from eighty-four million tons to fifty million over the same interval. Technological innovations and the ongoing development of new fields in southern Appalachia increased surplus productive capacity. Coal prices fell through the twenties and into the thirties, shaking out weaker firms. In the decade after 1923, the number of soft-coal mines in the United States declined by 40 percent.[1]

Always unstable, employment in coal mining grew perilously undependable. From 1926 to 1932, more than 200,000 workers lost their jobs. Where mines shut down, permanent displacement often befell bituminous and anthracite workers. New technology also portended banishment from the industry. Marked improvement in mechanical loaders meant that tens of thousands of men would never shovel coal again. For those remaining on the payroll, uncertainty of employment grew more severe. The typical anthracite mine operated 162 days in 1932, and the typical bituminous mine only 146 days. In 1931, one-third of West Virginia's miners had no job and another third worked less than three days a week. Although the brutal combination of mechanization and slack demand for coal accounted for most unemployment and underemployment, strikes and lockouts also cut into earnings.[2]

These wild fluctuations impoverished much of the mining workforce. Although families maneuvered to maintain themselves, the combination of wage cuts and unemployment drove a substantial share of miners to seek public and private aid. More than 20 percent of the population in such mining centers as Birmingham, Alabama, and the anthracite region of Pennsylvania received some form of relief in 1935. The inadequacy of welfare assistance left much deprivation. Miners and their families often lacked the necessities of life. Inadequate nutrition undermined resistance to infectious disease. Some starved. Miners' children missed school because of their lack of clothing. In isolated coal communities, widespread, prolonged destitution fostered a sense of having been abandoned. "The sufferings of our people have been indescribable," Thomas Kennedy told the National Recovery Administration in November 1933. "The limits of human endurance have long since been passed."[3]

Among those who suffered most in the economic cave-in were aging coal workers. Breathless old men often became the first casualties of industrial distress. In 1934, economist Homer Morris surveyed the depressed labor market in West Virginia and Kentucky: "It is certain that . . . the old and inefficient miners will be crowded out of the industry first. The industry has made no provision to care for these superannuated workers. They are cast upon society to be supported after having spent their best years digging coal." Growing use of medical examinations to weed out partially disabled employees deepened rank-and-file pessimism about their long-term prospects in a declining industry.[4]

In this bleak situation, miners sought help from the state. Following the lead of the thousands of workers from various industries who were suing their former employers for silicosis, some miners sued for damages caused by occupational exposure to mine dust. Others sought legislative aid. Often heedless of the neat, categorical boundaries between welfare programs, coal workers and their sympathizers pressed intertwined demands for old-age pensions, unemployment benefits, and workers' compensation benefits as patchwork solutions for the crisis of subsistence Beleaguered coal operators viewed these desperate propositions with dread.[5]

In the context of the upheavals of the depression, workers' compensation amendments became a relatively tractable type of governmental intervention on behalf of the insecure poor. In the nation's leading coal-producing state, new sympathizers bolstered the perennial demands of the United Mine Workers for disease compensation. With the added impetus of a deluge of silicosis lawsuits, Pennsylvania Governor Gifford Pinchot, a long-time Republican Progressive, became receptive to broadening the compensation statute of 1915. Failure to win changes in the 1931 legislative session sent the Pinchot administration looking for additional support.[6]

Pinchot enlisted expert guidance to help subdue this thorny problem. In an address before the Pennsylvania Safety Conference on May 13, 1932, he dwelled on the "fearful spectre" of industrial disease and on the necessity of social insurance as a spur to prevention. Tellingly, his overview of the state's major work-related disorders included anthracosis, as well as silicosis, lead poisoning, and other well-known conditions. In view of the complexity of the issues to be resolved, the governor called for a "careful, impartial, and scientific study to determine what form of legislation is most desirable and most practicable." In the next breath, however, Pinchot indicated that he sought not dispassionate, objective, neutral authorities but a judicious balancing of opposing interests. To this end, he signaled his intention to create a advisory body of "experts, with all sides represented."[7]

In September 1932, Pinchot appointed the Commission on Compensation for Occupational Disease. As promised, the appointees included the major parties to the contest: employers, employees, the medical profession, and insurance carriers. As the sole labor official on the commission, Thomas Kennedy represented the coal miners and all other Pennsylvania workers. At its initial meeting, the commission divided into three working committees to examine legal issues, medical issues, and the scope and cost of compensation.[8]

The medical committee, chaired by R. V. Patterson, dean of Jefferson Medical College in Philadelphia, tried to compile a list of compensable conditions. Patterson's group appears to have given no consideration to extending coverage to all work-induced diseases. Following the British model of scheduling a small number of specific conditions (starting with classic intoxications such as lead poisoning and mercury poisoning), the committee struggled to limit employers' liability for the adverse effects of work on employee health.[9]

The first tough question, of course, was whether or not to list the pneumoconiosis of coal workers. Scheduling of silicosis was a foregone conclusion; coal miners with that disorder would be assured compensation. But the real issue involved those whose exposure to coal dust and mixed mine dust produced effects that differed from silicosis. In the spirit of scientific government, the medical committee conducted a rapid survey regarding miners' asthma. If the phenomenon were not a sizable one, it could perhaps be set aside. However, in response to the commission's questionnaire, seventy-eight physicians in the hard-coal region reported that they had 10,214 patients with "well-developed" cases among the 45,207 miners under their care. If the disease were not debilitating, it need not be scheduled. But most clinicians familiar with the disorder reported that in some instances it became disabling. Rather than problematize the slippery concept of disability, the commission chose to accept the conventional definition of the time. Disability meant occupational disability: the crucial criterion was a loss of ability to perform one's usual work assignment. The notion of benign miners' asthma found little corroboration among the scores of practitioners closest to the condition, including many who were paid by anthracite operators. The findings of this survey contributed substantially to the case for the compensability of miners' asthma.[10]

Prevailing scientific thinking and potent economic interests made the decision less than straightforward, however. One member of the committee, Anthony Lanza, assistant medical director of the Metropolitan Life Insurance Company, initially wanted to dodge miners' asthma "on account of its general prevalence, the difficulty of establishing the matter of disability, and the fact that there might be filed under this heading such a vast number of claims that would cause utter confusion." As a cautious insurance professional, Lanza sought not to underwrite risk but to avoid it as much as possible. In this perverse view, victims of a work-induced disabling disorder deserved no compensation not because their disease was so rare as to fall below the threshold of public concern but rather because it was so commonplace. At this moment, however, the insurance carriers' fears did not control the formation of social policy. Overlooking the uncertainties surrounding this condition, the medical committee held that it could not overlook a highly prevalent illness associated with one of the commonwealth's major industries. The committee's first tentative schedule, drafted in late 1932, covered "chronic incapacitating asthma, the result of anthracosis in miners." Reluctantly joining the consensus, Lanza defended this choice in terms of popular understanding, not the scientific state of the art: "It was felt that the term 'miners' asthma' represents a perfectly definite clinical entity, well known to coal company physicians and physicians practicing in coal mining communities and also having a definite meaning for coal miners themselves." In a sense, this acknowledgment demonstrated that the promotional campaign to exonerate coal dust had not extirpated the preexisting concept of miners' dust disease: the reductionist view was dominant but not hegemonic. The Metropolitan Life official also deemed inclusion of miners' asthma necessary in order to placate the UMW. Lanza and his fellows spurned the advice of Henry Pancoast, who reportedly felt that to grant compensation for miners' asthma meant "in effect to pass an old age pension bill for coal miners."[11]

Despite its specialization, the medical committee was not insulated from the financial implications of its plans. In seeking "some common sense" from his former colleague Daniel Harrington as the contest heated up,

Lanza reminded the engineer that, besides the medical controversies involved, "the matter has very important economic phases as well." Heedless of the delicate political and economic situation, Harrington advised Lanza that the dust-disease crisis was even bigger than commonly thought because it extended to bituminous miners as well as anthracite miners. Harrington had no doubts about where to assign the costs: "If the coal mining industry or any other industry is so conducted as to injure the health of those engaged in it, that industry should bear the burden of such injury rather than throwing it on the shoulders of the unfortunates who are afflicted." Against this logic, employers and insurers repeatedly warned that, in the depths of a depression, any added expense would be unbearable. On December 13, 1932, commission chairman T. Henry Walnut told Pinchot that wrestling with the task of estimating the cost of disease benefits had already had a chilling effect, as business interests expressed cataclysmic fears of bankruptcy and wider ruin.[12]

Thomas Kennedy and Henry Walnut pursued their own agenda in the legal committee. Lacking a clearcut charge, this pair set out for higher ground. At the urging of John Andrews of the American Association for Labor Legislation, both devoted much time to fashioning a proposal to compensate all occupational diseases. Despite its superiority over the piecemeal approach in terms of equity and simplicity, this formulation received no serious consideration from the other members of the commission. The strength of British ideas kept the medical committee from embracing such a policy; the insurance agents who ran the cost-and-scope committee recoiled from the notion of underwriting unnamed, innumerable risks.[13]

Under pressure to deliver immediate guidance, the Commission on Compensation for Occupational Disease submitted its report to the governor in March, well into the 1933 legislative session. The document reflected a negotiated settlement of many of the deep differences among its authors. By a series of compromises, the commission's diverse membership had come to a number of tentative decisions on coal workers' respiratory ailments.[14]

Despite reservations, the Walnut Commission endorsed the schedule method of coverage. It rejected the AALL's blanket approach as financially imprudent and constitutionally problematic, though "most desirable from theory." The working group on costs declared that a broadly conceived occupational-disease insurance program might "amount, for all practical purposes, to old age compensation or to insurance against unemployment." In line with the guiding principle of cost containment, the commission opposed scheduling anthracosis. Upholding the predominant biomedical view that anthracosis itself indicated only discoloration, the medical committee found a "lack of definite information as to the disabling effects such as would justify its inclusion." With this safeguard against posthumous claims supported by autopsy evidence of blackened lungs, the conservative side of the commission was prepared to concede the compensability of some other miners' respiratory complaints.[15]

Miners' asthma appeared on the list. Somewhat defensively, the commission characterized the term as not rigorously scientific. Nonetheless, it maintained that the designation remained meaningful to many in the coalfields, including physicians, and that it aptly described a debilitating condition caused by work. The commission also went so far as to countenance the notion of the pathogenicity of coal particles. In the face of the reductive preoccupation with silicosis, it is remarkable that the largely discredited lay term miners' asthma survived the commission's deliberations to receive this sort of validation.[16]

The commission made no estimate of the cost of compensating those incapacitated by miners' asthma. As part of its balancing act, the report allowed the operators to vent their apprehensions on this matter. Pinchot's advisors passed along without comment one coal firm's estimate that miners' asthma benefits would cost it more than two million dollars per year. Other employers contended that their workers' compensation outlays would double or triple if coverage were extended to this condition.[17]

The Walnut Commission made its commitment to the compensability of miners' asthma contingent on further corroboration, however. Despite its own survey research among physicians and despite the major federal investigation in the Wilkes-Barre area less than a decade earlier, the commission regretted the "lack of any precise information as to the exact nature and the prevalence of this disease." It strongly urged another study by the federal government in the anthracite region. With the incorrigible scientistic optimism of an unreconstructed Progressive, Walnut privately assured Pinchot of the value of the proposed inquiry: "It should clear the way for occupational disease compensation in Pennsylvania. A Pennsylvania act that did not make provision for miners' asthma would be a travesty and in our present state of knowledge on the subject I do not believe anyone knew how it ought to be handled." Further, the commission proposed comparison of the findings in anthracite with those from a mass screening project already under way among bituminous miners in West Virginia. The commissioners hoped that further knowledge could override inevitable conflicts of interest and guide public policy. Of course, in the short run, the request for additional research aided the opponents of reform by delaying legislative consideration of asthma compensation.[18]

For all its equivocation, the report of the Walnut Commission did contribute to public understanding of the coal diggers' plight. Within four months of its publication, the state had distributed 1,000 copies of the document. Upon its release, the governor issued a statement to the press calling attention to the finding that more than one-fifth of hard-coal workers were at least partially disabled by miners' asthma.[19]

The miners' asthma investigation moved quite rapidly. On April 22, 1933, Surgeon General Hugh Cumming notified Pinchot that he was sending R. R. Sayers to do the study. Three weeks later, the United Mine Workers and the hard-coal operators formally agreed to cooperate in its administration. As was conventional before the acceptance of the principle of a worker's right to know about his or her own medical records, the union acquiesced in a plan under which the PHS withheld diagnoses and other individual medical information from study participants. Less than two months after the commission made its recommendation, federal public health workers were engaged in epidemiological field work in eastern Pennsylvania.[20]

The PHS inquiry was far more sophisticated than its venture into anthracite in the twenties. The biggest departure in research design was the systematic attempt to relate individual health effects to individual dust exposure. Moving from descriptive to analytical epidemiology, the investigators calculated the cumulative dust exposure for each study participant. These estimated doses rested on the questionable but defensible assumption that current job-specific particulate concentrations were essentially unchanged over the past thirty years, so that dust data from the summer of 1933 could illuminate working conditions from the beginning of older miners' careers. To this end, federal industrial hygienists drew 283 air samples from across the spectrum of worksites in and around the mines.

As expected, the chemical composition and concentration of dust varied greatly among these locations.[21]

Sayers's team performed a thorough medical evaluation of 2,711 active employees at three mines to assess the outcomes of dust inhalation. Taking a detailed occupational history from each miner enabled the investigators to calculate an individual exposure profile for each subject. The PHS physicians obtained a medical history from each subject, did a physical examination, took chest X-rays, and put the subject through a simple exercise test to determine respiratory health status.[22]

In a decision that had significant implications for calculating the magnitude of the dust-disease problem, the investigators chose to segregate from their sample of active employees a much smaller number of ex-miners for a separate study. These totally disabled men were studied in a different manner, defeating comparability with their still-employed counterparts. This group of 135 former anthracite workers was hospitalized and subjected to more intense study. In particular, susceptibility to tuberculosis among advanced cases of pneumoconiosis came under special scrutiny. Whether the decision to sever the active from the inactive workers in this manner aimed to deflate the prevalence estimate is, unfortunately, unknown.[23]

Correlation of environmental and medical data posed the central analytical challenge in this study. In search of an exposure-response relationship, the average dust concentration for every job assignment of each study participant was multiplied by the total years of exposure per assignment, yielding a cumulative exposure to mine dust. On the outcome side, the investigators assessed not merely the presence or absence of pneumoconiosis but also its stage of development. In this diagnostic task, they drew on a three-stage scheme taken directly from recent work on silicosis, yet another way in which understanding of that disorder framed perception of the issues in the anthracite region.[24]

In November 1934, the Pennsylvania Department of Labor and Industry issued a preliminary report prepared by the PHS. The federal epidemiologists found that 23 percent of the hard-coal miners examined suffered from chronic disease brought on by dust inhalation. Even though the population under investigation had been restricted to active employees, the more rigorous federal study had found exactly the same prevalence as had the commission by its survey of clinicians, whose patients included individuals who had left the mines due to disability. (Obviously, if Sayers and his team had taken a more comprehensive approach and sampled former miners, they would have obtained a higher prevalence rate.) The magnitude of the pneumoconiosis problem in anthracite was now undeniable.[25]

The inquiry's findings also substantiated the severity of this disorder. More than a matter of discomfort, the hard-coal miners' ailment in most cases decreased their ability to perform labor. Sixty-three percent of those diagnosed as pneumoconiotic were deemed to be disabled. However, straining to keep its balance on the political high wire, the PHS hastened to grade incapacity: "If for the moment slight disability for which the worker is able to compensate is disregarded, it will be noted that moderate and marked degrees of disability were found in 129 (20.9 percent) of those with anthraco-silicosis." This willingness to discount "slight disability" starkly illuminates the disjuncture between impairment, the result of biological processes, and disability, the product of political, economic, cultural, and social influences. Of course, a study design that excluded former miners from the main study guaranteed understatement of the extent of disability. These flaws notwithstanding, the report made clear that pneumoconiosis in hard-coal workers was hardly an innocuous concomitant of the aging process.[26]

Beyond its descriptive aspect, the PHS epidemiologists analyzed the impact of inhaling varying amounts and types of particulate matter. They identified a large group of employees whose working environment contained dust that had only a very small proportion of free silica. Quite strikingly, among the 1,435 mine employees who regularly breathed dust that averaged less than 5 percent free silica, respiratory impairment frequently followed long and intense exposure. Among the subgroup that had been exposed to a mean concentration of three hundred million or more particles of dust per cubic foot of air for a period of fifteen to twenty-four years, more than half had pneumoconiosis. Among the subgroup exposed to that dust concentration for twenty-five or more years, 89 percent had dust disease.[27]

The presence of pneumoconiosis in the virtual absence of silica exposure did not resurrect the fading concept of anthracosis as the distinctive dust disease of coal mining, with miners' asthma as its vernacular synonym. Instead, the imploding forces of reductionism yielded a fresh name for this illness. The interim report on the hard-coal study bore the title *Anthraco-Silicosis (Miners' Asthma)*. Sent into the field to study miners' asthma, the PHS took it upon itself to alter the conceptualization of the disease to fit its preconceptions and the needs of the powerful mine operators. Even where workers had undergone only minimal exposure to silicious rock dust, Sayers and his colleagues explained their ailment in a way that placed silica at the center of attention. Choosing to ignore evidence that silica played at most a minor role in this condition, federal authorities imposed an oblique interpretation on the data.[28]

The Walnut Commission unanimously endorsed the Public Health Service bulletin as the authoritative answer to its questions. In its letter of transmittal to the governor, the commission took no cognizance of the shifting conceptualization of the phenomenon under consideration. The UMW raised no objection to the changing definition of disease in pre-publication discussions with the report's authors. Proponents of compensation for coal miners' respiratory disease apparently assumed that confirmation of the wide prevalence of a debilitating disorder would suffice to justify compensation, regardless of the nuances in naming that disorder. In this vein, state Secretary of Labor and Industry Charlotte Carr complimented the PHS on its work: "Pennsylvania, with the publication of this preliminary report, becomes thoroughly and reliably informed on the scope and gravity of occupational disease hazards due to dust in the anthracite field." In her view, the document "should serve as the basis for early action looking toward compensation for occupational diseases and the inclusion of miners' asthma among those classified as compensable." The subsequent politics would not be so straightforward, however.[29]

The campaign to shrink the disease down to silicosis continued unabated. In December 1935, the PHS issued the final account of its anthracite investigation. Miners' asthma was not dignified as a synonym for anthraco-silicosis, as it had been the previous year. Public Health Bulletin 221, *Anthraco-Silicosis among Hard Coal Miners*, sent a strong message that traditional lay ideas had no merit for the Public Health Service. The bulletin shifted emphasis at a number of points to reinforce the narrower construction. In a contradictory manner, this reinterpretation characterized miners' asthma both as a disease and as only a symptom of disease. Federal revisionists also gave more weight to radiological evidence in making diagnoses, a suggestion that predisposed them toward identification of silicosis. Appropriation of a silicosis staging scheme recently developed by the American Public Health Association had the same practical effect. In addition, the PHS offered cases of conditions that local practitioners had mistakenly diagnosed as miners' asthma. National authorities redrew the boundaries of dust disease to exclude miners' asthma as commonly understood.[30]

In the culture of medical science in this period, the paramount issue in disease conceptualization remained the specification of an etiologic agent. Federal experts could not bring themselves to declare that coal particles might, under certain frequently encountered circumstances, induce chronic respiratory disease. The PHS investigators might have been allowed some evasiveness on this difficult matter in their hastily prepared preliminary report, but the failure of their final analysis to address the arresting evidence of coal dust as a major factor in the bulk of pneumoconiosis cases under study was truly glaring. Indeed, the skittishness of Sayers, who was intimately aware of Meriwether's findings in Alabama and Kentucky, seems particularly negligent. Needless to say, unwillingness to discuss in any depth broader ideas of disease causation fallaciously left silica, by default, as the culprit in dust disease.[31]

The reticence of the Public Health Service stood in stunning contrast to the boldness of another federal agency at this moment. In a brief pamphlet based on the findings of the hard-coal project, the U.S. Department of Labor did not hesitate to claim that anthraco-silicosis was "caused by breathing excessive amounts of coal dust." Unabashed in its advocacy of workers' health, the Department of Labor gave a far-reaching warning: "Although anthracite coal dust is probably the most hazardous, all coal dust is hazardous, and workers should be protected against breathing excessive amounts." The pamphlet urged limiting the dust concentration in coal mines to less than fifty million particles per cubic foot of air.[32]

In its original research agenda, the Walnut Commission anticipated making a comparison of the findings from the anthracite study with those of an inquiry already under way among bituminous miners. The U.S. Bureau of Mines carried out a study of dust conditions and their impact on health in Powellton, West Virginia, beginning in the summer of 1932. BOM representatives conducted environmental monitoring in at least three mines in that locality. Dr. Albert Russell, another PHS physician lent to the mining bureau, spent several months in central West Virginia, performing physical examinations and chest X-rays on hundreds of bituminous employees.[33]

Yet neither in its 1935 bulletin nor at any other subsequent opportunity did the PHS offer any comparisons between the findings in anthracite and those from the Powellton study in bituminous, which it had helped to staff. Nor did the Bureau of Mines come forth with any data or any analysis from that study. When an executive at one of the nation's leading soft-coal producers inquired in 1936 as to the results of the West Virginia project, he was given no substantive information and told that "no report has ever been made of this study." At the same time, the PHS boasted to a congressional committee that over the past quarter century it had issued more than eighty publications dealing with the dust diseases.[34] Although the reasons for nondisclosure remain unclear, a coincidental occurrence probably contributed to the quiet interment of this piece of research. Powellton was about ten miles from Gauley Bridge, West Virginia, site of an extraordinarily disastrous episode of acute silicosis stemming from the construction of a tunnel through a mountain of silica in 1930–31. Former tunnel workers and their surviving kin were filing hundreds of damage suits while the nearby bituminous study took place. Litigation over dust disease was just the sort of controversy that both the PHS and the BOM made a habit of avoiding, wherever possible. The Gauley Bridge affair may well have increased federal hesitance to publicize additional dust hazards. Whatever the rationale for the nonreporting of the Powellton findings, the failure to complement the work in eastern Pennsylvania served to reinforce the growing assumption that pneumoconiosis in the coal industry occurred only in the anthracite fields.[35]

The Bureau of Mines missed another golden opportunity in the mid-thirties to raise awareness not only of the findings from Powellton but also, more importantly, of the buried findings from Meriwether's study of the previous decade. To help inform the compensation debate in the coal states, the BOM made an exhaustive review of the literature on dust disorders, published first as a series of information circulars in 1935–36 and then compiled as a lengthy bulletin in 1937. Because Daniel Harrington coauthored this review, scattered suggestions that nonsilicious dusts might also induce pneumoconiosis offset somewhat the expected obsession with silicosis. However, neither in the section on the epidemiology of pneumoconiosis nor elsewhere in this encyclopedic work did the stub-

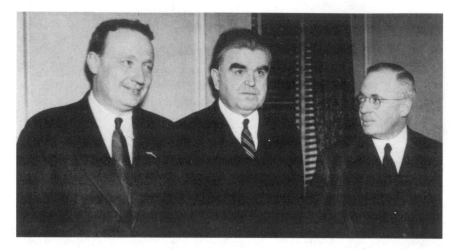

Left to right: George Earle, John L. Lewis, and Thomas Kennedy, 1937. (Courtesy of the United Mine Workers of America)

bornly dissident Harrington dare to shed light on the investigations in West Virginia or in Alabama and Kentucky. The bibliography of BOM Bulletin 400, whose 527 entries encompassed such skimpy sources as one-page newspaper articles, left out Meriwether's "The Effects of Mine Dust on Health," which was published in the proceedings of the National Safety Council. Thus banished from the literature, Meriwether's work stood no chance of influencing policymaking at this key juncture. Given the nature and strength of Harrington's opinions on this topic, it is not unreasonable to surmise that he had orders not to cite or discuss these incendiary findings.[36]

Despite the strangling circumscription of coal workers' disease, Pennsylvania mining capital continued to hold out against redistributive measures. The election in 1934 of the liberal Democrat George Earle as Pennsylvania's governor, with former breaker boy Thomas Kennedy as his lieutenant governor, seemingly ensured that social insurance for occupational lung disease would become law. The UMW, which now had more than a quarter million members in the state, escalated its lobbying in Harrisburg. Despite the changed climate, conservatives managed to repel compensation again in the 1935 legislative session.[37]

When the 1936 elections sent Earle and Kennedy more legislators who supported their Little New Deal, the balance finally tipped in favor of disease compensation. The coal industry resigned itself to some form of social insurance. Aided by federal reframing of the issue, the operators shifted from obstruction to containment. The Occupational Disease Compensation Act signed by Governor Earle on July 2, 1937, accommodated the interests of sick capital to a much greater extent than it did the interests of sick workers. In a departure from the conventional financial mechanism of workers' compensation, the act called for Pennsylvania's taxpayers, not the compensation claimant's employer, to pay part of the dust-disease benefit costs for the first ten years after the plan took effect. Under the phase-in formula, during the first year of the program, the employer bore only one-tenth of the costs. Thereafter, the employer's share increased by 10 percent each year. This provision aimed to help allay the operators' well-founded fears that the passage of reform would bring forth a flood of claims from displaced workers. In a further concession to the mine owners, the legislature let them choose whether or not to participate in the compensation program. In addition, the law relegated victims of pneumoconiosis to second-class status by limiting their total benefits to $3,600, a limitation not imposed on beneficiaries suffering from any other type of compensable injury or illness.[38]

The Pennsylvania statute fenced off eligibility for benefits in ways desired by the mine owners. When even the UMW backed away from plans to cover any and all illnesses contracted as a result of employment, the policy of enumerating eligible diseases became a foregone conclusion. The short schedule of compensable conditions excluded miners' asthma. Instead, in line with the advice of federal authorities, the Occupational Disease Compensation Act covered only those coal miners who had silicosis or anthraco-silicosis. Leaving no doubt that anthraco-silicosis did not encompass the outcomes of exposure to coal dust, the act strictly required "direct contact with, handling of, or exposure to dust of silicon dioxide (SiO_2)."[39]

Mine managers in Pennsylvania immediately grasped that they could safely ignore all respiratory hazards except one. Bituminous operators in particular realized that they had gotten off the hook. In October 1938, one of the state's largest firms, Pittsburgh Coal Company, asked the BOM whether soft-coal extraction involved a silica hazard. When Daniel Harrington, still chief of the bureau's Health and Safety Branch, replied with general information regarding dust hazards in coal mining, Pittsburgh Coal expressed impatience and reiterated its very specific concern with silica. Harrington refused to drop the point. In support of his conviction that a sufficient dose of any mine dust could be deleterious, he pointed out that the material he had sent discussed recent British discoveries that were especially cogent. To the BOM engineer, these discoveries "indicate very definitely that in numerous instances coal miners, not only anthracite but also non-anthracite, have dust disease, call it what you will or designate whatever cause you may wish." Harrington also offered a glimpse of the long-suppressed Meriwether report on Alabama and Kentucky. Straining against the bonds of his employer's policy of nondisclosure, Harrington complained that "the report is confidential and I cannot divulge the name of the author or other decidedly interesting data." Then he quoted an excerpt from Meriwether's conclusion that bituminous coal particles could induce pneumoconiosis. As further assistance, he provided the citation for Meriwether's presentation at the National Safety Congress in 1927. This faceful of provocation did not pique the curiosity of Pittsburgh Coal management, however.[40]

Implementation of the act distorted understanding of miners' disease in other ways as well. At some operations, the statute led to X-ray surveillance. When the law took effect in January 1938, the Philadelphia and Reading Coal and Iron Company, a leading anthracite firm, began systematic radiological examination of job applicants, rejecting those who displayed abnormalities. As always, reliance upon radiographic images hindered recognition of conditions other than silicosis. The imposition of mass screening and discharge forced the UMW to oppose the gathering of medical information on its members. No longer free to concentrate solely on illuminating illness among the rank and file, the union now also had to try to curb the abuse of pre-employment examinations and periodic re-examinations.[41]

The Pennsylvania legislature revisited the issue following Republican gains in the 1938 elections, including recapture of the governor's office. The bill signed by Governor Arthur James in June 1939 made it even harder for miners to obtain compensation. Under the amended law, in order to qualify for state benefits, a totally disabled worker had to prove that he had undergone at least six months' exposure to free silica in the period after October 1, 1939. This clause effectively denied aid to disabled men who had already left the workforce, further protecting employers against the backlog of pneumoconiotic claimants. Moreover, by its prejudice in favor of certain types of medical expertise, this measure tightened still further the imperative that only clear-cut cases of silicosis be compensated. The 1937 law had set up a Medical Advisory Board to resolve disputes over diagnosis or other medical questions. But whereas the original act was silent regarding the composition of the board, the 1939 statute required that one of the three members be a radiologist and that one be a pathologist. The way in which the radiologist's orientation predisposed toward the silicosis-or-nothing view needs no further elaboration, but it must be noted that the reorientation of pathology also disfavored recognition of pneumoconioses that did not fit into the silicosis mold. With the exhaustion of the nineteenth-century tradition of clinico-pathological correlation, pathological examination had turned away from identifying the source of melanoptysis and, instead, focused on finding silica deposits in the lung tissue of deceased miners.[42]

The 1939 revisions, albeit in a single parenthetical reference, readmitted to official discourse the old term miners' asthma. Specifically, the law now granted compensation for "anthraco-silicosis (commonly known as Miner's Asthma and hereinafter referred to as anthraco-silicosis)." However, because of the requirement that workers establish past silica exposure, miners' asthma in this context became no more than another name for silicosis.[43]

Despite its constrictions, the more conservative law did not satisfy Pennsylvania's mine owners. Almost all the bituminous and anthracite companies in the state refused to participate in the revised compensation plan. In 1941, Lester Thomas, state secretary of the Congress of Industrial Organizations, told his former coworkers at the anthracite tri-district convention, "We now have on the statute books of Pennsylvania an occupational disease law that means actually nothing to the anthracite miner." The following year, Mary Lawler desperately appealed to R. R. Sayers for guidance in winning benefits for her husband for what she characterized as a case of "chronic, far advance Pneumoconiosis." Lawler vented her frustration at her spouse's long-time employer: "Glen Alden Coal doesn't have to [pay compensation], if they don't want to." Sayers was no help. Claimants in the soft-coal regions of central and western Pennsylvania faced an especially steep uphill battle against the assumption that anthraco-silicosis was limited to anthracite mining.[44]

The unavailability of social insurance left many stranded in humiliation.

Some sick men turned their frustrations on themselves. One former coal worker and relief recipient committed suicide at home:

> Believed to have been driven to despair by miner's asthma, of which he was suffering, Adam Szalack, 61, of Shenandoah, ended his life on March 24 [1942]. He blew himself to bits with a charge of dynamite. The explosion, set off in a second floor bedroom, tore a hole through the ceiling of the kitchen below and also caught Mrs. Szalack, 56, who had just come in from hanging clothes out to dry. Mrs. Szalack was seriously injured.[45]

Their hopes for social insurance dashed, many disabled miners sued their former employers for damages. But in the judicial arena, as in the legislative one, the tyranny of silicosis remained absolute. Rather than simply decide whether a plaintiff had suffered respiratory damage as a result of his employment, the courts confined themselves to two smaller questions. First, the plaintiff, who invariably lacked scientific data on past working conditions, had to prove a long history of exposure to silicious rock dust. Second, the former miner had to have a fully documented diagnosis of silicosis, together with a medical assessment of total disability. Very few litigants managed to surmount these obstacles. As Hudson Coal Company prepared in 1942 to oppose the suit brought by Guiseppe Prattico, it enlisted the services of six physicians, including two radiologists. By the early forties, the promise of relief held out a decade earlier with the appointment of the Walnut Commission remained unfulfilled.[46]

In other coal-producing centers, the compensation contest came to different outcomes. But beneath the differences lay the essential commonality of little or no protection for most coal workers with respiratory disability. In Illinois, where silicosis litigation catalyzed legislative measures that extended to other conditions as well, Chicago compensation attorney Walter Dodd observed the mounting alarm of downstate mining interests. "The problem of compensation for silicosis is somewhat actively at issue," Dodd noted in February 1934, "and, from a political standpoint, is involved with miners' asthma and other diseases likely to develop from bituminous coal mining." In these particular circumstances, the Progressive plan for coverage for all work-induced illnesses won acceptance. The Illinois legislature granted overarching protection to victims of occupational diseases in 1936.

But as in Pennsylvania, this statute was hamstrung because employer participation was elective. In 1937, Indiana's Workmen's Occupational Diseases Act followed this model of blanket coverage at the option of the business owner.[47]

Mining states south of the Ohio River made even less provision for victims of dust disease. Tennessee, Virginia, and Alabama did nothing. Kentucky granted compensation for silicosis in 1944. In West Virginia, a tightly drawn insurance plan cut off the litigation stemming from the Gauley Bridge disaster. To allay not only the fears of the coal industry, which viewed any form of disease compensation as an entering wedge, but also similar anxieties of other dusty industries, the West Virginia statute made silicosis the state's sole compensable disease in 1935. Other restrictions included a severe statute of limitations for claims, the employer option as to participation, and the adjudication of disputed claims by a medical board, two of whose three members had to be radiologists.[48]

Some states outside southern Appalachia reached the same policy destination as West Virginia. Ohio, Maryland, and Utah all scheduled silicosis after 1935, while ignoring disease induced by non-silicious dust. Five years' experience in Maryland's statutory straitjacket left UMW leader John Jones disenchanted. "Although thousands of coal miners in western Maryland are daily threatened . . . by exposure to health-endangering bituminous coal dust," Jones informed the state legislature in 1944, "the law provides no coverage for those afflicted." Accordingly, he continued to argue that coverage for all occupational diseases constituted the appropriate remedy for this injustice.[49]

The Utah compensation law of 1941 rested on additional epidemiological research as well as the accumulated precedential legislation. In 1939, the Public Health Service, in cooperation with the State Board of Health, studied three bituminous mines in Carbon County, Utah. The United Mine Workers welcomed this inquiry, in hopes of building momentum for some sort of legislative relief. At the District 22 convention in July 1939, union leader Albert Roberts uncritically encouraged delegates to cooperate with the investigators: "If we have an impartial report from the Federal government, I believe the report would not be subject to doubt from either side. This investigation has been made in the state of Pennsylvania by the miners and the operators and they have been able to place an occupational disease law on the statutes of their state." Executing a research design similar to that deployed six years earlier in anthracite, the PHS conducted both air monitoring and more than 500 medical examinations. The federal investigators still suffered from tunnel vision. They analyzed no pneumoconiosis hazards other than free silica, even though few Utah coal workers were exposed to much silica. No disease entities other than silicosis received consideration. The PHS allowed only active employees to participate in the screening, thereby guaranteeing that few of the very few silicotic miners were deemed severely disabled. This approach concealed the wider range of respiratory effects of working in soft coal. Moreover, with the routinization of these field inquiries, a process that Thomas Kuhn termed "normal science," the possibilities dwindled for insights that would disrupt the dominant paradigm. This study did, however, admit the possibility that silicosis might arise in bituminous mines. The investigators applied the term anthraco-silicosis to this condition, contradicting the growing misconception that pneumoconiosis in coal extraction occurred only on the anthracite side of the industry.[50]

In late 1941, the Public Health Service reported on its inquiry in Utah. This report informed readers that "coal dust in itself usually does not contain sufficient silica to be considered as producing a silicosis hazard," without raising the possibility of other deleterious outcomes of inhaling coal particles. The PHS bulletin called attention to a project just completed in southern Appalachia, in which B. G. Clarke of Harvard and C. E. Moffet of MIT found that only 1 percent of bituminous miners at one firm had silicosis. Like Clarke and Moffet, the federal investigators emphasized the value of radiological testing of the mining workforce. They specifically recommended pre-employment examinations, including a chest X-ray, for all job applicants and annual examinations, including a chest X-ray, for all mine employees.[51]

In finally making public an account of a sizable study of soft-coal workers, the PHS in its lengthy bulletin made no reference to its own previous work on this population in conjunction with the Bureau of Mines. The agency missed another opportunity to resurrect, for purposes of comparison, the data gathered and the analysis made in the Alabama-Kentucky study and in the Powellton, West Virginia, study. The body of information accumulated since the early twenties thus continued to be neglected. The sort of institutional amnesia displayed in Public Health Bulletin 270 obviously helped to perpetuate silicosis reductionism. Less obvious but per-

haps equally effective for this end was the revisionist interpretation imposed at this juncture on other preceding federal work. In a distillation of
their Utah report appearing in *Industrial Medicine* in 1942, Robert Flinn and
two of his PHS co-workers skipped over the Alabama-Kentucky project
but paused to integrate into their article material on both the previously
published Wyco study and the previously unpublished Powellton study.
Despite the fact that the PHS had not originally reported the Wyco miners'
fibrosis as associated in any way with silicosis, Flinn and his colleagues announced that "generalized pulmonary fibrosis indicating early silicotic
changes was found" in that inquiry. To reinforce this distortion, they cited
private correspondence as the source for the claim that "unpublished observations by Russell in 1932 in another section of West Virginia confirmed
these findings." The federal public health officials thus not only failed to
make available all extant information relevant to this subject but also se-
lectively recalled work that could be manipulated to buttress the conventional interpretation.[52]

The net result of the decade-long compensation drive was to stymie disabled mine workers seeking remuneration for their diminished respiratory capacity. Only those few who could fit through the eye of the needle
to establish an irrefutable case of silicosis gained a measure of financial relief through the social insurance laws enacted during the New Deal years.
For the masses who could not, the suffocatingly tight definition of occupational disease caused only frustration. Moreover, as the definitional battles
wore on, coal workers and their leaders became intimidated by the abstruse discourse of medical differentiations without human differences.
The paralytic effects of mystification surfaced at a convention of West Virginia unionists in 1943. When one delegate demanded extension of compensation to miners' asthma, a defensive UMW district president offered
yet another discouraging indication of the obsession with silicosis: "You
men know and I know that the question of silicosis and occupational diseases is a question that a bunch of laymen cannot draw up a bill that is eq-
uitable, because doctors even disagree on whether a man has silicosis or
not, and what silicosis is and the different names of comparative diseases."
Confusion served some parties better than others. By the 1940s, the miners' organization sorely needed more sympathetic expertise to decipher
the complex, changing ideas in play in politics and science and to help
assert the interests of the victims of conceptualizations such as anthraco-

silicosis. Even in the heyday of the liberal New Deal, it certainly could not rely on governmental health expertise to protect its members' wellbeing.[53]

Faced with a genuine threat of redistribution, coal mine owners successfully contained their liability. Unable to standardize labor costs in general, either through their own efforts or through government intervention, the operators saw it as an economic imperative that the disease costs of production remain an object of interstate and interregional competition in a sagging industry. In 1944, Thomas Kennedy looked back on the inhibiting dynamic set in motion by the war among the mining states: "When we endeavored to have legislation enacted, of course we ran into the competitive situation. The operators in Pennsylvania had taken the position that if they compensated for miner's asthma, silicosis or [other] occupational diseases in the mining industry in that State, and if they did not compensate in other states that were in competition with their coal, automatically they would be put out of the markets." The resulting minimal accommodation meant that only totally disabled workers who had held a few specific silica-exposed jobs within one segment of the industry had much probability of recovering compensation. Like the strategic response of British mine operators to nystagmus and, of more direct relevance, like the response of U.S. employers in several competitive industries to silicosis, the bituminous and anthracite mine owners in this country impeded access to social provision to the point that dyspneic employees often had more incentive to hide their symptoms in order to keep their jobs than to seek redress through the compensation system.[54]

Alongside the main battle over compensation, political conflict broke out on another front during the Roosevelt administration. With a rash of mine disasters at the end of the thirties, the longstanding, gross inadequacies of state-level mine regulation came under heavier criticism from the United Mine Workers. As a remedy, the union and its New Deal allies sought intervention by a renovated U.S. Bureau of Mines. In this scenario, the BOM would give priority to improving underground health and safety conditions. Such a reorientation entailed deemphasizing the bureau's customary role of helping mine operators to maximize productivity, often without regard for the human consequences.[55]

The Neely-Keller bill, introduced in May 1939, promised action to prevent both explosions and work-induced diseases. This Democratic proposal sought to empower the Bureau of Mines to make annual inspections of coal mines and to publicize its findings. Actual regulatory power would still reside with the states, which would presumably upgrade their performance under the stern gaze of federal oversight. In addition, the BOM could launch investigations of occupational diseases and suggest preventive measures. In Senate hearings in June 1939, Thomas Kennedy testified that the plan for disease studies "in itself fully justifies and makes imperative the enactment of this legislation." In hearings before the Committee on Mines and Mining of the House of Representatives the following year, Kennedy reminded legislators that "too many mine workers are afflicted with miners' asthma" and claimed that "little or nothing has been done by any mining state with regard to the prevention of occupational diseases." The UMW leader also looked to federal investigations to show that disabling miners' asthma occurred outside the anthracite workforce. "Bituminous miners are affected," he told the House committee, "but we have never had a real honest-to-God investigation in the bituminous field." (Kennedy was apparently among those left ignorant by the wall of silence surrounding federal field work in soft coal since the twenties.) Senator James Davis, a Pennsylvania Republican, endorsed this initiative. "Miners asthma and silicosis must be studied intensely and adequately," Davis declared on January 19, 1940, "as they can be if we mobilize the scientific resources of the Federal government."[56]

That the Neely-Keller bill relied upon the weak and pliable Bureau of Mines did not appease mining capital. Although the operators saved their most strenuous objections for the proposed annual inspections, they also opposed the possibility of expanded investigatory activity. B. P. Manley of the Utah Coal Operators Association told Congress in 1940 that the federal-state project currently under way in his state obviated the need for additional studies of pneumoconiosis in coal mining. The National Coal Association agreed that the industry already knew enough about occupational disease. Employers worried that a minimal investigative intrusion could explode into more onerous impositions. To western Pennsylvania operator Byron Canon, enactment of the proposal would "eventually lead to an inspection bureau which will . . . lead to a Federal Compensation Act and a Federal Occupational Disease Act."[57]

Congress passed the Coal Mine Inspection and Investigation Act, and President Roosevelt signed it on May 7, 1941. Perpetuating scattered responsibility, the law ignored the Public Health Service and gave the Bureau of Mines the right to make "investigations in coal mines for the purpose of obtaining information relating to health and safety conditions, accidents, and occupational diseases." These investigations would serve as "the basis for the preparation and dissemination of reports, studies, statistics, and other educational materials pertaining to the protection and advancement of health and safety in coal mines." The act left all enforcement of healthful and safe conditions in the hands of state inspectors.[58]

As implemented, the Coal Mine Inspection and Investigation Act did not realize the UMW's hopes for a major epidemiological inquiry in the bituminous fields. After all, the act granted no new authority to the PHS, the only federal agency with the expertise to do such studies. Instead, the BOM stuck to its accustomed function as a management consultant, carrying out dust studies at the request of individual firms and quietly reporting to these clients. Firm-level data were not compiled, analyzed, and disseminated in such a way as to present a national picture of the dust hazard and its effects. In the same vein, the bureau refused to make any strong recommendation regarding a standard for permissible daily exposure to non-silicious mine dust.[59]

To be sure, with Daniel Harrington in charge of its Health and Safety Branch, the Bureau of Mines did take some advantage of the wider opportunities to prevent disease. The agency took steps to advise the industry of the mounting evidence that coal dust, even in the absence of silica, posed a threat to employees' lungs. Perhaps most remarkably, even R. R. Sayers, long an influential proponent of the silicosis-only approach and after 1941 the director of the BOM, began to publicize, if not embrace, the British findings. In its capacity as a center of engineering expertise, the bureau also consistently and insistently prodded managers to abate mine dust by wet methods and better ventilation.[60]

The reductionist paradigm emerged from the turmoil of the depression very much intact. If anything, it became more secure by adapting in response to political challenges. The rise of anthraco-silicosis served to incorporate the undeniable lung illnesses in coal into the dominant dust-disease framework.

Just as they enjoyed no Progressive Era with regard to occupational disease reform, breathless coal miners had no New Deal. They were not aided by policies that strove to create what Irving Bernstein called a "caring society." There was no nationalization of the profoundly inequitable state-level workers' compensation plans. In contrast to the unemployment insurance system, no federal standards for administration of state compensation were developed. The inspection and investigation law of 1941 kept the national government in the minor role of technical consultant on disease prevention. In part, weak federal policy reflected the entrenched division of responsibility under federalism. But beyond the perennial structural problems, it also reflected the historical accumulation and dissemination of a body of official misinformation. Taken together, fragmentation of public responsibility and strong, ideologically shaped preconceptions foreclosed any fresh insight into the causes of the coal workers' predicament.[61]

CHAPTER SIX

FRIGHTENING FIGURES

The path toward understanding of the health effects of coal mine dust became especially circuitous in the two decades after World War II. Decisions to privatize and to ignore the pneumoconiosis plague stimulated a campaign to illuminate the problem. After much delay, labor forced the state to conduct the epidemiological research crucial to revealing that a dust-induced disorder other than silicosis plagued the coal industry. A small group of physicians associated with the UMW Welfare and Retirement Fund (WRF) played a pivotal role in pressing the federal bureaucracy to generate knowledge.

By the forties, the United Mine Workers was left virtually alone with the dust-disease issue. North American medical scientists and practitioners, still enthralled by the specious rigor of radiological depictions of silicosis, were not ready to rethink the varieties of dust disease in the coal-mining workforce. In 1942, for example, Eugene Pendergrass gave the Wayne County Medical Society in Detroit a demonstration of reductionist gymnastics: "There will be instances in which a careful history fails to show any exposure to silica-containing dust and yet abnormal shadows will be seen on the roentgenogram. In such cases, one is at a loss to know what to call the condition. My present plan, when absolute data are lacking other than the occupational record and physical findings, is to make a diagnosis of *'modified silicosis'*" (italics in original). The medical literature consistently reinforced the dictum that inhaled coal dust carried little or no risk. The pneumoconiosis issue in coal mining was seemingly settled and, therefore, intellectually uninteresting.[1]

Medical schools in the mining centers, specialized professional associations in pulmonary and industrial medicine, and other health institutions turned their attention elsewhere. The spectacular expansion of governmental capacity to study disease, embodied primarily in the National Institutes of Health, brought very little attention to occupational disease in general or coal miners' respiratory disease in particular. Instead, growing concern over cancer and heart disease served to trivialize the disorders endemic to one industry.[2]

The Mine Workers could not so easily forget the issue. Unionists at the local level remained face to face with a sizable contingent of dyspneic men, struggling to stay on the job or struggling to survive after becoming too debilitated to work. Despite decades of failure, the UMW never abandoned the quest to extend workers' compensation to respiratory diseases beyond silicosis. With the federal government taking on a bigger share of the responsibility for social protection, the miners' organization also began to look to Washington for disability insurance and for more liberal old-age pensions. At the 1940 international convention, for instance, Local 781 from Wharton, West Virginia, argued that because miners' asthma and silicosis drove most aging coal workers into premature idleness, there was a need for federal benefits "for disabled miners regardless of their age." After 1935 the rank and file demanded that eligibility for retirement pensions under Social Security begin at age fifty or fifty-five, not sixty-five. The UMW considered any form of social insurance that might support disabled members.[3]

By the mid-1940s, however, it became clear that there would be no federal assistance for out-of-breath coal workers. No new income-maintenance initiatives were at all likely. Daunting restrictions surrounded existing categorical programs. R. B. McCray's plight epitomized that of many men who were stranded beyond the reach of the welfare state. After loading coal for the Elkhorn Coal Company in Kentucky for twenty years, McCray had severe enough miners' asthma to be forced out of work. His former employer blocked his claim for unemployment insurance with the contention that he had not been laid off because of lack of work but had quit voluntarily. Adding insult to injury, Elkhorn management informed the forty-five-year-old worker that in twenty years he could collect Social

Security. "It reminds me of some men who buy a horse, work him till he gets too old to work, then turn him out to starve and die," concluded McCray. Repeated defeats and illusory victories on the workers' compensation battleground fed the same bitterness. In 1946, the *United Mine Workers Journal* derided occupational disease compensation as "a joke." By the end of the Second World War, both the inadequacies of existing societal provision and the dim prospects for extending entitlement were manifest to the miners.[4]

Cut off from public benefits, coal workers set out to forge a private welfare system. Such a course suited the ideology of union president John L. Lewis. A conservative who usually supported the Republican party, Lewis had made an acrimonious break with Franklin Roosevelt in 1940. The UMW leader relished the chance to construct a private security plan that went beyond the partial protections afforded by the New Deal and promised by the Fair Deal of Roosevelt's successor, Harry Truman. No visionary in the realm of health and welfare, Lewis reacted to mounting rank-and-file anger.[5]

Beginning in the bituminous bargaining sessions in 1945, the UMW demanded a far-ranging, employer-financed welfare plan. Although this proposal aimed to address many misfortunes and grievances unrelated to industrial disease, it also rested to a significant extent on the claim that employers should pay for the damage done by work-induced disease. In March 1945, Thomas Kennedy told the soft-coal operators that the widespread occurrence of "that dread disease of the mines, miner's asthma," justified an industry-wide fund. This bargaining foray met implacable resistance and went nowhere.[6]

Undeterred, the union tried again the following year, in both the bituminous and anthracite negotiations. On March 12, 1946, Lewis demanded a fund to care for those "scrapped with silicosis, miners' asthma, chronic rheumatism, arthritis, blindness, and scores of other occupational ailments." The union brief for privatization contended that workers' compensation had proven a disastrous failure. To drive home its point, the Mine Workers publicized cases like that of West Virginia miner Floyd Cowan, recently discarded by the Island Creek Coal Company after twenty-eight years of service. Despite numerous symptoms of dust disease, Cowan could not prove that he had silicosis, so he did not qualify for workers' compensation benefits. Instead, the union reported, he was driven to a humiliating dependence on relatives in order to support his wife and four young children. In the view of rank-and-file activist Allen Croyle, the lack of social insurance left no alternative to private arrangements:

> Neither the State nor the Federal Government has enacted legislation to compensate the miner for disabilities caused by occupational diseases. . . . Should the coal industry support its workers in accordance with the American standard of living? The coal operators must protect the workers and be held accountable for the victims of occupational diseases. A health and welfare fund would be security and freedom from fear.[7]

The UMW strategy for winning private benefits depended crucially on government intervention. The union leadership may well have realized from the previous year's failure that they would need outside assistance to gain this ambitious objective. Certainly, with the war over, but with the industry still controlled by a wartime agency for the 1946 bargaining round, the canny Lewis knew that this would be the last opportunity to wrest from the Coal Mines Administration a concession that he could not extract directly from the mine owners. In the collective bargaining agreement with Secretary of the Interior Julius Krug on May 29, 1946, the union made a historic, if somewhat nebulous, advance, in what the agreement termed a "health and welfare program in broad outline" for the bituminous fields. From this beachhead, the UMW in subsequent contracts with the mine owners themselves gained a comprehensive union-controlled welfare plan. It also won adequate financing to carry out this plan, generated by a royalty on coal production. By 1950, the United Mine Workers of America Welfare and Retirement Fund became a firmly established, if still controversial, institution in the soft-coal industry.[8]

The Krug-Lewis Agreement also committed the Coal Mines Administration to make "a comprehensive survey and study of the hospital and medical facilities, medical treatment, sanitary, and housing conditions in the coal mining areas." Under the direction of Admiral Joel Boone, investigators mounted a study of 260 mines that assessed both health services and hazards to wellbeing. With its broad scope, Boone's orientation toward preventive medicine, and the union's recent claims as to the burden of occupational disease on its members, the Medical Survey Group might well have looked into working conditions as a factor in ill health. But rather than monitor the dust risk underground, the investigators made a conventional sanitary survey of water purity, sewage treatment, garbage disposal, and similar concerns. With the work environment still artificially separated from the community environment of the mining localities, another opportunity for recognizing the dust hazard passed. The narrowness of his approach did not stop Boone from noting the prevailing medical ignorance of hazardous conditions, however. In a critique appearing in the November 30, 1946, issue of the *Journal of the American Medical Association*, he complained, "There is no affirmative evidence, except in rare instances, that the company doctor or the practicing physician in mining communities goes into the mines for the express purpose of observing at first hand the working environment of his patients."[9]

Boone amplified this theme in his final report, published in March 1947. The Coal Mines Administration found only a "negligible number" of mine physicians knowledgeable of the risks that existed underground. The report recommended that company medical personnel familiarize themselves with mining conditions in order to help prevent occupational illnesses and injuries. Dependent on company doctors for evidence of industrial hazards and their effects, Boone knew only that he was in the dark. "Medical records of the bituminous-coal industry," he lamented, "do not disclose the presence or incidence of various occupational diseases." He called on management to undertake "industry-wide studies and investigations of the nature, occurrence, and control of occupational diseases and disabilities peculiar to the industry" to repair this deficiency. Besides its stunning naivete, this recommendation is remarkable for its presumption that a private party, not the government, should perform this elemental public health task. The Boone report vindicated John L. Lewis's view that miners themselves would have to improve conditions, for salvation by state intervention was not imminent.[10]

The federal report also sharply criticized the United Mine Workers for its want of leadership on health issues. This widely disseminated document, a copy of which went to every UMW local, pushed the union toward a comprehensive, public health approach to understanding and safeguarding its members' wellbeing. The Boone Report had a seminal influence on the miners' embryonic welfare plans. In particular, the consequent attempt to transform health services for coal workers would have powerful ramifications for the recognition of dust disease.[11]

While program development under the bituminous fund awaited sub-
jugation of many intransigent employers in the late 1940s, the Anthracite
Health and Welfare Fund moved quickly to address pneumoconiosis. As
in the simultaneous soft-coal negotiations, the union sought private benefits for hard-coal miners to make up for the absence of societal protections,
especially given the obstacles to receiving workers' compensation benefits.
Following its establishment in 1946, the anthracite fund granted pensions
to elderly members, including many with chronic respiratory disorders,
and embarked on an innovative medical treatment and research project. In
this venture, the fund responded to pleas such as that of Stanley Sluzalis,
who had lost his father and seven other relatives to what he called the
"Black Plague." Sluzalis in June 1946 excoriated opponents of the welfare
fund who had "never served the death watch with a victim of miner's
asthma." Similar concerns animated a UMW local from Shenandoah,
Pennsylvania, which encouraged a search for a cure or at least "aid to the
suffering caused by occupational diseases."[12]

The Anthracite Health and Welfare Fund contracted with Jefferson
Medical College of Philadelphia in 1947 both to study and to care for victims of dust disease. Through a regimen centering on administration of
oxygen, the Jefferson program gave symptomatic relief and a measure of
hope to a large number of pneumoconiotics. It also developed pulmonary
function tests with which to evaluate more accurately the degree of disability in dyspneic miners. Driving this inquiry into pulmonary physiology was the belief that X-ray images often gave a misleading indication of
the underlying state of a coal worker's health. The fund expended over two
million dollars for research and for treatment of more than two thousand
cases of pneumoconiosis during the two decades after its founding.[13]

In its educational activities with clinicians in eastern Pennsylvania and
in the numerous publications flowing from the Jefferson project, the anthracite fund unfortunately reinforced the tenet that only silicosis merited
scrutiny and remedial action. Thomas Kennedy, chairman of the fund's
board of trustees and himself a victim of miners' asthma, boasted at the
1952 union convention of the strides made toward curing "the great evil of
silicosis," making reference to no other disorders. However, the Philadelphia program never seriously pursued its stated objective to gather data
on the incidence of anthraco-silicosis.[14]

While their counterparts in anthracite plunged into action, architects of
the bituminous fund spent much of the late forties in a thorough assess-

ment of the needs of approximately a third of a million members. Several of the medical administrators for the ten geographical areas within the Welfare and Retirement Fund came to their assignments with a broad vision. Exponents of social medicine brought the progressive legacy of the New Deal into the conservative era of postwar privatization. Experience in the Farm Security Administration's pioneering medical program for migratory workers and in the Pepper Committee's deliberations on health reform prepared this cohort of activist physicians for their adventures in the coalfields. This radical perspective would shatter not only pre-existing notions of miners' respiratory ailments but also long-standing practices of managing these illnesses.[15]

In their initial observations, the WRF medical staff wrought no revolution in the identification of bituminous miners' dust disease. Early reports from the field commented on the occurrence of "silicosis" in the mining population. Nonetheless, the accumulation of disquieting experiences began to raise doubts. Sent to Morgantown, West Virginia, in 1949 to serve as an area medical administrator, former Public Health Service officer Lorin Kerr was unsettled by contradictions to the dominant paradigm: "I was beginning to see miners who had respiratory disability. And their disability was of such a nature that it didn't fit the definition of silicosis. And the definition of silicosis was laid down by what appeared in the X-rays." Another medical officer for the fund instantly decided that the dust disease problem would "have to be solved by the environment hygiene approach" and expressed his desire "to get into that aspect of preventive medicine" some day.[16]

The fund deliberately set forth to subvert the status quo. Picking up where the Boone Report left off, the WRF considered physicians under the control of mine management unequal to the task of detecting occupational disease. This condemnation rested on close observation of the ways in which dependence upon mining corporations compromised professional judgment in cases involving mine employees.[17]

As an alternative, the fund aimed from the outset to integrate recognition of occupational disease into the practice of primary-care and secondary-care medicine. To this end, it conducted considerable educational work in the medical community and spent untold millions of dollars to identify and treat pneumoconiosis in the quarter century after its founding. By the early fifties, the miners' health plan was making two types of institutional change that especially improved diagnosis and treatment of dust disease. Through the Miners Memorial Hospital Association, the fund built and operated ten acute-care hospitals in Kentucky, Virginia, and West Virginia. These institutions developed considerable expertise in radiology, pulmonary physiology, and other specialties relevant to handling pneumoconiotic patients. In addition, the fund sponsored a number of group-practice clinics in mining communities. By virtue of their innovative structure and expansive preventive-medicine perspective, these multi-specialty groups were able to recruit high-caliber medical talent to small, often remote, localities and to make effective use of this talent. The clinics devised protocols for thorough evaluation of suspected cases of industrial lung disease. Essential to this evaluation was a complete occupational history. To prepare its physicians to take such a history, the Russellton Miners Clinic, near Pittsburgh, required that they all spend a day underground. Michael Micklow, a rank-and-file miner who served on the governing board of the Russellton clinic in its early days, recalled that the board discussed pneumoconiosis "all the time." Another local activist, Ted Venesky, appreciated the ways in which the staff at the Miners Clinic not only identified respiratory illnesses as work-induced but also readily shared information with their patients, in contrast to the secretive, adversarial style of company doctors. Moreover, the fund subtly changed the atmosphere of medical practice for clinicians outside its hospitals and clinics by promoting higher standards of care and by bolstering autonomy from employer influence.[18]

As the Welfare and Retirement Fund began to explore the question of dust disease in the late 1940s, the problem was already undergoing profound conceptual change. Over the preceding decade, British scientists presented cogent evidence of the existence and prevalence of a pneumoconiosis in coal workers that could be distinguished from silicosis. In 1936, S. L. Cummins noted "the gradual realization of the fact that, especially in the South Wales coalfield, cases of more or less disabling lung conditions are frequently met with which cannot conscientiously be fitted into the category of silicosis," despite "dyspnea on exertion, which marks them out as quite unfit for work." Cummins naturally recalled the work of Edgar Collis and J. C. Gilchrist on Cardiff coal trimmers, i.e., laborers who shoveled coal into ships. As Collis and Gilchrist's seminal article had revealed in 1928,

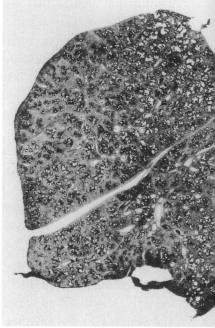

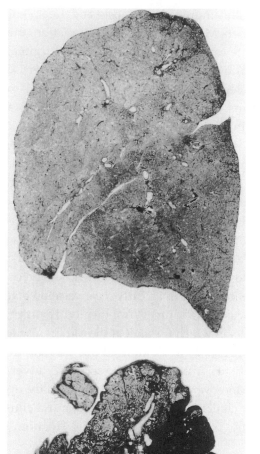

Gough sections of lung tissue:
Top left. Lung tissue of a ninety-year-old tea
Top right. Simple coal workers' pneumocon
Bottom left. Complicated coal workers'
pneumoconiosis.
(Reprinted from U.S. Senate, *Coal Mine Hea*
and Safety)

coal trimmers displayed pneumoconiosis even in the absence of silica exposure. Curiosity grew as to whether more than one disease afflicted coal miners. The obsession with silicosis came into doubt.[19]

Opponents of reductionism soon struck a devastating blow. In September 1940, Jethro Gough, a pathologist at the Welsh National School of Medicine in Cardiff, reported, from autopsies on coal trimmers, the existence of small fibrotic lesions that differed unmistakably in structure from the nodules present in silicosis. Moreover, shortly thereafter, a multifaceted inquiry by the British government's Medical Research Council (MRC) brought to light the widespread extent of non-silicotic lung illness in South Wales. From radiological screening of more than two thousand Welsh coal workers, investigators for the MRC noted the frequent occurrence of fine, diffuse reticular markings among miners with respiratory symptoms. The pathology component of the MRC study reinforced Gough's findings. As a result of these discoveries in the laboratory and in the field, the British set apart a new disease entity, originally called pneumokoniosis of coal workers but soon commonly called coal workers' pneumoconiosis (CWP). In 1943, Great Britain added this entity to its schedule of compensable conditions.[20]

In the years after 1943, a stream of confirmatory studies poured forth, particularly from the Pneumoconiosis Research Unit in Cardiff, which was founded by the MRC in 1945. With CWP acknowledged in law, British researchers aimed to refine understanding of the disorder through further pathological, clinical, and radiological investigation. Gough's innovative methods of sectioning lung tissue allowed a fuller description of the coal macule, the characteristic lesion of this disase. Work also continued on the difficult task of differentiating the radiographic pattern of this disease from that associated with silicosis. To this end, Charles M. Fletcher, the first director of the Pneumoconiosis Research Unit, and his colleagues developed a novel classification scheme. In 1950, the Third International Conference of Experts on Pneumoconiosis adopted this scheme to standardize the interpretation of pneumoconiosis X-rays. Leaving no doubts as to his view of the North American preoccupation with the silica component in mine dust, in 1951 A. G. Heppleston, a pathologist at the Cardiff research unit, attacked Sayers's anthracite study and Flinn's bituminous study in Utah. Heppleston bluntly urged that the term "coal workers' pneumoconiosis" replace "anthraco-silicosis." In a return to a much earlier focus of interest, the British researcher noted the presence in the lungs of some deceased pneumoconiotics of necrotic areas filled with thick black fluid, which he compared to ink.[21]

Medical scientists and practitioners in the United States did not rush to reconsider coal miners' lung ailments, despite the evident rigor of the British work. Only in Alabama was the new science put to immediate use. Indeed, the struggle over recognition of and compensation for pneumoconiosis in the coalfields surrounding Birmingham had begun before the diffusion of these Welsh and English advances.[22]

In the 1940s, the workers' compensation law in Alabama gave no coverage to any type of occupational respiratory disease, excluding even silicosis. Initially, that policy pleased the state's coal operators, the most prominent of which remained the Tennessee Coal, Iron and Railroad Company (TCI). As of 1945, this U.S. Steel subsidiary carried on its tradition of medical paternalism, employing a staff of forty-four full-time physicians for its 29,000 steel workers, coal miners, and iron miners. Most coal companies in the Birmingham area provided health care, either through direct employment of physicians or, more often, through contractual arrangements with private practitioners. The local medical community "for all practical purposes denied the existence of coal workers' pneumoconiosis," according to the UMW attorney William Mitch, Jr. In the view of Allen Koplin, the medical administrator for the Welfare and Retirement Fund in Alabama from 1949 to 1964, company doctors who diagnosed most respiratory conditions among miners understood that their employers opposed acknowledgment of a distinctive disabling respiratory illness in their industry and, therefore, that it was not good for one's medical career to propound any such notion. Along the same lines, TCI and other operators in the district routinely performed both pre-employment examinations on prospective employees and periodic re-examinations on active employees. TCI management did not inform those screened when it made a diagnosis of pneumoconiosis. Thus, despite the maturation of the Alabama coal industry, which entailed a large cohort of career employees with long dust exposure, and despite the relentless mechanization of these operations, which increased the dust hazard, pneumoconiosis remained a matter of quiet individual suffering, obfuscated by confusion and ignorance.[23]

After 1945, this situation changed dramatically. Louis Friedman, an independent specialist in pulmonary medicine new to Birmingham, began to diagnose cases of what he came to label "pneumoconiosis in soft-coal workers." Friedman averred that patients with this disorder were truly disabled, sometimes totally, and that their disability originated not in a defective personal lifestyle but in their work experience underground. He devised his own system for classifying X-rays, in an attempt to come to grips with images other than the markings exhibited by prototypical silicosis. Friedman also began to send samples of lung tissue to Jethro Gough at the Pneumoconiosis Research Unit. The young solo practitioner thus threw down a direct challenge to corporate power and medical authority in the Birmingham district.[24]

In the absence of workers' compensation allowances, victims of pneumoconiosis in Alabama could sue their former employers at common law for negligence for failing to prevent this condition. In the late 1940s, the United Mine Workers sponsored a large number of lawsuits by disabled miners. In fact, District 20 President William Mitch welcomed the opportunity to address an injustice he had long recognized. Mitch, who had led the drive to rebuild the union from virtually nothing in the mid-thirties, hoped that forcing mine owners to internalize more of the health costs of production would induce them to do more to control coal and rock dust. Friedman, unintimidated by the coal industry and its physicians, served as the star witness in many of the union-supported suits.[25]

Plaintiffs began to win cases. Sympathetic juries in mining communities generally awarded pneumoconiotics a few thousand dollars in damages. In response, the operators started to settle cases out of court for smaller amounts. The dialectics of litigation also served to educate some mine managers. When, for example, an official of one prominent Alabama mining company requested information on dust hazards from the U.S. Bureau of Mines in 1949, he was referred to the report of the Medical Research Council's study of South Wales, which had catalyzed the recognition of coal workers' pneumoconiosis.[26]

Friedman based his assessment of patients on a workup that included an occupational history, chest X-rays, and pulmonary function tests. Such an elaborate evaluation was prohibitively expensive for a sick, usually unemployed miner, who had no guarantee that he would ultimately recover any damages from his former employer. The transformation of the health care financing system at this very moment proved a godsend for men in this difficult circumstance. The union Welfare and Retirement Fund reimbursed Friedman for his diagnostic services in aiding lawsuits, although not for serving as an expert witness in the courtroom. Such assistance would have been unthinkable under the old regime of employer-controlled benefits.[27]

With the floodgates opened, the wave of damage awards and settlements rolled on. By 1951, TCI and the other major bituminous enterprises were ready to work out a deal to contain costs. William Mitch, Jr., and his legal partner Jerome Cooper negotiated amendments to the state compensation law with attorneys for the coal operators. The amendments passed the legislature without difficulty and became law in June 1951.[28]

The statute threw a blanket over various forms of dust disease. As defined in the act, "the term 'occupational pneumoconiosis' shall include, but without limitation, such diseases as silicosis, siderosis, anthracosis, anthra-silicosis, anthraco-silicosis, anthraco-tuberculosis, tuberculo-silicosis, silico-tuberculosis, aluminosis, and other diseases of the lungs." This profuse enumeration captured the underlying complex interactions among diverse working and living conditions and the resulting complicated forms of disease, such as the possibility of coal mine dust exposure combining with a low standard of living to foster anthraco-tuberculosis. Its many variations notwithstanding, this list still centered around silicosis in a way that reflected that condition's pre-eminence at mid-century. Along the same lines, the statute neglected to identify and thereby legitimate coal workers' pneumoconiosis as a distinct entity.[29]

With the patronage of district president Mitch, Allen Koplin gave important assistance to the effort to extend workers' compensation in Alabama. In general, however, the staff of the bituminous health and welfare plan lacked an unequivocal authorization to take on the dust-disease problem as it unfolded in the forties and fifties. Both the basic structure of the fund and its particular financial arrangements served to inhibit activism. The UMW Welfare and Retirement Fund was, under the provisions of the collective bargaining agreement of March 5, 1950, an irrevocable joint trust. The three trustees consisted of one union representative (Lewis), one management representative (Charles Owens in the early fifties), and one neutral trustee agreed upon by the other two. From 1950 on, Josephine Roche, a Lewis loyalist, occupied this key position. Roche also directed the fund's operations, so that she had both policy-making and administrative functions. Moreover, revenue for this health and welfare program came

from a royalty on each ton of coal produced. It was objectionable to operators to have to pay an assessment on production for any purpose; it was especially galling to have the royalty used for medical services that gave
their employees the evidence to sue them or, in some circumstances, to file
compensation claims. Employers did not hesitate to voice their grievances
regarding what they perceived as double jeopardy.[30]

In this context, Roche, herself a former coal operator, made known early
on that WRF staff would refrain from certain types of advocacy. In the recollection of one long-time subordinate, "Miss Roche got upset about it
when we tried to do anything that would be contrary to what the operators wanted." Members of the fund's staff were not to testify in lawsuits or
in workers' compensation claims proceedings. They were not to lobby for
or testify on behalf of pending compensation legislation. The resources of
the bituminous fund, unlike those of the anthracite fund, were not to be
used to support research into occupational disease. Medical officers and
other WRF administrators had to walk a tightrope when it came to encouraging any form of redistribution related to pneumoconiosis.[31]

Within these confines, a small group of medical activists waged an in-
defatigable, often subterranean, campaign to expand awareness of coal
workers' pneumoconiosis. The WRF launched a multi-faceted educational
campaign to show conclusively that CWP was a discrete entity. As its immediate objective, this effort sought to enlighten the medical community,
coal operators, and union leaders as to the hazards of coal mine dust and
to the nature of coal workers' pneumoconiosis. In attaining this objective,
fund officials intended to set in motion a process that would culminate
in disease prevention. The strategy was that growing awareness of CWP
would lead to an epidemiological study to ascertain the prevalence of the
condition. Determination of the magnitude of the problem would catalyze
revision of workers' compensation laws to cover CWP. The financial burden imposed by compensation would, in turn, compel mine operators to
institute dust controls, which would effectively eliminate the respiratory
hazard in the mines. Pursuit of this strategy took the miners' fund on a
convoluted journey in the 1950s and 1960s.

Shortly after the enactment of the Alabama compensation amendments,
William Mitch went to Europe for a series of meetings of international
labor groups. Louis Friedman arranged for him to visit Cardiff and tour
the Pneumoconiosis Research Unit. The District 20 president discussed his

trip at the UMW executive board meeting in October 1951. Coming after Thomas Kennedy's report to the board on the rising interest in prevention of pneumoconiosis on the part of the Coal Mines Committee of the International Labor Organization, Mitch's revelations prompted John L. Lewis to request that he "relate some of those medical matters to the people in our Welfare Department." Mitch agreed to do this and underscored a critical political point:

> If I would write up what I have in mind on this silicosis and pneumoconiosis situation, and quote what they put in their report [at the Miners' International conference in Luxembourg], it might be helpful to all of us, because I don't think enough of us understand this matter. They point out definitely for years and years, as long as they have had industry over there, men have died progressively, and the result is the doctors would invariably report tuberculosis, lung condition, anything they could think of, but everything was a subterfuge to keep from paying compensation. Now they are getting compensation.[32]

Within a week, Mitch sent a long letter to Josephine Roche and her executive medical officer, Warren Draper, recounting not only his European experiences but also the passage of compensation reform in his own state. Perhaps most important, he asserted that the advent of social insurance had already stirred greater interest in dust control among Alabama's mine managers.[33]

Thus apprised of encouraging developments at home and abroad by a reputable senior leader within the union, the Welfare and Retirement Fund raised its commitment to addressing the dust disease issue. In what proved to be a major decision, Warren Draper assigned his assistant, Lorin Kerr, who had recently been transferred from West Virginia to the Washington headquarters, to become the fund's expert on occupational respiratory disorders.[34]

Kerr instigated a campaign to introduce British scientific advances to the U.S. medical and public health community. In an era before the advent of readily available, inexpensive photocopying, the circulation of reprints of journal articles and other scholarly publications remained important to the dissemination of medical knowledge. Throughout the fifties, Kerr coordinated the acquisition and distribution of countless thousands of copies of reports from British authors and other sources. For example, each of the fund's area medical administrators received ten copies of Joseph Martin's path-breaking article on his study in West Virginia, published in the *American Journal of Public Health* in May 1954. In the accompanying memo, Draper suggested that "this paper might be of assistance to you in overcoming the reluctance of American physicians to properly diagnose and identify coal workers' pneumoconiosis." In addition to passing along the work of others, in 1956 Kerr himself surveyed the literature on CWP in *Industrial Medicine and Surgery*. The primary objective of this exercise, in fact, was to produce a short summary suitable for widespread reprinting. Kerr distributed 25,000 copies of the article, with the aim of giving a copy to every doctor in the Appalachian coalfields. Moreover, this broker of subversive ideas supplied professional colleagues with numerous eye-opening Gough sections of lung tissue, many sets of the ILO standard X-rays for classification of pneumoconiosis, and copies of the occupational history and clinical evaluation forms used at the Welsh pneumoconiosis unit. In the distribution network that developed after 1951, information flowed through the fund's area offices to front-line clinicians and to researchers at nearby academic institutions.[35]

Kerr helped bring British authorities on pneumoconiosis to the United States on several occasions. He also prevailed upon visitors who came to this country under other auspices to participate in additional educational sessions. In the course of explaining their methods and findings, British researchers had ample opportunity to take on skeptics. The first round of meetings came in the fall of 1952, when Kerr arranged for Charles Fletcher and Philip Hugh-Jones to discuss CWP with chest physicians in Washington. More important, WRF staff introduced British medical workers into mining districts far from the academic medical centers of the East Coast. John Gilson of the Pneumoconiosis Research Unit toured Ohio, West Virginia, Kentucky, Tennessee, and Alabama in 1955. When Jethro Gough came in 1958, his lecture in Pittsburgh, according to one member of the audience, "presented the story of coal workers' pneumoconiosis as only the father of the entity as developed in Britain could. His presentation was complete with a review of the epidemiology, the pathogenesis and very expertly presented pathologic evidence."[36] Sustaining these connections through regular correspondence, Kerr also elicited comments from his British colleagues on the situation in this country. In 1955, John Rogan, chief medical officer of the National Coal Board, reacted to an idea that was being taken seriously by some North American specialists in occupational medicine: "You told me that there was a feeling in the States that coalminers became breathless because of emotional problems, particularly at home and at work. This seems to me absolute nonsense." The North American habit of blaming the victim looked ridiculous from across the Atlantic.[37]

The dissemination of information gradually made the medical profession and health scientists aware of CWP. To be sure, considerable ignorance and denial persisted. Although Rutherford Johnstone and Seward Miller identified "coal miners' pneumoconiosis" as a major type of dust disease in 1960, their textbook still cast it as a "clinical entity . . . unfamiliar to most American clinicians." In the Birmingham area, where only a decade before Louis Friedman stood alone, by the mid-fifties several physicians were prepared to diagnose CWP. Adolph Kammer of the University of Pittsburgh used the Second Symposium on Coal Workers' Pneumoconiosis at the Golden Clinic in 1955 to try to explain the gap between British and North American understanding of occupational lung disease in the mines. Kammer reasoned that "exaggerated reliance upon animal experimentation" and other factors served to perpetuate an outdated preoccupation with silica dust in this country. Thus, within a short time a self-critical attitude began to replace complacency.[38]

One of the main lessons of the British experience for Kerr and his colleagues was the importance of epidemiology in guiding public policy. Just as social insurance coverage for byssinosis and asbestosis had awaited evidence of their prevalence in Britain, the compensability of CWP had depended upon demonstration of the extent of the disease across South Wales. Although the absence of quantitative data on coal workers' pneumoconiosis in the United States comparable to that available abroad was manifest to WRF administrators, British investigators themselves underscored this deficiency during the formative days of the fund's pneumoconiosis program. When Charles Fletcher requested data on the number of pneumoconiosis cases in this country in August 1952, Warren Draper had to reply that extant statistics were "so fragmentary as not to be of value." A month later, Fletcher gave a paper on British epidemiological work at a major conference on industrial disease in Saranac Lake, New York.[39]

Under this goading, the UMW welfare fund began to press the Public Health Service to undertake a field study. In October 1952, Draper asked

Surgeon General Leonard Scheele to tackle the subject, challenging him with the estimate that approximately 50,000 of the nation's bituminous miners suffered from the disease. Draper reminded the surgeon general of the unique capability of the PHS to handle this assignment. "We know of no private group to which we can turn," he pleaded, "for a scientific unbiased investigation of this disease." This appeal won an assurance of cooperation. In April 1953, Kerr told a colleague that federal officials had informed the fund of their intention "to conduct a detailed research project on pneumoconiosis . . . 60,000 to 80,000 bituminous coal miners will be extensively examined." A prevalence study appeared to be imminent.[40]

Such optimism seemed warranted not only by discussion at the executive level in Washington but also by pressure for action emanating from the coalfields. Upon arrival in Knoxville, Tennessee, in 1949, John Winebrenner, the fund's medical officer for Tennessee, eastern Kentucky, and Virginia, encouraged the founding of the Miners' Chest Group, later the Knoxville Chest Group. Although modeled after the anthracite specialists' organization at Jefferson Medical College, the Knoxville physicians adopted a broader perspective on pneumoconiosis. With the support of the WRF, the pulmonary group raised awareness of dust disease in the coal workforce through its delivery of medical care and its pursuit of clinical research. These efforts soon led the Tennessee Department of Public Health to request the assistance of the PHS in assessing the severity of the problem.[41]

To underscore its concerns, the Knoxville Chest Group put on a conference in May 1953. Allen Koplin, who brought a dozen Alabama practitioners to the event, came away with the sense that at this point future progress required "statistically unchallengeable data." To Koplin, "This type of data cannot be developed from clinical practice but requires a research project with adequate controls, proper selection of sample population for study, etc. Only in this way can conclusions be drawn capable of withstanding prejudicial attacks." The movement within the medical community to recognize CWP had reached a stage where it seemed imperative that the next step be epidemiological inquiry. Because the union and everything it touched were deemed to be contaminated by partisan bias, it was essential that federal authorities intervene to carry out this work.[42]

With the concerns of the Knoxville group and the WRF in mind, Tracy Levy and Henry Doyle of the Public Health Service surveyed the records of eight clinics in southern Appalachian mining districts. Levy and Doyle examined the files of approximately 7,000 bituminous miners with symptoms of respiratory disease and discussed the situation with local clinicians. They found evidence that a chronic pulmonary condition was common among soft-coal workers. Moreover, they tentatively concluded that coal dust alone or coal dust mixed with silica probably caused this condition. These provocative findings strengthened the case for a full-scale effort to gather original data. Strangely enough, Doyle didn't see it that way. On September 18, 1953, he told Kerr that "as a result of this preliminary survey, we are of the opinion that a field study of chest disability in soft coal miners is premature at this time." Primary among the reasons Doyle gave for delay was that "no disease entity has been clinically defined." Doyle's superior, Seward Miller, told Warren Draper that rather than rush into the field, "a more basic scientific approach to the problem should be made through environmental studies, medical studies, and animal experiments." Miller gave no indication how the proposed studies would surpass the British work his agency was disregarding.[43]

To promote better radiological interpretation and thereby help lay the groundwork for a sounder prevalence survey, the fund brought Robert Ian McCallum, a prominent English radiologist, to the United States later in 1953. (Of course, improved X-ray reading was seen as valuable for reasons beyond mass screening, principally in diagnosing individual patients in the clinical setting.) McCallum spent a year instructing physicians in mining centers throughout the nation in the use of the ILO system for classifying chest X-rays. In the course of his presentations, he described British mobile X-ray units used for large-scale screening projects. McCallum found other ways to pique curiosity. In Pittsburgh on December 8, 1953, he asked his audience of local practitioners and biomedical scientists what proportion of U.S. coal workers were disabled with pneumoconiosis. No one knew. Besides helping with McCallum's travel expenses and arranging his appearances, the Welfare and Retirement Fund supported his work by distributing several sets of the standard films exemplifying ILO categories of dust disease.[44]

Despite rising expectations, at the end of McCallum's extended visit a prevalence study seemed no closer to reality. The publication in May 1954 of Joseph Martin's criticism of the lack of epidemiological work, accompanied by his estimate that as many as 58,000 bituminous workers suffered from CWP, apparently left the federal bureaucracy unmoved. At Kerr's urging, McCallum met with PHS officials on October 4, 1954, to try to get things going. McCallum learned that in the name of a holistic approach, the Public Health Service was preparing a massive, encyclopedic inquiry into coal workers' health status, rather than a study focused solely on occupational lung disease. For reasons of expediency, advocates of broader recognition of pneumoconiosis sought a relatively narrow investigation, which would rely heavily on radiological methods of disease detection. Because PHS officials in Cincinnati had previously warned him that coal management's opposition was holding up the proposed pneumoconiosis inquiry, McCallum took this response as a disingenuous stalling tactic, given the patent impossibility of finding the resources to mount such an ambitious project. Both McCallum and Kerr inferred that pressure from the coal industry, not real concern over the multi-factorial nature of disease and the multiplicity of diseases afflicting miners, had blocked the prevalence study.[45]

Kerr continued to call in foreign authorities to combat embedded resistance. In 1955, he brought John Gilson, who had succeeded Fletcher as director of the Pneumoconiosis Research Unit, to address the annual conference of the International Association of Industrial Accident Boards and Commissions, the U.S.-Canadian organization of state workers' compensation agencies. This presentation stimulated the compensation administrators to pass a resolution, drafted by Kerr and WRF coworker Kenneth Pohlmann, urging the PHS to conduct a prevalence study. Based on an informal estimate made during the course of discussion at the conference, the association suggested that "in excess of fifty thousand coal workers are afflicted with this disease." Warren Draper made sure that the surgeon general received a copy of the resolution. The fund sent Gilson to speak in more than a dozen cities before he returned to Wales. Buoyed by this visit, Kerr wrote to Charles Fletcher that he was "very optimistic about being able to move forward rather quickly on a prevalence study."[46]

Federal officials remained deaf to these appeals and to unflattering comparisons with British action, however. Their unresponsiveness made the reformers shift tactics. In late 1955, physicians at the Centerville Clinic in western Pennsylvania, one of the group-practice clinics sponsored by the Welfare and Retirement Fund, began to prepare their own investigation. The Centerville doctors, who were soon joined by colleagues at two other

clinics in the area, intended to develop a data base directly from their patient population of sick miners. These practitioners aimed first "to confirm
the British work" and then to help build a case for revision of the state
compensation law. In addition, the project sought "a valid rational method
of treatment" as well as dust suppression in the workplace.[47]

The clinics' study never got off the ground because state officials were
induced to preempt it. The proposed project attracted the attention of Jan
Lieben, head of the occupational health unit in the Pennsylvania Department of Health. Lieben agreed first to provide a mobile X-ray van and then
to take over administration of the whole venture. The state stepped in not
merely because of its customary responsibility to investigate major public
health problems but also because, despite the circumscribed entitlement to
benefits, expenditures for pneumoconiosis under the Occupational Disease Act of 1939 were escalating. The Centerville doctors welcomed this
turn of events because they knew that the state commanded greater resources, including a reputation for rigor and impartiality. In contrast, the
group-practice physicians associated with the UMW were considered
dangerous renegades by many in the medical community. Hence, when
Lieben in June 1957 announced plans for a state investigation, the miners'
fund signaled its readiness to cooperate. During the preliminary planning
process in the winter of 1957–58, the union stressed that "results of the
study should be published and made readily available to all interested
groups and individuals as soon as feasible." Expecting the state to produce
strong evidence substantiating their views, the proponents of CWP sought
to ensure that this evidence rapidly reached a wide audience.[48]

The Pennsylvania study began in 1958 by resurveying the anthracite district. The principal finding was that approximately 30 percent of a sample
of 1,300 working hard-coal miners had definite or suspected pneumoconiosis. In addition, about three quarters of the 428 retirees examined
showed X-ray evidence of dust disease.[49]

In 1959, the health department team moved on to their main interest, the
soft-coal fields in the central and western regions of the state. There,
Lieben noted, frank skepticism persisted: "The bituminous coal industry
still questions that the pneumoconiosis problem in its mines is of major
significance." With the assistance of UMW locals and mine owners, his
group examined more than 16,000 active and retired soft-coal workers.
Although their protocol encompassed occupational and medical histories

and pulmonary function tests, the primary diagnostic tool remained the chest X-ray. In a coup for partisans of CWP, Lieben got Eugene Pendergrass of the University of Pennsylvania, the dean of industrial radiologists, to read the radiographs. Pendergrass, who had recently come to accept CWP as a discrete entity, employed the ILO classification scheme, i.e., the nosology that federal officials feared to adopt. On the other hand, the overall design of this study, like that of the concomitant anthracite study, took a step backward from previous work in this country and abroad. Both investigations were merely descriptive: the epidemiologists made no attempt to correlate cumulative dust exposure to the severity of disease.[50]

The results of the Pennsylvania study exploded the notion that soft-coal dust was innocuous. Among working bituminous miners aged forty-five through sixty-four, 23 percent had radiological evidence of pneumoconiosis. Over one third of retirees presented signs of dust disease on X-ray. Most disturbingly for those committed to the indispensability of radiology, the investigators reported that "no correlation between subjective symptomatology and roentgenographic diagnosis was found." These striking findings were widely promoted in the medical literature. A concomitant analysis of death certificates by the state vital statistics bureau demonstrated that dust disease remained a significant primary or contributory cause of death for bituminous miners even where underground silica exposure was minimal. Nonetheless, indicative of the difficulty of embracing a still-controversial concept, Lieben and his coworkers shied away from the term "coal workers' pneumoconiosis."[51]

Its inertia illuminated by the Pennsylvania research, the U.S. Public Health Service had no choice but to conduct its own belated investigation. In proposing a prevalence study in 1962, the PHS took cognizance of Lieben's work. It also finally made use of British discoveries, noting that pneumoconiosis in coal workers "differs in considerable detail from the classical silicosis and anthraco-silicosis found in this country." The research proposal allowed that "most authorities agree that coal pneumoconiosis [sic] is a significant occupational disease problem in the United States at this time." During the fall of 1962, both the UMW and its bituminous welfare fund took part in planning this national study. At the insistence of the WRF, federal epidemiologists defined the population at risk as all current and former bituminous workers. Concerns over confidentiality of records led the PHS to promise that neither study participants nor their employers would have access to individual medical findings. (An exception was made for notification of the subject's personal physician if cancer or another lethal condition were discovered.) Although this policy assuaged the fears of miners that their employers would learn their diagnoses and fire them before they could file compensation claims or lawsuits, it protected confidentiality in a way that denied workers a right to know their health status.[52]

Finally, in 1963, a decade after the Mine Workers' fund broached the subject and two decades after Britain certified CWP as a compensable disorder, the Public Health Service began to examine a randomly chosen cross-section of active and inactive soft-coal workers in several mining states. During the next two years, federal agents screened 3,740 individuals, relying primarily on chest X-rays. As had been the case in Pennsylvania, the PHS made no attempt to relate the quantity of dust inhaled to individual health outcome.[53]

After collecting a mass of data, the Public Health Service refused to divulge its findings. As of 1967, three years after field work ended, the agency had published only one brief, superficial account of the project. Most glaringly, this brief article failed to indicate the total number of cases of CWP in the United States. Lorin Kerr came forward to fill this void. In collaboration with Jan Lieben, Kerr analyzed the PHS data, together with the Pennsylvania prevalence figures, data from WRF records, workers' compensation statistics, and other evidence. Fittingly, the Public Health Service provided the forum for presenting the fruits of this analysis. As a result of congressional interest spurred by its epidemiological work, the PHS established the Appalachian Laboratory for Occupational Respiratory Diseases at West Virginia University. At a conference sponsored by the laboratory in May 1967, Kerr claimed that at least 125,000 current and former miners were suffering from dust disease. That total included 100,000 victims of coal workers' pneumoconiosis, with the other 25,000 cases attributed to silicosis or mixed-dust pneumoconiosis. The assertion caused heated debate. In Kerr's view, management physicians at the conference "tried to lynch us."[54]

As expected, this estimate provoked further discussion. In March 1968, public-interest advocate Ralph Nader challenged Secretary of the Interior Stewart Udall with the claim that 100,000 miners had what he termed "coal pneumoconiosis." In an article in the *American Review of Respiratory Disease* in August 1968, W. K. C. Morgan of the PHS Appalachian Laboratory attempted to fix attention on regional differences in rates of dust disease and to explain these in terms of variations in the chemical properties of coal across regions. Although Morgan's article was titled "The Prevalence of Coal Workers' Pneumoconiosis," he advanced no specific estimates of the national or regional prevalence of CWP. In any event, the union had won the war of numbers, not by precisely determining the magnitude of miners' pneumoconiosis but rather by creating a sustained, open debate in which all parties assumed that this disease claimed many thousands of victims. CWP had gained recognition as a substantial enough problem to be unavoidable for public policy makers. The production of quantitative data placed the issue on the reform agenda.[55]

Unlike previous investigations whose findings were shelved, the work of Lieben and his associates fed directly into sustained political deliberations. Confirmation of widespread dust-induced lung disease in the bituminous fields set in motion a campaign to expand Pennsylvania's workers' compensation protection. After Eugene Pendergrass expressed to Governor William Scranton his shock at the "amazing amount" of dust disease discovered by the Department of Health, Scranton called for a conference to discuss remedial measures. Reformers undoubtedly took encouragement from the fact that, in contrast to the secret machinations of the gubernatorial commission of 1932–33, the forum chosen for policy debate in Pennsylvania would be an open one.[56]

The Pennsylvania Governor's Conference on Pneumoconiosis (Anthraco-Silicosis), as its very name made clear, was both a product of and an exercise in the negotiation of disease. Acceptance of CWP remained incomplete. In his introductory remarks on November 30, 1964, state Secretary of Health C. J. Wilbar, Jr., set out "to clarify terminology" but clarified little. Wilbar refused to define, or even to mention, coal workers' pneumoconiosis as a disease entity. Instead, he explained that anthracosis was "a disease condition caused by coal in the lung." Wilbar then attempted to salvage the embattled category of anthraco-silicosis by defining this disorder as the result not simply of silica inhalation in a coal mine but instead as the result of mixed dust inhalation. This was a last-ditch effort to uphold anthraco-silicosis, the object of derision among the British innovators and their North American followers, as the dominant conceptualization of dust disease.

Indeed, none of the senior state officials who opened the conference uttered the phrase "coal workers' pneumoconiosis." The secretary of mines and mineral industries left room for doubt as to whether pneumoconiosis was even a type of disease: "The term pneumoconiosis was proposed in 1867 to include all pulmonary manifestations of dust inhalation, whether the dust is injurious or harmless." Governor Scranton also avoided the alien concept, but seemed more concerned with solving the unmistakable underlying problem than with labeling it. Scranton pressed for disease prevention, while freely acknowledging that "we have great gaps in our knowledge of these conditions." He also tried to break the deadlock by appealing to common sense: "You don't have to be a physician to know there is something wrong when a man forty to fifty years old, who should be in the prime of life, is unable to walk up a small hill without stopping for breath. When a man acts like this, . . . nine times out of ten he has 'miners' asthma.'" The governor signaled that imperfect biomedical knowledge would no longer suffice to block corrective action.[57]

Through three days of deliberation, the three hundred conferees pondered ways to assess, prevent, and compensate cases of dust disease in the mines. With neither Lieben nor any representative of the UMW welfare fund's office in Pittsburgh on the program, it fell to Henry Doyle to broach the subject of CWP. Doyle made a cursory survey of European implementation of dust-suppression measures, a reminder that this was a preventable condition. Then he made the fundamental point that the predominant, if not unanimous, expert opinion was that "coal pneumoconiosis is a distinct clinical entity, resulting from inhalation of coal dust." In what must have been an unpleasant moment for the management representatives in the room, Doyle announced that "coal workers' pneumoconiosis is recognized as a compensable disease in each of the European coal producing countries and in most the compensation cost for coal pneumoconiosis is greater than all other occupational diseases combined." He then traced the growth of an indigenous biomedical literature since the early fifties, including the recent work of Lieben's team. Only one other speaker, Eugene Robin of the University of Pittsburgh, joined in reviewing the abundance of evidence for the existence of CWP.[58]

Despite pervasive reticence and persistent resistance, one group at the conference did move toward embracing the new designation. The chairman of the Special Session on Disability Evaluation, Leon Cander of the

Hahnemann Medical College, reported that his session had produced a decisive proposal: "Since there is a large body of evidence from Great Britain and from recent studies by the USPHS in this country that inhaled carbon particles containing little or no free silica may produce disabling pneumoconiosis, it is recommended that the term anthraco-silicosis be abandoned in favor of the more inclusive term 'Coal Workers' Pneumoconiosis.'" Cander's group also attacked the privileged status of radiological data: "Since the relationship between the x-ray stage of Coal Workers' Pneumoconiosis and the degree of disability is frequently poor or nonexistent, it is recommended that less emphasis be placed on the x-ray stage of the disease and more emphasis be placed on functional evaluation in disability determination." Participants in the disability evaluation session proposed to remove the statutory limitation of claims to those whose last exposure to mine dust was less than four years before filing their claim, in light of the long interval between dust exposure and total disability.[59]

In contrast, the Special Session on Workmen's Compensation Legislation brought forth no concrete substantive recommendations. After noting that much division of opinion existed on this topic, the chairman of this session finished his report with the dithering suggestion that "the individual as well as collective appraisals and opinions be made known to the proper authorities." The conference failed to meet the expectations of the UMW and, presumably, of disabled miners. On the strength of the state's epidemiological discoveries, the miners' union had hoped to make the conference a forum on compensation reform.[60]

Despite its failure to make recommendations on social insurance, the governor's conference did raise the visibility of miners' respiratory disorders, and reformers took advantage of the sense of urgency it created. The next session of the Pennsylvania legislature immediately took up proposed amendments to the Occupational Disease Act of 1939. At the urging of Joseph Yablonski, president of UMW District 5, and other union officials, the legislature changed the act to cover coal workers' pneumoconiosis and explicitly broadened the definition of the dust hazard to include bituminous and anthracite coal particles as well as particles of free silica. After decades of denigrating vernacular conceptions of this disorder, the lawmakers felt obliged to indicate that this condition was still "commonly known as Miner's Asthma." Popular awareness of the varying degrees of disability caused by this condition did not translate into public policy.

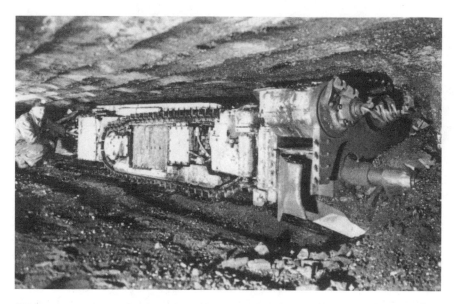

Continuous mining machine, ca. 1952. (Courtesy of the United Mine Workers of America)

Despite vigorous lobbying by the union, the 1965 amendments did not extend benefits to those partially disabled by dust disease and did not loosen the statute of limitations.[61]

In the wake of the Pennsylvania legislation, Virginia legislators revisited pneumoconiosis compensation. This state had previously opened and then closed off an entitlement. In 1952, Virginia made workers' compensation available to victims of "all occupational diseases arising out of and in the course of employment," including the pneumoconioses of coal mining. With the development of specialized expertise under the auspices of the UMW Welfare and Retirement Fund and especially with the founding of the Kentucky-Virginia Pneumoconiosis Society in 1956, the number of successful benefit claims by former coal miners in the southwestern corner of the state increased, and the prospect of much larger outlays loomed ahead. In 1958, mining interests and their allies secured legislation that gave employers the option to assume liability for compensation for all work-induced diseases or to be responsible only for disability from a schedule of diseases. This list included silicosis but excluded CWP.[62] UMW District 28 lobbied subsequent legislatures for the reinstatement of protection for CWP, but to no avail. In 1968, the reforms in Pennsylvania, together with the weight of medical evidence pointing to a pneumoconiosis beyond silicosis, tipped the balance. Virginia augmented its schedule to provide compensation for "coal miner's pneumoconiosis" stemming from workplace exposure to coal dust.[63]

The Welfare and Retirement Fund's strategy for extending recognition and control of dust disease had its contradictions and limitations. The most fundamental contradiction was that the payment of tonnage royalties to such a benevolent cause as the fund served to muffle criticism of a dramatic rise in the mechanization of coal extraction in the postwar years. Without question, the virtually unrestricted introduction of mechanical loading and continuous mining equipment during this period greatly increased the dust hazard underground.[64] Thus, internalization of the health and welfare costs of production perversely led to more disease.

From the formative days of the WRF, John L. Lewis understood that the spread of continuous mining equipment and other forms of mechanization caused many more cases of respiratory disease among his members. Yet the cynical labor executive chose not to probe too deeply into this matter, tacitly accepting a decline in working conditions as part of the price of the fund and, beyond that, as part of the price of the survival of the industry. As Lorin Kerr put it, Lewis "wished to God that he didn't know anything." But he did know the fundamental elements of the pneumoconiosis situation, in part because Kerr told him. Others forced the issue to his attention. Although Lewis asked William Mitch to apprise fund administrators of developments in Europe and Alabama in 1951, Mitch sent a copy of his lengthy report directly to the union president as well. In addition, Benjamin Golden sent Lewis a personal invitation to the Second Symposium on Coal Workers' Pneumoconiosis at his clinic in Elkins, West Virginia, in 1955. Golden reminded his long-time acquaintance that "several years ago you and I discussed miners' asthma." Then he suggested that anyone interested in this subject would profit from attending the upcoming symposium. Going straight to the main point, Golden informed the UMW president, "Today we recognize the so-called miners' asthma as a truly debilitating disease but unfortunately the industry as a whole is attempting to fight this recognition." Lewis did not attend the conference in Elkins.[65]

To be sure, with coal losing out to petroleum and other rivals, the UMW had relatively little leverage on this issue in the 1940s and 1950s. The share of the nation's energy provided by coal fell from 51 percent in 1945 to 28 percent in 1959. That Lewis and the leading coal operators considered productivity gains from advanced, dusty extractive techniques crucial to meeting the competitive challenge cut down the options available to prevent occupational disease. In fact, miners' leaders had always encouraged or at least acquiesced in mechanization: the Lewis administration merely upheld the organization's longstanding policy on this perennial question. Moreover, no massive groundswell of rank-and-file opposition to ongoing mechanization for health reasons arose to chasten the UMW hierarchy. Nonetheless, in negotiating the postwar accord with management, the union could have tried to make implementation of new technology contingent upon the use of improved ventilation and other feasible methods of dust control, even if this meant cutting royalties to the fund a few cents per ton to cover the costs involved.[66]

Elitism further diminished the fund's effectiveness. By the 1960s the organization had locked itself into a highly bureaucratic approach. Instead of educating rank-and-file mine workers, the fund generally pursued a trickle-down strategy in which it conveyed news of British biomedical advances to U.S. scientists, public health officials, and medical practitioners. A sizable share of the information distributed in this way never reached the dust-breathing population. Further, the fund gave miners themselves no significant, active role in the struggle to gather more information on the problem. Mass mobilization of CWP victims to pressure the federal bureaucracy was unthinkable. The WRF looked upon sick workers and former workers en masse primarily as material for epidemiological research. The quest for a prevalence study, however worthwhile, entailed a dehumanizing objectification. With the exception of a few officials, miners were patients, beneficiaries, or statistics from the fund's perspective.[67]

Lorin Kerr's appearance at the United Mine Workers convention of 1968 encapsulated some of the principal strengths and weaknesses of the Welfare and Retirement Fund's handling of the problem. By this time, UMW president W. A. Tony Boyle was anxious to begin to reverse a long period of lethargy by top union officials on the occupational disease issue. But just arranging for Kerr to address the convention took considerable maneuvering, given the structural separation between the fund and its parent. In his overdue address, the WRF's expert on dust disease emphasized the long history of medical observations and studies of miners afflicted with

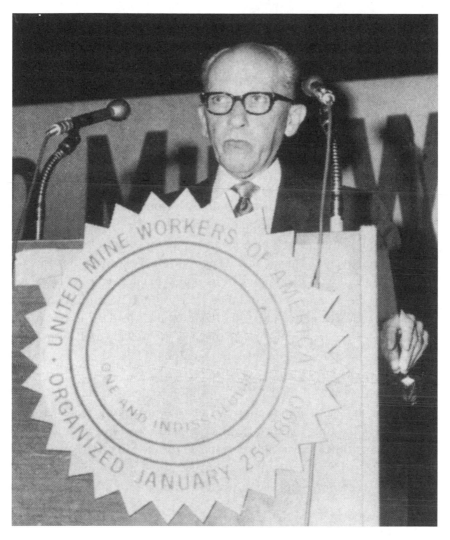

Lorin Kerr addresses the UMW convention, September 10, 1968. (Courtesy of the United Mine Workers of America)

the all-too-familiar syndrome of coughing, gasping, and spitting. He described the definition of CWP by the British a quarter century earlier, and the granting of compensation to thousands. "In Great Britain coal miners' pneumoconiosis accounts for more deaths than do all other forms of dust diseases combined," Kerr announced, after suggesting that recent epidemiology in this country yielded a "grisly repetition" of British findings.

He alluded to one of his own skirmishes: "In 1956 the concern of some physicians about management attitudes effectively blocked the publication of a paper of mine on coal workers' pneumoconiosis in the most widely circulated medical journal in the United States. One can only wonder how many times other medical information vital for the protection of workers has not been published for the same reason." To buttress the miners' sense that this disease pervaded all coalfields, not just the anthracite region, Kerr offered the "frightening figures" that at least 125,000 bituminous and anthracite workers had CWP and that in the past two decades at least 1,000,000 miners had incurred daily exposure to coal dust. Doubtful that much further enlightenment would flow from ongoing federal activity, Kerr characterized the Appalachian Laboratory for Occupational Respiratory Diseases as not the hoped-for vibrant center of expertise but rather as "relatively dormant" and disappointing. Following this brief direct involvement with the union and its policy-making process, however, Kerr resumed his circumscribed duties at the fund in the autumn of 1968. Although neither designed nor authorized to take a leadership role in the prevention of occupational disease, the UMW Welfare and Retirement Fund had pursued for two decades an ingenious, if flawed, strategy to this end. But it could carry the issue only so far.[68]

Kerr's speech moved the UMW convention to demand more inclusive respiratory disease compensation in all coal-producing states. In the union's view, the time for corrective action had come. But in at least one major mining center, it was already too late for the Mine Workers leadership, discredited by decades of inaction and mired in habitual unresponsiveness to its members, to lead any reform campaign.[69]

EXTREME SOLIDARITY

At the end of the 1960s, an angry insurgency overcame much of the ignorance and misunderstanding created by decades of denial and obfuscation. The insurgent movement mobilized not only masses of dust-disease victims but newfound professional support as well. This community of challengers transformed public policy on coal miners' respiratory disease.[1] By 1970, federal responsibility encompassed not only compensation but also the emerging priority of prevention.

The lack of provision for disease victims propelled the initial phase of the reform campaign of the late sixties. Just as their inability to obtain public benefits had pushed miners toward private arrangements in the 1940s, so disappointment with their negotiated scheme sent them back into the political arena two decades later. Conflict over social insurance began at the state level and escalated to the national level. With heretical audacity, the movement strove to restore the legitimacy of discredited facets of coal workers' lung ailments. Dissemination of harsh facts on the consequences of underground work gave political leaders, medical authorities, and the general public a grasp of what came to be known as black lung.

When the United Mine Workers declared its intention to rewrite the workers' compensation statutes in order to accommodate victims of coal workers' pneumoconiosis, it faced a steep challenge. As of 1968, the compensation statutes in all major mining states except Alabama, Pennsylvania, and Virginia were highly restrictive, and had remained virtually unchanged over the preceding quarter-century or more. Moreover, an accretion of administrative restrictions made social insurance benefits even more difficult to obtain. For example, applicants were required to prove the precise chemical composition and concentration of dust inhaled twenty or thirty years earlier, which posed an impossible obstacle. Operators energetically controverted claims, causing long delays in their adjudication. In 1965, half the claimants in one coal state died prior to resolution of their claims. To qualify for benefits, the dyspneic coal miner still virtually always had to obtain a diagnosis of silicosis. As a practical matter, this meant presenting X-rays displaying the shadows cast by silicosis. Conversely, compensation administrators routinely discounted clinical evidence of disability.[2]

Breathless bituminous workers fared worst in West Virginia, by the 1960s the nation's leading coal-producing state. The 1935 legislation covering silicosis had not been broadened to accommodate other respiratory diseases. Except in the most extraordinary instances, such as when autopsy evidence supported the claim of a deceased applicant, no compensation existed for CWP in West Virginia. The defeat of innumerable claims embittered miners across the state. In 1964, UMW Local 5869 in Dehue called on union leaders to "make all possible efforts to get the State Compensation laws amended to include any chest ailment or disease that may be contracted while working in a dusty or damp atmosphere, be it miners asthma, pneumocosis, empyema or any other associated disease." Four years later, another local demanded social insurance for emphysema, asserting that the "compensation laws of West Virginia were written by the coal company for the coal company's benefit with little change for many years." The benefits for the small fraction of miners with silicosis were skimpy. Although radiographic images correlated poorly with underlying disability, West Virginia relied on the interpretation of X-rays to decide whether a miner had first-stage or advanced silicosis. Claimants judged to have the disease in its first stage received a lump-sum payment of one thousand dollars, not regular, periodic payments and reimbursement of health-care expenses.[3]

By the end of 1968, disparate developments knitted together to launch a militant campaign for compensation reform in West Virginia. One vital component in this explosive mixture was a cohort of outside agitators. High rates of poverty, especially in rural areas, brought community development workers to the state as part of the Great Society's War on Poverty. More than one hundred members of the Volunteers in Service to America (VISTA), a domestic version of the Peace Corps, resided in the mining districts of West Virginia in the late sixties. The VISTAs brought the attitudes, tactics, and ideals of the civil rights and anti-war movements to the coalfields. Perhaps the most crucial attitude was the volunteers' respect for the people they were trying to help. VISTA workers overcame rural West Virginians' distrust of outsiders by their willingness to listen carefully to problems and to accept priorities set by those in need. Taking on elemental issues like bad roads, some VISTA organizers became thoroughly familiar with the plight of former bituminous workers. These largely upper-middle-class college graduates immersed themselves in a desperate world of suffering and deprivation. From a modest beachhead in community organizing around infrastructural issues, a small crew of activists set out to help repair injustices heretofore largely hidden in the hollows of the state.[4]

The poor people's movement in the West Virginia coalfields began with those denied private, not public, benefits. The vicissitudes of the coal industry and major errors in the management of the UMW Welfare and Retirement Fund forced periodic restrictions in access to fund benefits. Resentment festered as the fund jettisoned widows, individuals with long term disabilities, those displaced by permanent unemployment, and other vulnerable beneficiaries. The miners' private welfare state, seen as a panacea in the years after World War II, was unraveling. In 1966, the Association of Disabled Miners and Widows (ADMW) formed to regain wider eligibility for union benefits. From the outset, the association received assistance from W. W. Garber and other VISTA volunteers assigned to southern West Virginia.[5]

Along with reform of the Welfare and Retirement Fund, the ADMW began to press for changes in public entitlements. Like those dislocated by the Great Depression, disabled miners in the late sixties cast about for the means of bare subsistence. As one close observer put it, "People were searching for some kind of income security." When VISTA worker Rick Bank, a recent law graduate from the University of Pennsylvania, came to Beckley in the summer of 1967, he took on the needs of welfare recipients. Bank soon identified the occupational origins of dependency: "Almost everybody that I worked with who was on welfare was a former miner; and most of them . . . had been disabled in the mines, and many of those people had been disabled by black lung." Beyond representing individuals in disputes over eligibility for public assistance, Bank and other VISTA volunteers helped organize a campaign for state legislation to increase welfare provision.[6]

In West Virginia, as elsewhere across the nation, the welfare-rights movement became ever more forceful and participatory. Reliance on legal expertise and legalistic tactics gave way to disruptive direct action. In May 1968, the Mountaineer State sent a large delegation to Washington for demonstrations organized by the Poor People's Campaign. On June 1, more than a hundred members of this contingent held a rally at the home of Senator Robert Byrd in Arlington, Virginia. When Byrd failed to meet with protesters, he was denounced as responsive only to the interests of the rich. The indignant senator, in turn, derided the demonstrators as "riff-raff" who disgraced the state. Simultaneously, the Ad Hoc Committee for the Poor, Unemployed and Disadvantaged Citizens of West Virginia set up camp on the lawn of the state capitol in Charleston. The committee demanded the convening of a special session of the legislature to provide jobs and relief for the unemployed. Although the campers obtained no concessions through their week-long demonstration, they managed to publicize their concerns and to practice confrontational tactics. Moreover, this statewide effort aided future pneumoconiosis organizing by forging an activist network that transcended local rivalries and other parochialisms. The campaign also overturned some barriers of racial separation and antagonism. The burgeoning movement developed indigenous leaders, including some African Americans, with administrative and communication skills.[7]

In 1968, the Association of Disabled Miners and Widows, which doubted that the union welfare plan would ever meet its needs, proposed changes in West Virginia's tightly drawn workers' compensation law. These proposals included survivor's benefits for widows of silicosis victims. In the course of refining their critique of the existing legislation, the association concentrated on the lack of coverage of most coal miners' respiratory disorders. VISTA Craig Robinson, who worked with the ADMW at this time, gravitated to the issue after "meeting so many disabled men and listening to their stories about how they were 'beat out of compensation' and left with nothing but a stack of medical reports." Besides casting specific demands, organizers were helping to germinate what Bank called "a sense of righteousness in people, that they were entitled to compensation for what was happening to them." As E. P. Thompson and other scholars have argued, protest movements depend critically on the articulation of legitimating notions of right, which when raised to the level of group or community consensus, overcome fears and feelings of inferiority and help build group identity.[8]

In mid-1968, the incipient movement gained a charismatic leader, Isidore Buff. A long-time critic of the state's overbearing coal industry, Buff took part in the Poor People's Campaign, where he saw the potential for elevating other grassroots grievances. By flamboyant, often outrageous, methods, this Charleston cardiologist promoted the issue of work-related lung disease in ways that intensified the miners' belief in the righteousness of their cause. He took the coal diggers' intuitive sense that the mines wrecked their health and brought it to a focus on the miseries of respiratory impairment. In the summer of 1968, he began to call for workers' compensation not for silicosis but for something called black lung.[9]

Buff began entirely on his own. Barnstorming the bituminous communities of southern and central West Virginia, this independent activist framed his explanation of respiratory disease in populistic terms. He damned the coal operators, company doctors, state political leaders, West Virginia University, and the leaders of the UMW as uncaring or worse. No specialist in pulmonary disease, he promoted the concept of black lung. This graphic, nonscientific label perfectly suited the purpose of popular education. Although he showed slides of lung tissue as in a conventional medical lecture, Buff dwelled on the signs and symptoms familiar to his audience. His stark clinical picture spared miners the abstruse Latinate terminology: "Tell me, you there, brother, how much longer do you think you're going to live? You got the black lung. You can't walk ten steps without resting. You can't breathe. You spit up black juice. But the company says you just got compensationitis." Tellingly, this description featured melanoptysis, the lurid black sputum, which had all but faded into invisibility during the reign of radiology. Miners greeted Buff as a prophet. Here, at last, was a physician who spoke plain English. Black lung, the descendant of miners' asthma in the vernacular tradition, became a rallying cry for the disinherited of the Appalachian coalfields. The term attained this status in large part because of its simplicity but also in part because of the forthright, forceful manner in which it was originally propounded.[10]

No epidemiologist, Buff melodramatically exaggerated the size of the issue. "You've all got black lung," he would routinely shout into a crowd of miners. "You're all gonna die." A measure of the power of this blunt rhetoric was that those sentenced to death would respond with cheers. Away from rank-and-file audiences, he variously claimed that half or four-fifths of West Virginia's 40,000 mine workers suffered from the condition.[11]

However crude, Buff's agitation immediately bore fruit. In mid-September 1968, disabled miners and their survivors opened a formal drive to modify the compensation law. This initiative sought not just to ease eligibility requirements in silicosis cases but to recognize a new disease entity, black lung. Activists in the Kanawha Valley may have drawn some inspiration from an editorial in the state's leading newspaper. On August 27, the *Charleston Gazette* voiced "outrage that an incensed public has not demanded that pneumoconiosis be listed among those diseases for which compensation is awarded." The editorial insisted that "one of the first orders of business at the next regular session of the West Virginia Legislature must be passage of legislation that provides for compensation to coal miners suffering from pneumoconiosis, or as it is more commonly referred to, black lung disease."[12]

Buff made connections despite his prickly individualism. In the fall of 1968, he formed a partnership with two other dissatisfied physicians. Both Donald Rasmussen and Hawey Wells had conducted studies in connection with the Public Health Service but were not content to wait for the federal bureaucracy to take care of dust disease. Rasmussen and Wells complemented Buff with real expertise in occupational respiratory disease. Rasmussen, a pulmonary specialist, gave sober professional summations of current medical knowledge on CWP. Based on his own original physiological research, Rasmussen underscored the fundamental point that the X-rays so sacrosanct to the compensation system provided poor guidance to the underlying state of impairment. The pathologist Wells, who had performed many autopsies on coal workers, shocked audiences by displaying samples of blackened, dessicated lung tissue. With his own flair for the dramatic, Wells crumbled tissue specimens between his fingers and informed horrified witnesses that their lungs would end up in this state. Beyond validating an ailment that coalfield medical authorities had trivialized, the black lung physicians emphasized the right to workers' compensation for this condition. To this end, they regularly compared the compensation plan in West Virginia with that in neighboring Pennsylvania.[13]

The three dissident doctors spoke out in coal towns across the state in the autumn of 1968. On many occasions, Craig Robinson and other VISTA workers worked with local unions to set up public meetings, commonly held in churches, schools, courthouses, and community centers, as well as union halls. In this proletarian public sphere, indignant discussion of work-induced disease replaced the atomizing, victim-blaming discourse of private exchanges. For years, in clinical encounters, compensation claims transactions, and personnel interviews, coal managers and company doctors told mine workers that they deserved neither work nor benefits. But now a different message prevailed. As their reputations spread, the doctors' presentations sometimes drew crowds of several hundred. With Buff always speaking first and setting the tone, these events took on the flavor of evangelical revival meetings. Heretofore isolated victims of chronic disease instantly gained an awareness of their numbers and of the commitment of sympathizers. The decision of the UMW convention to fight for compensation further fueled excitement.[14]

For a century, spectacular mining catastrophes overshadowed and thus hindered recognition of the unspectacular occurrence of respiratory disease. But in one peculiar set of circumstances, loss of life through traumatic injury had the opposite effect. On November 20, 1968, an explosion killed seventy-eight workers at a Consolidation Coal Company mine in Farmington, West Virginia. Although, obviously, no one died of pneumoconiosis in the Farmington disaster, events in its immediate aftermath served to accelerate the black lung movement. With casualties trapped underground and no way of immediately confirming their deaths, scores of representatives of the news media camped in West Virginia for several days. The army of journalists from the major television networks and other national news organizations turned their attention to other facets of the coal miners' dismal plight. Arriving in Farmington the day after the explosion, Isidore Buff wasted no time explaining to the media the evils of inhaling coal mine dust.

Another figure who appeared on the scene on November 21 was UMW president Tony Boyle. In an astonishingly callous display, Boyle exonerated Consolidation Coal for this preventable catastrophe. When, in the presence of the victims' families and co-workers, Boyle praised the firm's safety record and recited threadbare truisms about the inevitability of risk, groans and curses could be heard. The union executive, by a single blunder, forfeited what remained of his credibility as the miners' champion. To many miners and others in the coalfields, it was now inescapably clear that two decades of cozy accommodation with corporate management had left the top leadership of the Mine Workers hopelessly out of touch with the on-the-job experience of its members. At approximately the same time, district officials appointed by Boyle indicated to local unions in West Virginia that they were in no hurry to pursue compensation amendments. As Donald Rasmussen put it, District 29 officers in Beckley ordered a delegation of concerned miners to "mind their own damn business." The union hierarchy completely discredited itself on the pneumoconiosis question.[15]

Official negligence provoked independent self-assertion. During the formative interval following the Farmington disaster, dissidents took decisive steps to push the black lung issue. In Davitt McAteer's memory, at this moment "the pot was boiling." Buff, Rasmussen, and Wells constituted themselves the Physicians for Miners' Health and Safety, which remained an organization with three members, and increased their inflammatory educational work. Buff became more critical of the Boyle administration; UMW officials counterattacked.[16]

VISTA organizers helped to devise a legislative remedy. Collaborating with local union officers, Craig Robinson arranged meetings between miners and the physicians' committee. Group discussions focused more closely on flaws in the existing workers' compensation law and the legislative changes that miners would support to correct them. Based on this dialogue, Robinson and Rick Bank drafted amendments to the compensation law in December 1968. Most crucial among these was a proposal that any claimant with respiratory disability who had worked for a long period in the mines would be presumed to have a compensable disorder. A reaction to innumerable anecdotal accounts of frustrated claims, the principle of presumption originated with Bank. Miners immediately grasped the concept and wholeheartedly endorsed it, as did Donald Rasmussen and other sympathetic physicians.[17]

Presumption aimed to transform the concept of work-induced disease. In a truly revolutionary approach to the question of the relation of work to health, the principle of presumption threw aside the medicolegal hairsplitting exercises that had always dominated the field. The new perspective assumed that miners were not laboratory animals who inhaled a single air contaminant that gave rise to a singular disease. Instead, many cases of respiratory illness defied easy categorization. The presumptive approach proceeded directly from the miners' traditional empirical notion that underground work inexorably devoured labor power, including respiratory capacity. Appalachian coal diggers thus placed dust disease in a wider context that conferred entitlement. Needless to say, such an audacious stance guaranteed all-out resistance from the coal operators.

UMW rank-and-file dissidents gave up on international and district officials and began to chart their own course. Indeed, a foreshadowing of such rebellion preceded the Farmington affair. In October 1968, the Boyle regime renewed the national collective bargaining agreement with the Bituminous Coal Operators Association. The contract granted unionized miners a wage increase and other economic gains. However, despite bland assurances and some negotiation on dust controls, the agreement did nothing to prevent pneumoconiosis. Upon announcement of the settlement on October 15, Isidore Buff lambasted it as a betrayal of the workers' health "for a few pieces of silver." Wildcat strikes broke out at several West Virginia mines. This action, though short-lived, marked the first collective rank-and-file protest against the UMW leaders' irresponsibility on the dust-disease issue.[18]

Independent of the VISTA initiative, UMW local leaders made their own plans to alter the compensation statute. In early January 1969, they formed the West Virginia Black Lung Association (BLA). In light of the antipathy of the union hierarchy to any such self-help endeavor, this undertaking took a great deal of courage. The association elected Charles Brooks, an African American local union president, as its first president. Brooks mortgaged his home to help the group raise ten thousand dollars to hire Paul Kaufman, a liberal former state senator, to edit and lobby for a black lung compensation bill. Kaufman immediately consulted with Bank and Robinson in refining the BLA plan. At this juncture, the insurgent movement was loosely decentralized and quite inchoate. In fact, while the BLA was retaining Kaufman, Bank and Robinson independently prevailed on legislator Warren McGraw to carry their bill (without paying him ten thousand dollars). The Black Lung Association relied on an entirely conventional special-interest legislative strategy, hiring a lobbyist to win passage of a piece of legislation.[19]

Armed with concrete proposals, the black lung insurgents accelerated their organizing in January 1969. Craig Robinson and local union leaders set up a series of meetings in southern West Virginia. At the same time, the Association of Disabled Miners and Widows, the BLA, and other grassroots groups sponsored meetings in the northern and central parts of the state. Sometimes traveling to more than one rally per day, the Physicians for Miners' Health and Safety addressed the medical issues related to dust exposure. Whereas Rasmussen concentrated on coal workers' pneumoconiosis, Buff elaborated an expansive construction of black lung, which extended to chronic bronchitis and emphysema. The rampaging populist expressed exasperation with the whole question of disease definition, buttressing the presumptive approach to compensation. "It doesn't matter what the damn thing is called," he declared. "The man can't work, he's disabled." Hawey Wells, whose postmortem dissections provided an ample supply of tissue specimens, continued to shock audiences by crumbling blackened lung tissue. Advertisements for a meeting on January 11, 1969, in Chelyan in the Upper Kanawha Valley promised an exhibition of diseased lungs. Pathological anatomy had returned with renewed political force.[20]

By this time, black lung rallies devoted as much attention to legislative agitation as to health education. Buff took every opportunity to connect illness to injustice. On January 4, he told a large crowd of coal workers in Vivian, "You work in the mines fifteen years and get black lung, then they throw you out like dirty dishwater." Like the original Progressive proponents of social insurance a half-century earlier, Buff maintained that requiring the mine owners to make compensatory payments would lead them to prevent dust exposure. Craig Robinson had the job of explaining the details of the planned compensation amendments, emphasizing the key principle of presumption. UMW local presidents also spoke out at these gatherings, sometimes declaring that it would take a strike to force any fundamental change in the law. Organizers promoted a demonstration planned for later in the month in Charleston. At the close of the rally at Vivian, for example, the 450 miners in attendance voted to join the upcoming statewide protest.[21]

These careful preparations paid off. More than 3,000 protesters appeared at the Charleston Civic Center on January 26. This massive turnout in itself sent a strong message to legislators, as did numerous signs in the crowd demanding an end to "black lung murder." The rally began with a song written by James Wyatt, a sixty-year-old pneumoconiotic. Despite evident difficulty breathing, Wyatt sang "Black Lungs" himself:

> A young miner's lungs may be hearty and hale
> When he enters the mine with his dinner pail
> But coal dust and grime
> In a few years time
> Fills up his lungs and they begin to fail.
> Black lungs, full of coal dust
> Coal miners must breathe it or bust.
> Black lungs, gasping for breath
> With black lungs we are choking to death.

Building on this testimonial by an unsuccessful compensation applicant, Paul Kaufman described the major features of his bill, which was already before the legislature. Buff excoriated medical subservience to corporate interests. "Most of the doctors in West Virginia who deal with black lung are paid by the coal operators," he asserted, "and the coal operators would rather let their miners die than recognize the problem and do something about it." Donald Rasmussen criticized continued medical resistance to pneumoconiosis recognition. "If it takes too long to educate the doctors," Rasmussen suggested, "we will educate the miners and the legislators." The medical establishment had had its chance; now there would be a democratic approach.[22]

The Charleston rally, like the Farmington disaster, did much to publicize the controversy over miners' respiratory disease. Ralph Nader sent a message of support, which was read to the protesters. Nader reiterated criticisms of the negligence of the national institutional players, including the union hierarchy. Ken Hechler, a member of U.S. House of Representatives from West Virginia whose district included mining areas, also confronted the most powerful opponents of reform. Taking note of a coincidental meeting of the executive council of the West Virginia Medical Association at a nearby hotel, Hechler facetiously told the miners that the physicians' association had asked him to relay a message to them. At this point, he held up a placard that read "black lung is good for you." The crowd went wild. Hechler warned the assemblage of their adversaries' tactical resourcefulness:

Now the coal operators and some doctors who seem to be close to the coal operators say that there is no such thing as black lung, or if there is, maybe it won't hurt you. But if it does hurt you, we'd better not compensate you for it. But in case we do compensate you for it, we had better study this subject scientifically. We'd better refer this whole question to an impartial board of other coal company doctors. Then we'll study it for five, or ten or fifteen years, and by that time either the problem will go away or your lungs will go away.

The renegade congressional representative finished his characterization of the opposition by waving a twelve-pound hunk of bologna. The miners roared with laughter.[23]

The rally ended with a march to the state capitol, where the protesters held a prayer meeting. The event as a whole thrilled participants. "People's emotions were sky high," in Rick Bank's view, "and this was an escalating kind of excitement." The Charleston rally marked a major step for the black lung movement. It gave both participants and sympathizers who learned about the event through media coverage an understanding of their own numbers and determination. It also confirmed that the rank-and-file movement had medical and political experts willing to make a strong commitment to their side. Donald Rasmussen heard wary miners openly express skepticism that he and his colleagues would stick with their cause for very long. The Charleston demonstration did much to overcome such suspicions.[24]

Miners had no shortage of objects for distrust. In large measure, the task of black lung activists was to put that distrust to use. In a speech in Matewan on February 1, Buff warned of duplicitous lawmakers who posed as the miners' allies while conniving to stall meaningful reform. He also advised the Matewan miners that real reform depended on their own efforts, that he could not be their savior. Two days later, Hechler sounded the same theme, urging the discontented to "rise up and demand effective action by . . . the state legislature." Besides attacking recalcitrant politicians, Buff never tired of condemning the mine owners. He reminded 400 miners in Fayetteville on February 9 that the operators "care nothing" about them.[25]

Buff's florid rhetoric and hyperbolic claims infuriated the coal industry and its allies. The medical establishment rallied around coal workers' pneumoconiosis as a delimited alternative to the sprawling notion of black

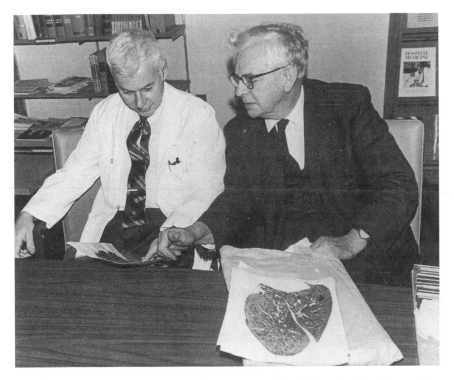

Murray Hunter and Jethro Gough confer prior to testifying before the West Virginia leg-islature, February 1969. (Courtesy of Murray Hunter)

lung. Charles Andrews, provost for health science at West Virginia University, took exception to including emphysema and bronchitis under this rubric. "If black lung means anything in a medical sense," Andrews stated flatly, "it means coal workers' pneumoconiosis." Conservatives identified cigarette smoking, not dusty working conditions, as the most frequent cause of chronic bronchitis. Herbert E. Jones, Jr., president of the Logan Coal Operators Association, observed that many aging miners had bronchitis, asthma, lung cancer, and other respiratory difficulties. Jones was concerned that he and his fellow mine owners "might end up paying . . . for lung infections caused by other health factors unless the claim could be incontrovertibly proven to have originated in West Virginia coal mines." Moreover, Jones, like many other opponents of the insurgent movement, argued that CWP could cause significant disability only when it progressed to its complicated phase, progressive massive fibrosis; simple CWP, which occurred more frequently, constituted no real threat. As in the

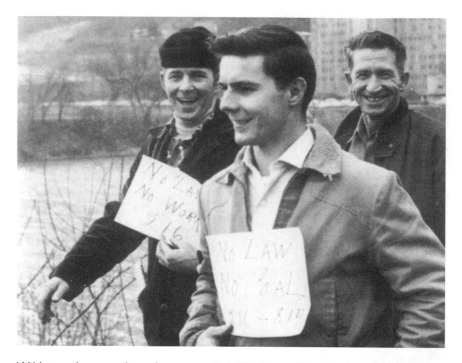

Wildcat strikers march on the state capitol, Charleston, West Virginia, February 1969. Photograph by Douglas Yarrow. (Courtesy of Douglas Yarrow)

1930s, when vested interests could no longer deny the existence of a disorder, they fell back to defining it in the narrowest terms as a second line of defense. A number of county medical societies passed resolutions declaring that pneumoconiosis affected relatively few miners. Stephen Young, vice president of the West Virginia Coal Association, decried attacks on the state's politicians as well as such indecencies as "the flamboyant displaying of so-called diseased lungs." Young urged that legislation rest on "the solid medical facts of coal workers' pneumoconiosis, not sensationalism and emotionalism." Thus, the rise of black lung fostered belated acknowledgment of CWP, which had become the lesser evil.[26]

Young and his colleagues were about to face an inundation of medical facts, few of which served their purposes. On February 11, the Judiciary Committee of the West Virginia Senate held a joint hearing with its counterpart in the House of Delegates. It was a wholly extraordinary session. On very short notice, Murray Hunter, medical director of the UMW welfare fund's clinic in Fairmont, assembled a panel of expert witnesses.

Presenting a united front, the Physicians for Miners' Health and Safety agreed to cooperate with the union leadership on this occasion, despite their extremely hostile relations.[27]

Thousands converged on the capitol on February 11. Coal miners across the state abandoned their jobs for the day to make the trip to Charleston. The crowd overflowed the galleries and corridors of the capitol and spilled outside the building. Not mere spectators, the demonstrators articulated their demands. Many carried signs warning "No Law, No Work." The Black Lung Association let it be known that failure to make satisfactory legislative changes might well precipitate a statewide shutdown. Miners paraded with black coffins.[28]

Hunter introduced the panel supporting expanded access to compensation. His prefatory remarks looked past his own objections to Buff's unscientific thinking and undignified manner. He began by tackling the idea most in dispute: "Black Lung, as a term, has no medical standing but is a valuable and useful term. Were it not for this term, I doubt if we would be having these hearings this afternoon. Black Lung to me means breathless coal miners and encompasses a variety of conditions." After many years of fastidiousness on the matter of disease definition (and many years taking care of sick miners), Hunter had concluded that there were worse things in the world of medicine than imprecise, lay concepts of disease.[29]

Two intertwined themes ran through the testimony of the proponents of reform. First, they felt obliged to demonstrate that work-related lung disorders besides silicosis afflicted coal miners. In this endeavor, the star witness was Jethro Gough, who flew in from Cardiff for the occasion. Gough traced the development of medical knowledge of coal miners' respiratory disorders in Britain, culminating in the definition of coal workers' pneumoconiosis. In addition, he entered the opinion (which he shared with Donald Rasmussen, among others) that simple CWP could be disabling. Following Gough's statement, Eugene Pendergrass, long a silicosis reductionist, modestly and somewhat self-effacingly characterized American biomedical science as "Johnny come lately" regarding coal workers' pneumoconiosis. Other witnesses echoed this view. Except for Buff, who disapproved of "fancy terms we don't understand" and held forth on black lung, all the medical advocates of reform addressed themselves to CWP.[30]

The second theme that emerged from this panel was the inadequacy of radiology to the task of determining disability. Here the testimony of the eminent radiologist Pendergrass became especially cogent. Pendergrass indicated that for simple CWP the chest X-ray "does not provide any information that can be used as reliable evidence for evaluation of pulmonary function." Leon Cander of the University of Texas Medical School argued, "There is almost no correlation between the functional impairment, that is, the change in lung function associated with the inhalation of the dust, disability, that is, the ability of the man to continue to work, and the X-ray changes." These presentations helped to justify a presumption in favor of breathless miners, even in the absence of clear-cut X-ray evidence of pneumoconiosis. Speakers acknowledged the need for flexibility in crafting a presumptive clause. In fact, at this juncture it was not fully apparent that a policy of presumption followed more directly from the expansive, elusive concept of black lung than from the narrower one of CWP.[31]

Opposing medical witnesses had a hard time in this unexpectedly hostile setting. Rowland Burns, a particular nemesis of the insurgents, fell into a defensive stance after cross-examination revealed that the coal operators' association was paying him to testify. Boisterous heckling and derisive laughter from the gallery also unsettled another operators' ally, W. K. C. Morgan of the University of Maryland. Moreover, following the review by Gough and his teammates of the extensive research already conducted, the argument for further scientific study, to avoid an error of haste in making public policy, rang hollow.[32]

The protesters' hopes that their experts' performance on February 11 would clear the way for progress proved short-lived. In the aftermath of the hearing, the compensation plan remained bogged down in committee. Impatient with obstructive tactics of the opposition and aware that it would take more than superior medical knowledge to effect change, miners took matters into their own hands. On February 18, a wildcat strike by approximately 400 men erupted at a mine near Beckley. Because the presence of a single picket sufficed to stop employees from going to work, the strike spread rapidly. Some of those freed from their jobs drove to Charleston to lean on recalcitrant lawmakers. By the weekend of February 22–23, the dispute had shut down the coal industry across the southern portion of the state and had begun to advance northward.[33]

Though the result of no formal planning, the strike grew out of much informal preparation among the West Virginia miners. The critical preparatory effort was to build a rank-and-file consensus on the importance of the movement's aims and on the necessity of confrontational collective action to achieve them. Hence, although the black lung walkout was, in a sense, a spontaneous uprising, it was also the culmination of a protracted process of communication and of estimating collective willingness to take the risks a walkout entailed. The forbidding language of the labor-management agreement made administering a wildcat strike a dangerous affair. For the past twenty years, top UMW officials had vigorously put down intracontractual stoppages. As the black lung stoppage gained momentum, the West Virginia operators demanded that the miners' union use all means at its disposal to return its members to their jobs. Rank-and-file leaders endorsed illicit action, nonetheless. Consider this statement by BLA president Charles Brooks at a meeting of more than a thousand on February 23: "Now, as president of my local union, I can't tell my men to strike. You know that. But if it takes pressure, put it where it belongs. Now if you men want to go on vacation, I'm with you a hundred percent." Another rebel leader cleverly traded on the impotence of high union officials. Asked to intercede to get the miners back to work, BLA Secretary Raymond Wright replied, "If the district and international can't control them, we certainly can't." UMW local officers also signaled their support by allowing the use of union halls for strike meetings. With rank-and-file miners taking the initiative, VISTA workers and the physicians' committee played a very small part in this protest.[34]

Having staked out a position in favor of a broad presumption of the ill effects of their work and having pressed this position by disruptive tactics, the strikers had to justify themselves to the public. Somewhat surprisingly, criticism from an important ally increased the need for self-justification. "I don't believe," Ken Hechler warned on February 20, "that endless bitter and disorganized strikes and walkouts will either solve the problem or result in good legislation." Miners replied by declaring themselves hard-working citizens, deserving of special assistance. "We support the state and the federal government with our taxes," one coal worker told the *Charleston Gazette*. "It's time we did something for our benefits." Ernest Riddle, treasurer of the BLA, confronted Governor Arch Moore at a news conference on February 25 with the contradiction between Moore's willingness to spend millions on welfare and his unwillingness to establish a state medical facility to study coal workers' diseases. In this view, miners had earned an entitlement not from their employers but from the government.[35]

In its second week, the black lung strike grew in scope and intensity. Picketing closed mining operations throughout the northern section of the state. With proposals still stuck in committee despite legislators' repeated assurances that their emergence was imminent, impatience turned into outrage. Plainspoken miners made no pretense of diplomacy as tensions heightened. The BLA's Wright warned that in the event of disciplinary sanctions against protesters, "The state of West Virginia may never have another coal mine again." On February 26, about 3,000 miners and their supporters again marched on the state capitol. Ken Hechler apologized for opposing the wildcat and donated $1,000 to the cause. (This donation exceeded by $995 that of West Virginia Secretary of State John D. Rockefeller IV.) "The national searchlight is on West Virginia," Hechler reminded the demonstrators. "The hopes and prayers of many people throughout this land are with you." Governor Arch Moore addressed the rally on the capitol steps. The crowd booed Moore's suggestion that the enactment of compensation amendments might have to wait for the next legislative session.[36]

The West Virginia Coal Association kept up its opposition to any presumptive provision. On February 26, Stephen Young decried proposed changes as inappropriate "social legislation" that amounted to a "signed blank check" for nonoccupational lung ailments of all sorts. Only two days later, the mine owners made a still gloomier assessment. Paul Morton, president of the coal association, described the bill approved by the House of Delegates as "not just social legislation but galloping socialism in one of its purest forms." Morton reiterated his group's fears of unbounded responsibility for such widespread conditions as chronic bronchitis and emphysema. As an alternative, the operators held out for a tighter plan to compensate radiologically confirmed cases of advanced coal workers' pneumoconiosis. At the same time, the mine owners sought an injunction and damages of more than one million dollars per day to quell the convulsive protest.[37]

No court order stopped the strike, however. By the weekend of March 1–2, more than 40,000 miners had suspended work. The black lung strike had become the largest work stoppage caused primarily by an occupational health issue in the history of the United States. It was also the biggest political strike in the nation's history. The coal industry in West Virginia stood still. Most remarkably, sympathetic miners in neighboring states left their posts as well. Because some of these workers were employed by firms that also operated in West Virginia, this gesture was not purely symbolic. Adding moral weight to the cause, a delegation of widows of victims of the Farmington disaster joined in a mock funeral procession at the statehouse on March 7. Against the recurrent charge of mob intimidation, the Black Lung Association invoked such sober scientific authorities as Eugene Pendergrass on the fallacy of relying too heavily on X-rays. As the strike entered its third week, its leaders successfully marshalled both material and ideological resources.[38]

Bowing to popular pressure that threatened further economic and political disruption, the legislature in Charleston scurried to produce amendments before the winter session adjourned. Finally, a settlement emerged. On March 11, Governor Moore signed a workers' compensation reform bill.[39]

The new law gave the protesters much of what they had sought. Echoing the Alabama statute, West Virginia defined compensable conditions quite broadly:

> The term 'occupational pneumoconiosis' shall include, but shall not be limited to, such diseases as silicosis, anthracosilicosis, coal worker's pneumoconiosis, commonly known as black lung or miner's asthma, silico-tuberculosis (silicosis accompanied by active tuberculosis of the lungs), coal worker's pneumoconiosis accompanied by active tuberculosis of the lungs, tuberculo-silicosis, asbestosis, siderosis, anthrax and any and all other dust diseases of the lungs and conditions and diseases caused by occupational pneumoconiosis which are not specifically designated herein.

Lawmakers curbed this definition by excluding any "ordinary disease of life to which the general public is exposed." Confused irresolution seemed the order of the day, as one provision seemingly reached out to the victims of chronic bronchitis and emphysema, but another provision denied benefits for disorders that were not peculiarly occupational.[40]

In a significant victory for dust-exposed miners, the measure permitted a diagnosis based on clinical, physiological, or other data beyond radiological findings. Specifically, the law declared that "X-ray evidence shall not necessarily be held conclusive." To Donald Rasmussen, among others, adoption of this language marked an enormous advance for disabled mine workers seeking financial relief. The long tyranny of radiology had ended in the leading coal state.[41]

The legislation struck a compromise on the matter of presumption. When the claimant had worked ten of the last fifteen years in a job that involved dust exposure, his respiratory disorder was presumed to be occupational in origin. This standard fell short of the BLA proposal to require only five years' mining experience. The presumption was not ironclad, but rebuttable, with controverted cases handled by a newly created Occupational Pneumoconiosis Board. Despite these limitations, the presumptive approach represented a historic breakthrough.[42]

Miners voted to return to work upon learning the provisions of the law. To be sure, the shortcomings of the measure troubled some. From decades of bitter experience with the Silicosis Medical Board, West Virginia coal workers looked askance at the board that would administer the program. Nonetheless, to most bituminous workers, especially those already afflicted with shortness of breath, this legislation promised a much better chance to qualify for compensation.[43]

The movement for social insurance spread rapidly to other states. The message spread by aggressive proselytizing forays, as well as media attention. Another significant factor in the diffusion of reform was the decision by the upper echelon of the United Mine Workers to work in partnership with grassroots activists.

In a number of states, including Illinois, Tennessee, and Ohio, the UMW drafted and lobbied hard for changes in workers' compensation laws. The day after the signing of the West Virginia legislation, leaders of District 6, which took in the mines in eastern Ohio, announced intentions to attain a similar plan there. The union proposal sought a presumption of compensability for all those disabled by respiratory maladies who had had dust exposure in five of the last eight years preceding their claim. Desperate to place the union (and himself) at the forefront of the crusade, Tony Boyle obtained Josephine Roche's permission for Lorin Kerr to testify on behalf of the union's bill. On May 6, Kerr informed the Ohio legislature that CWP was "not a new unknown disease" but one long recognized by medical researchers and mine workers alike. Kerr treated black lung as a lay synonym for coal workers' pneumoconiosis and refrained from deploying the term. In contrast, Murray Hunter, in testimony delivered the same day, unabashedly embraced the concept. Hunter testified that coal miners aged forty-five to fifty-four died of respiratory disorders at four times the expected rate for the general population and that miners aged fifty-five to sixty-four succumbed to these diseases at six times the expected rate. He emphasized not just the occurrence of CWP but also the elevated incidence of emphysema, chronic bronchitis, and unspecified impaired lung function in the bituminous workforce. Milton Levine, Hunter's long-time partner at the Bellaire Clinic, underscored the "frequency of recurrent bronchitis" among miners. District 6 arranged a mine tour to give legislators a better grasp of the intensity of the hazard.[44]

Hunter's policy point was that the presence of diverse work-related disorders, however indistinct, warranted a broad-brush legislative response. While conceding the inexactitude of his recommendation, he cited past mistakes to justify covering more than CWP:

> If it is truly the intent of the Ohio State Legislature to fully do justice to the
> coal miner, it ought to take into account the high frequency of chronic bron
> chitis and emphysema in coal miners and while these conditions are not
> unique to coal miners, they occur with such an increased frequency that
> I personally would favor inclusion of such disorders. . . . I would favor the
> inclusion of these diagnostic terms in the law in the form of a presump-
> tion . . . which, while admittedly creating an error in favor of the coal miner,
> would be an error of relatively small magnitude and one that would effec-
> tively redress the errors of past years that have operated against the miner.

In contrast, Kerr's statement made no endorsement of the principle of presumption and could have been taken to support the compensability of CWP alone. In any case, the shrunken and precarious state of the coal industry in Ohio and the consequent diminished political clout of the miners' union precluded any tranformative legislation, despite the shock waves from neighboring West Virginia. When the moment of excitement faded, miners won a circumscribed concession, albeit a significant one. In August 1969, the legislature passed a measure adding CWP to its schedule of compensable conditions. The law required that a diagnosis of

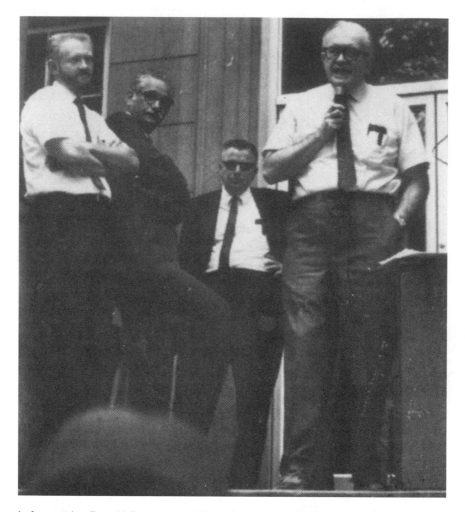

Left to right: Donald Rasmussen, Allen Koplin, UMW District 19 president William Turnblazer, and I. E. Buff, Harlan, Kentucky, May 4, 1969. Buff told the crowd at the county courthouse, "I am convinced that the incidence of black lung is as high here as in West Virginia. Most of the victims are living on charity. It is not their fault they got sick. It is the industry's and the industry should pay." (Courtesy of the United Mine Workers of America)

occupational disease rest on radiological, pathological, or other medical evidence, not on tenure underground.[45]

Whereas in Ohio the UMW acted as a conventional interest group, without resort to alliances or unruly demonstrations, in Kentucky the campaign adopted a more aggressive strategy. During their adventures promoting black lung, Buff, Rasmussen, and Wells made numerous visits to the bituminous fields in the eastern part of the state. As in West Virginia, VISTA workers set up meetings, often with the cooperation of local unionists, during the formative stage of organizing. On April 27, 1969, Buff stirred up a rally of approximately 400 miners in Hazard. Initially, UMW officials responded coolly to this agitation. In early May, District 30 President Carson Hibbitts boasted, "Our people can get black lung legislation passed in Kentucky . . . without shutting down a mine one day and causing loss of wages." Buff and his colleagues hammered away at the inequity of legislation that denied benefits for work-related illness. They also sharply criticized the failure of their medical colleagues to make correct diagnoses. Buff suggested to a crowd of 250 in Hindman that physicians who performed compensation evaluations should be barred from owning stock in coal companies. To end dependence on company-oriented physicians, he resurrected a proposal, defeated in West Virginia, for a state diagnostic and research center.[46]

The movement soon reached a reconciliation with higher union officials. All three UMW districts in the state actively promoted the formation of the Kentucky Black Lung Association in June 1969. Like its counterpart in West Virginia, the association followed a participatory strategy, albeit with less transgressive tactics. In July, the Washington headquarters again dispatched Lorin Kerr, who had just taken a newly created position as the union's director of occupational health, to testify in legislative hearings in Frankfort. Shortly thereafter, the Kentucky black lung group named both Kerr and Buff to its medical advisory board. Throughout the fall the association held rallies to keep pressure on legislators, threatening to strike if no satisfactory remedies came from the upcoming legislative session. After the state enacted presumptive pneumoconiosis compensation in February 1970, Kerr addressed a celebration attended by 1,000. On the workers' compensation front, the union had returned to the forefront of leadership.[47]

By 1969 few activists, either inside or outside the union, believed that either the states or the device of social insurance could ultimately solve the problems surrounding miners' lung disease. Despite recent gains, the majority of coal states effectively excluded miners' respiratory disorders from compensation coverage. State inspectors had no authority to bring the concentration of mine dust within healthful limits. In its unending search for lower labor costs, the industry still played states off against one another. The inexorable dynamic of degenerative competition seemed to bar dramatic progress in any mining center. Accordingly, the black lung movement came to focus more intently on direct disease prevention on a uniform, nationwide basis.

Such a reorientation was long overdue. Certainly, a truly pragmatic attack on this problem would have placed much less emphasis on precise determination of the etiologic agent of disease and full explication of the pathological mechanism of disease. It was enough to know that dust in coal mines promoted various respiratory troubles in many workers who long inhaled it. A straightforward public health approach would have given top priority to finding and implementing effective methods of disease prevention. (Recall the prototypical intervention in which John Snow in 1854 prevented cholera by removing the handle of the pump that supplied contaminated water to Broad Street in London, even though he did not know the identity of the contaminating pathogen. Snow and his colleagues did not delay for three decades awaiting Robert Koch's description of the bacterium involved.)[48]

Indeed, from the turn of the century onward, dust control was not a utopian fantasy but a feasible objective. The technology of ventilation had progressed considerably by 1900. Electric fans could move huge volumes of air through mine workings. Elaborate systems of bratticework for channeling the flow of fresh air predated the onset of industrialization. Innovations in wet methods of dust control in the early twentieth century soon became widely known within management circles. Other technologies, such as devices that collected dust at the point of generation, appeared not long after the turn of the century. By the late 1960s, these engineering measures had undergone several decades of refinement.[49]

The coal industry understood the potential value of existing forms of dust suppression. Beginning in the Progressive Era, some firms controlled dust in order to avoid explosions. By the mid-twentieth century, a number of operators curtailed the particulate hazard in order to prevent respiratory disease as well. For example, in 1942, Pittsburgh Coal Company reported that spraying a mixture of water and oil into the kerf in coal cutting reduced dust by ninety-three percent.[50]

The U.S. Bureau of Mines long encouraged managers to adopt the best available practices to remove particulate matter from the working environment. Daniel Harrington doggedly promoted primary prevention of disease. In 1925, his observations on western advances left conscientious operators no room for evasion: "Trouble due to dust in the lungs of machine runners in coal mines has been known since about 1913 in Wyoming and Utah, and the remedy then applied and now largely used is the spraying of water on the cutting chain when the machines are working." Harrington scorned the denials used to forestall disease prevention: "Suggestions as to remedial methods or equipment such as sprinkling, or the use of water in drilling or in coal cutting, or the use of currents of fresh air to remove dust are held to be impracticable or are considered the dream of the theorist, even though these methods or devices are in thoroughly successful use in other mines or in other localities." As mechanization rolled on through the mid-twentieth century, others at the BOM joined in encouraging application of dust-killing techniques. However, the bureau lacked coercive power in this regard, and its recommendations were often disregarded.[51]

Although they, too, had easy access to the publications and statements of the proponents of dust control, the United Mine Workers did little to force management to alleviate the threat. Recurrent complaints from the ranks over unhealthy conditions, along with proposals for remedial action, alerted union leaders. The 1948 UMW convention, like subsequent union policy-making sessions, buried suggestions for hazard controls on loading and cutting machinery. The issue apparently never received serious attention in national contract negotiations before 1968, even though working conditions had been considered an appropriate subject of bargaining ever since the late nineteenth century. After World War II, centralization of labor-management negotiations left almost no opportunity to make changes at the local level. Moreover, John L. Lewis's determination to maintain labor peace and to prevent interruptions of production that would cut royalty revenue to the union welfare fund left miners with unresolved grievances regarding the dust hazard no recourse through strikes. To make matters still worse, the Safety Division established by the Lewis administration in 1947 remained preoccupied with traumatic injuries, devoting no resources to controlling respiratory diseases.[52]

In the face of a callous and sometimes hostile bureaucracy, local union safety committees waged an uphill battle to limit the dust hazard. First authorized under the 1941 bituminous agreement, safety committees tried repeatedly to upgrade conditions. As early as 1946, one committee proposed the installation of a "water system" to abate mineral dust, which it considered "an important health factor." Because committees could only recommend remedies, management's efforts to eradicate these hazards often were dilatory and inadequate when finally implemented. Nonetheless, some militant locals persevered. A few even struck to bring down dust levels. But absent a commitment by the UMW as a whole to a systematic national campaign, scattered local actions alone could not reduce coal mine dust to innocuous levels.[53]

Even while concentrating on fixing the workers' compensation system, black lung reformers raised the issue of disease prevention. In a polemical article in February 1968, Ralph Nader took as his basic premise that coal workers' lung ailments were preventable. Nader's manifesto concluded with a challenge to federal lawmakers: "Congress, which has displayed such staunch efforts to preserve tax depletion allowances for companies engaged in extractive industries, should have little difficulty persuading itself of the need for preventive measures to diminish the bodily depletion of their employees." By July 1968, Isidore Buff advocated giving miners supplied-air respirators. At the same time, Buff attacked UMW leaders' passivity and accused them of uncritically swallowing management's contention that protective measures cost too much.[54]

Prior to 1969, state mine safety agencies supposedly filled the regulatory vacuum. However, long accustomed to treating coal mine dust merely as an explosion hazard, state regulators generally did relatively little to reduce its health hazards. Lacking the capacity to develop their own standards for permissible exposure, they took guidance from the American Conference of Governmental Industrial Hygienists (ACGIH), a private professional group. In setting a "threshold limit value" for coal mine dust in the late 1940s, the ACGIH devised a set of formulae based on the silica content in the particulate mixture. The conference suggested that the value of twenty million particles of dust per cubic foot of air apply to dusts con-

taining between 5 percent and 50 percent free silica. Where silica constituted less than 5 percent of the dust, as it often did in coal mines, the
ACGIH considered acceptable an exposure of up to fifty million particles
per cubic foot, very approximately in the range of twenty-seven milligrams of dust per cubic meter of air. Impervious to subsequent revelations
regarding CWP and related disorders, this influential recommendation remained in place for three decades.[55]

The Farmington disaster provided an imperative for federal intervention in miners' safety that spilled over into adjacent areas. On December 9,
1968, the Department of Health, Education, and Welfare proposed a limit
of three milligrams of respirable mine dust per cubic meter of air. Though
promulgated as an "interim national standard," this recommendation was
merely forwarded to the Department of the Interior, where the toothless
BOM was to pass it on to the states. This proposal attempted to build on
a pending Johnson administration plan for federal occupational health
standards for mining, to be enforced by the Interior Department but based
on scientific criteria put forward by Health, Education, and Welfare. Ken
Hechler, for one, took the announcement of the three-milligram limit as an
authoritative endorsement of this level of protection.[56]

A number of bills introduced at the commencement of the congressional
session in January 1969 aimed to shift responsibility for health and safety
in the coal industry to the federal government. Some offered specific provisions for setting and enforcing restrictions on the concentration of hazardous mine dust. The UMW's plan, sponsored in the Senate by Jennings
Randolph of West Virginia, among others, sought to reach the objective of
three milligrams per cubic meter of air by requiring reengineering of continuous mining equipment. Behind this proposal lay the explicit threat to
seek abolition of this technology and reversion to older, less productive
methods of extraction. Ken Hechler's bill, introduced on February 6, 1969,
would establish national dust regulations irrespective of their economic
impact.[57]

After the spectacular black lung strike and subsequent compensation
legislation in West Virginia, those facets of health and safety reform related to respiratory disease rose in importance in Washington. In Donald
Rasmussen's recollection, congressional concern over disease prevention,
previously low except with the firebrand Hechler, soared immediately after the insurgency in central Appalachia. That forty thousand miners were

willing to lose pay and perhaps their jobs in order to address the lung disease issue startled Congress.[58]

Discussion of the extent of black lung also helped foster a sense of urgency among national political leaders. As early as September 1968, President Johnson cast his own proposal to improve coal health and safety in quantitative terms: "At the very least, one out of every ten active miners— and one out of every five retired miners—suffers from a serious respiratory disease. For the tens of thousands of miners so afflicted, the shortness of breath may shorten their lives." The difficulties of calculating precisely the toll of respiratory disease made agnosticism the safest course. For some, a lack of definitive statistics was no impediment to expeditious reform. To liberals like Senator George McGovern, the president's message represented "a clear and urgent call to action," even though "we are unable as yet to measure the cost of our coal in the sickness and death caused by such occupational diseases as coal miner's pneumoconiosis, or 'black lung.'" On the other hand, Walter Hickel, Secretary of the Interior in the Nixon administration, rejected extant epidemiological data as inadequate. On March 7, 1969, Hickel told Senate investigators that "at this stage we are not in a position to give even a reasonably accurate estimate of the extent of the problem." Taking any preventable loss of workers' health as indefensible, Murray Hunter dismissed the whole question: "I shall not indulge in a numbers game. I cannot make an accurate statement as to how many coal miners die or suffer with respiratory disability as a result of their occupation. Ethically and philosophically, it really doesn't matter."[59]

Other participants in this discussion unhesitatingly plunged into the numbers game, however. It was a spirited, confused contest. Wide disagreements arose even among those who worked directly from the PHS findings, that is, that dust disease affected roughly one in ten active employees and roughly one in five inactive miners. The National Coal Association believed that the ratio of active miners to inactive miners was four to one and concluded that approximately 15,000 individuals had pneumoconiosis. Surgeon General William Stewart believed that the ratio of active miners to inactive miners was one to four and put the prevalence at approximately 100,000. Stewart's subordinate Henry Doyle, probably without intending to undercut this estimate, estimated the number of inactive miners at 120,000 (i.e., slightly less than the total number of active employees) and concluded that the prevalence was 38,000. Politicians who entered the fray came up with differing misinterpretations of the PHS findings. Seeking to magnify the problem, Senator Harrison Williams construed the estimate of 100,000 as pertaining to the active employees alone and erroneously concluded that 70 percent of the coal-mining workforce had black lung. Seeking to minimize the problem as potential, not actual, Senator Robert Byrd took 100,000 to be the population at risk of disease, not those who already had it.[60]

Reliance on evidence beyond that gathered by the PHS gave rise to still higher figures. In his appearances before congressional committees, Lorin Kerr defended his revised estimate of 125,000 by citing the Pennsylvania studies and other unspecified sources of information, as well as the federal findings from 1963–64. Kerr pointed out that long ago the UMW Welfare and Retirement Fund had taken the prevalence question to public health agencies, where "no one was willing to even guess how many breathless miners were disabled by their jobs." Moreover, for many years the fund was "unable to get any help or information" from health officials. Ralph Nader privately advised Ralph Yarborough, chair of the Senate Labor and Public Welfare Committee, that "well over 150,000 miners, active and retired, have advanced black lung disease; tens of thousands more are affected to one degree or another." Nader did not explicate the basis for this contention. Isidore Buff apparently ignored the PHS data altogether in concluding that "about fifty percent of the miners eventually become disabled from this disease."[61] Less important for legislative purposes than the imprecision of much of this quantification and the failure to reach consensus on the exact size of the problem was the fact that the discussion came to center on six-digit numbers.

Mandatory dust limits remained the object of much congressional dispute. Ken Hechler in particular pressed this issue, based on his understanding that UMW leadership, despite threats to restore outmoded technology, was prepared to settle for federal legislation covering only safety hazards, sacrificing the interests of its members in protection against the greater threat posed by health hazards. Hechler advised the House Committee on Education and Labor on March 19 that "the most critical feature of the bill before you is the dust standard." Unwilling to begin from a weak proposal that alleviated the operators' anxieties over regulatory costs, he called for the three-milligram limit. He defended this position on unabashedly humanistic grounds: "We ought to find out what is necessary to protect the life, the health and the safety of these 144,000 human beings who work in the coal mines. And then we ought to go ahead boldly and take the measures necessary to protect these human beings. In other words, what is the level of coal dust which causes black lung?" From this perspective, the federal objective should be to ensure that workers could complete a career in the mines without significant disability. This stance disregarded adverse economic implications: Hechler was willing to let some firms go out of business if they could not meet the standard. The legislator pointed out the perversity of technological advance: "The coal miner has been watching the grandeurs of science and technology bring a new life to millions of Americans, gouge out twenty tons of coal per day per miner, while doing nothing to improve his health and safety. In fact, science and technology has brought greater hazards to the individual coal miner." Hechler wanted the public to understand that their air-conditioned comfort required a plague of respiratory disease.[62]

Diverse allies joined the campaign for a strict dust standard. Moving toward the ultimate objective of hazard eradication, Isidore Buff wanted no exposure at all to respirable dust. Buff confronted the threat of mine closings with a rhetorical question: "What is the price of a coal miner who chokes to death the last ten years of his life and leaves his family . . . to support him?" Activist pressure stiffened the resolve of the UMW hierarchy to seek immediate imposition of the three-milligram standard. Lorin Kerr told Congress that the best evidence indicated that CWP did not develop at a concentration of three milligrams per cubic meter of air but certainly did at higher levels. Kerr also pointed out that some U.S. mines already met the more stringent standard.[63]

Yet coal operators opposed three milligrams as unattainable or needlessly onerous. They rallied around the Nixon administration's proposal to permit exposure up to 4.5 milligrams. Defense of the slacker standard rested on a simple division of labor: government officials focused on technological feasibility, industry leaders on national economic wellbeing. Interior Secretary Hickel and other senior administrators held that current technology could not reach the lower standard. At the same time, Republican officials made little effort to defend the contention that extended exposure to the 4.5-milligram concentration did not result in pneumoconiosis. When, for example, Representative Patsy Mink inquired whether there existed "any relationship between the 4.5 and the health standards needed to prevent black lung among our coal miners," Nixon's lieutenants retreated. They defended this limit as "what we can get now," as Hickel put it. When a group of Farmington widows lobbied for strong legislation in February 1969, they pointed to the burgeoning space exploration program as proof of the nation's technological prowess. Widow Sara Kaznoski told Walter Hickel that, though she had no objection to the imminent mission to the moon, conditions on earth needed attention as well. At the apex of national ebullience over extraordinary scientific and engineering feats, others wondered aloud how the United States could split the atom and travel into space but could not remove dust particles from coal mines.[64]

For their part, the coal operators assailed the financial impossibility of compliance with drastic dust regulations. They tried to perpetuate the outmoded image of their industry as too fragile to withstand much federal rulemaking. Despite soaring demand for coal from electric utilities, some managers warned that the costs of strict dust limits and other proposed requirements would be catastrophic. The Harlan County, Kentucky, Coal Operators' Association opposed any mandatory dust limits at all. Only slightly more conciliatory, the National Coal Association offered as an interim standard the ACGIH threshold limit value of fifty million particles per cubic foot of air, a relic of the 1940s. Jennings Randolph articulated the operators' fears when he appealed for "a degree of flexibility" in setting standards. "The search always must be for the feasible alternatives to complete closure and to the payroll cutoff," Randolph advised. Thus, from the conservative perspective, infeasibility stood as the cardinal principle of health policy. A subsidiary theme that ran through the operators' critique of the stronger proposals was the need for careful consideration, further research, and avoidance of hasty rulemaking. Harlan County mine owners' representative Clowd McDowell called for "study of this problem in order to establish all the facts pertaining to it rather than setting an arbitrary limit." Obviously, a delay until after the commotion subsided served the operators' interests.[65]

The appearance of victims before congressional committees reasserted the need to stop black lung. To dramatize the consequences of this incurable disease, Hechler brought in a group of men to attest to their permanent disability. These ordinary workers resembled in no way the conventional parade of medical experts droning through the scientific literature. The demonstration by Otis Ratliff, a fifty-two-year-old former coal miner, before Senate investigators on March 20 proved to be particularly disturb-ing. After hopping up and down twenty-five times, Ratliff collapsed into a chair, gasping for breath. No one demanded to see his X-rays for confirma-tion of his ailment.[66]

Hechler's critique of misplaced economic concerns continued unabated. At a rally of 300 miners in Clifftop, West Virginia, on March 22, 1969, he derided the "backward thinking" of Herbert E. Jones, Jr., a coal executive who threatened that federal restrictions would all but destroy the state's economy. "Just how much," Hechler asked rhetorically, "is a human being worth?" In a speech the following month at West Virginia University, he reiterated the need to set more humane social priorities, especially in light of the healthy profitability of the coal industry. On July 8, he urged UMW president Boyle to do more to support a strong dust standard, regardless of economic consequences. Beyond cooperation on the immediate objec-tive of three milligrams, Hechler sought the unionist's endorsement of a limit of one milligram of respirable dust per cubic meter of air within five or six years and an ultimate limit of one-fifth of a milligram within eight years. "The cost to industry," the radical reasoned, "can never exceed the cost in human debris." This overture to Boyle undoubtedly took into ac-count his growing vulnerability to criticism. With Joseph Yablonski's re-cent announcement that he would run for the presidency of the union and emphasize health and safety in his campaign, the incumbent had further incentive to cover his flank on this issue. Under pressure from Hechler, Yablonski, and other critics, the Boyle administration could no longer un-critically accept and pass on to its rank-and-file members the mine owners' threats that a strong federal dust standard would kill countless jobs.[67]

The black lung partisans managed to shift the debate toward fuller con-sideration of the flesh-and-blood realities of suffering and diminished quality of life. BOM director John O'Leary's remarks at the National Coal Association convention on June 16, 1969, for example, reflected the influ-ence of the humanitarian perspective. "Our mining research to date has been preoccupied with one element of cost: those that we can list as eco-nomic," O'Leary candidly observed. "I think more and more, not because we want to but because we must, we are going to be forced to look upon human cost and environmental cost as well." O'Leary's apologies may not have appeased the unhappy mine owners, but they did convey to them that the old logic of efficiency no longer held in Washington. As this realization sank in, the operators began to adjust to their transformed political situation.[68]

The combination of the preponderance of evidence and the ongoing threat of a disruptive work stoppage compelled Congress to settle on tight limitations on miners' exposure to the dust hazard. The final version of the Federal Coal Mine Health and Safety Act of 1969 required that operators immediately provide a working environment with no more than three milligrams of respirable mine dust per cubic meter of air. Three years after the effective date of the act, employers had to reduce the particulate level to two milligrams. (This exposure limit remains unchanged a quarter century later.) Congress prefaced this regulation with a lofty statement of purpose: "To provide, to the greatest extent possible, that the working conditions in each underground coal mine are sufficiently free of respirable dust concentrations in the mine atmosphere to permit each miner the opportunity to work underground during the period of his entire adult working life without incurring any disability from pneumoconiosis or any other occupation-related disease during or at the end of such period." National policy thus embraced, albeit not without qualification, the principle that coal workers had a right to a career, if not a whole life, unimpeded by the effects of breathing at work.[69]

In large part, the more stringent dust standard passed because it paled in comparison with a still more disturbing Democratic proposition. Plans for federal compensation for individuals with black lung especially inflamed coal operators and their political allies. In fact, the prospect of massive, unprecedented, and possibly precedent-setting remuneration to casualties of production could only cause consternation in the business community as a whole.

Demands arose for a national compensation program despite the adoption of CWP compensation in several states. Even under those state laws with liberal statutes of limitation for filing claims, a sizable backlog of former miners fell outside the bounds of eligibility. Activists looked to the federal government for a supplementary plan to rectify this perceived inequity. In addition, dissatisfaction with employer-dominated compensation administrators and difficult rules of evidence at the state level prompted hopes that the federal bureaucracy would be more lenient in implementing social insurance. Interest in uniform national benefits and eligibility criteria also stemmed from the fear that differences among workers' compensation plans would confer a competitive advantage on firms operating in states with niggardly provision.[70]

Ken Hechler's bill of February 6, 1969, started the fight for federal black lung benefits. Again the lone visionary, Hechler began advocating a national insurance scheme for victims of dust disease in December 1968. In this daring plan, the modest principle of supplementation served as the entering wedge for federalization of social insurance. The Hechler bill proposed to make up the difference between state compensation benefits and those paid under the federal Longshoremen's and Harbor Workers' Compensation Act. Where state provision was limited in duration or by a ceiling on total benefits, the supplement would continue for the duration of disability, including periods of partial disability. Further reconstruing supplementation, this bold plan granted payments for respiratory disease claims denied by state officials.[71]

On March 27, 1969, very shortly after Isidore Buff took up federal black lung compensation in a speech in Washington, politicians close to the UMW officers presented a second bill. In introducing his coal health and safety bill only two months earlier, Jennings Randolph had maintained that workers' compensation was purely a state matter. But reportedly at the urging of W. A. Boyle, Randolph rethought federalism. Along with Robert Byrd, he offered a plan to aid those found ineligible for state benefits. Far from a takeover of workers' compensation, the Byrd-Randolph measure involved federal grants for benefits of no more than a meager twenty-five dollars per week. This bill left compensation administration and definition of black lung to the states.[72]

In the course of the subsequent legislative maneuvering, a seemingly unlikely champion of purely federal compensation emerged: Philip Burton, a member of the House of Representatives from San Francisco. On closer examination, however, Burton's involvement was not so unlikely; San Francisco had no coal mines, but it did have a port. There the federal system of injury and illness compensation for longshore and harbor workers, which Burton knew well, offered a precedent for further intervention. Unlike Hechler, he served on the Education and Labor Committee, an ideal vantage point for attacks on both the coal operators and the Nixon administration. In addition, he enjoyed the wealth of expertise on mining issues provided by Gary Sellers, a public interest attorney working with

Ralph Nader. In an exchange with Deputy Secretary of Labor James Hodgson on March 26, 1969, Burton complained that the administration's bill neglected many miners who had already fallen out of the workforce. When Hodgson agreed that "there is no ex post facto aspect to this bill," his bland legalism set off the volatile Californian. "That," Burton shot back, "is a very fine set of three Latin words to say that this proposal isn't going to provide any help to ninety-five percent of the workers affected." At moments like this, the San Franciscan served to make Ken Hechler look moderate. (During subcommittee deliberations over the dust standard, Burton blurted, "Why shouldn't it be zero?" At one juncture in the dealmaking, Burton advised a top official of the National Coal Association that failure to accede to far-reaching reform would lead to a government takeover of his industry.)[73]

Opponents of national compensation maintained two major lines of defense. Tradition was the first defense. In the evolution of federalism, it had long been customary to leave workers' compensation to the states (with a few exceptions). In addition, the Nixon administration correctly noted that because the individual states had been handling compensation for occupational injuries and illnesses for more than half a century, their long experience gave them considerable administrative expertise. Accordingly, the Nixon proposal allowed small federal grants to the states to upgrade their compensation plans to cover black lung.[74]

The second principle guiding opposition to compensation was containment. Much as they had done in the thirties, coal companies seized on the most minimal definition of the underlying substantive problem. The operators were understandably determined not to assume more than a fraction of the human costs of producing coal. In this view, progressive massive fibrosis, the advanced form of CWP, constituted the only appropriate object of redistribution. To this end, the operators denied that simple CWP entailed significant disability. Given that numerous medical investigators, including some influential British researchers, concurred in this assessment, the operators occupied a strong position on this front.[75]

Antagonists of reform also clung to progressive massive fibrosis as a distinctively occupational disorder in contrast to less clear-cut, multifactorial conditions. They singled out cigarette smoking as the most important etiological factor in bronchitis and emphysema and reiterated the nonspecific nature of the signs and symptoms exhibited in these disorders. Ian

Higgins of the University of Michigan, who had studied miners' respiratory maladies in both Britain and the United States, summarized the dilemma and his sense of its policy implications: "It is impossible in the individual to say how much his bronchitis and emphysema is due to his work or to his smoking or to other factors in the cause of these diseases. It is not practicable to compensate all persons who have bronchitis and emphysema." Denial of compensation, on the other hand, was eminently practicable.[76]

Proponents of federal compensation made a variety of rejoinders to these contentions. The more cautious insisted only on the compensability of progressive massive fibrosis, conceding the disputed border territory. Others stuck to the claims that simple CWP could disable its victims and that emphysema and bronchitis occurred with sufficiently higher frequency among miners to warrant inclusion under an insurance plan. Donald Rasmussen invoked Jethro Gough's conclusion that simple CWP did indeed cause disability. Murray Hunter argued that smoking posed a lesser respiratory hazard than mine dust.[77]

Advocates of wider federal responsibility also attempted to extend the range of redistributive possibilities. Hawey Wells called on Congress to restore to sick miners the right to sue their former employers for damages, given the illusory nature of workers' compensation. By mid-1969, Buff was denouncing the West Virginia compensation reforms as worthless and demanding a national pension system for coal miners. In one rendition, this system would have the Social Security Administration pay a monthly allowance to all twenty-year survivors of the industry, regardless of the state of their lungs, with financing through a tax on coal production.[78]

At the end of 1969, the legislative mill ground out a compromise that reflected the unresolved state of medical knowledge. Amazingly enough, the compensation plan carried the outrageous title "Black Lung Benefits," a vivid legitimation of the democratic upheaval in disease recognition. Behind this banner, however, lay a modest disease entity. Indeed, the term "black lung" appeared only once in the statute, in naming Title IV. Elsewhere, pneumoconiosis, "a chronic dust disease of the lung arising out of employment in an underground coal mine," constituted the problem. Work-related bronchitis and emphysema fell by the wayside. The final compromise also excluded from coverage individuals with less than total disability. The measure privileged radiological and pathological data in determining benefit eligibility, despite their limitations in disclosing disability.[79]

On the other hand, the legislation opened the door to a sizable share of those excluded from state protection. Individuals with ten years or more experience underground and a diagnosis of pneumoconiosis enjoyed a rebuttable presumption of eligibility for federal compensation. Claimants with ten years or more experience and a diagnosis supported by autopsy or biopsy evidence of "massive lesions" or radiological findings of complicated CWP had an irrebuttable presumption. Although the criteria for the irrebuttable presumption plainly applied only to the advanced form of dust disease, the plan nowhere explicitly disallowed claims based on simple pneumoconiosis. That any type of presumption arose and that any consideration was given to simple pneumoconiosis represented stunning departures in national policy.[80]

The mine owners could grudgingly accept this benefit program because it shifted much of the financial burden to the general public. Unlike state workers' compensation, which was funded by employers' insurance premiums, the federal black lung entitlement drew from general revenues of the national government during its first three years of operation. Ken Hechler helped to defend placing this obligation on the U.S. taxpayers rather than levying a federal tax on the coal industy. "The Federal Government is directly responsible for the coal miners having pneumoconiosis," Hechler contended, "because through inaction and neglect no coal dust standards have ever been set to prevent black lung." Given the very large backlog of potential claimants looming in 1969, this approach allowed the operators to avoid a considerable share of the costs entailed by the establishment of the program.[81]

Between compensation and primary prevention, a novel provision of the Federal Coal Mine Health and Safety Act addressed the gradual downward trajectory of workers with dust-induced, chronic disease. The law established the right of individuals with pneumoconiosis to transfer to less dusty locations, without suffering a loss in pay. Initially, the statute guaranteed jobs in which average exposure to respirable mine dust would not exceed two milligrams per cubic meter of air. Within three years of the effective date of this legislation, pneumoconiotic workers were to be reassigned to jobs where the dust concentration averaged no more than one milligram per cubic meter of air. Where this level of air quality could not be attained, the individual was to be given the least dusty position in the mine. This protection enabled those with incipient cases of CWP to remain in the workforce.[82]

The act introduced a program of medical surveillance that raised the likelihood that a miner would request a job transfer. The law called for periodic X-ray examinations of mine employees by the Department of Health, Education, and Welfare. In a quantum leap for workers' right to know what health professionals knew of their predicament, HEW had to supply miners with the results of their own examinations. Federal officials also had to advise workers of their rights under the act.[83]

The act ordered HEW to carry out epidemiological investigations to "provide information on the incidence and prevalence of pneumoconiosis and other respiratory ailments of miners." The resulting investigative program, the National Study of Coal Workers' Pneumoconiosis, which built upon a major study that had already begun in late 1969, continues up to the present. No other group of workers in the nation is subject to this level of scrutiny. The law further stipulated that the findings of these investigations and of related research activity be made available to the general public. Henceforth, federal policy would guard against the disappearance of research findings, such as occurred in the 1920s following the study in Alabama and Kentucky.[84]

At the end of the 1960s, marshalling of epidemiological evidence largely gave way to very different measures of the magnitude and intensity of the dust disease epidemic in the coalfields. Sick miners, previously atomized by clinical encounters and compensation claims procedures, collectivized their grievances and, in that process, redefined them. In a moment of what Rick Bank called "extreme solidarity," tens of thousands of coal workers, aided by a small group of conscientious experts, challenged those who had long dismissed their ailments. The mass movement restored to prominence the wholistic idea of miners' asthma, renamed black lung. Breathless coal diggers finally won a large measure of recognition and a modicum of justice.[85]

It took an exceptional confluence of forces not only to build such a solidaristic movement but also to make it effective in achieving change. Human agency was not the whole story. Underlying the black lung insurgency were shifts in two structural factors that had posed insurmountable obstacles to reform. After a brutal shakeout, the coal industry was enjoying a respite from the hypercompetitiveness that it had suffered for half a century. Second, amid the wide-ranging expansion of national governmental authority that prevailed in the 1960s, the long-established borders of federalism became subject to wide-open reconsideration with respect to such matters as income redistribution and workplace regulation. These structural changes opened the possibility for a national political accord to take unhealthful working conditions out of competition.[86]

An extraordinarily militant worker-centered movement made that possibility a reality. However indispensable they were to the cause of reform, leaders like Buff, Hechler, and other nonminers rode a wave of protest whose power ultimately derived from the determination of rank-and-file miners and their families to shut off the nation's principal source of energy if their demands were not met. The unparalleled strike in West Virginia won state compensation and sent out shock waves that proved decisive in winning federal legislation. The movement represented not so much a rejection of the United Mine Workers of America as a facet of the larger project of reconstituting the union on a more democratic basis. Local officers and other activists within the union played the critical parts in advancing the cause. Without question, the slow accumulation of scientific knowledge since the 1940s and the advocacy of conscientious experts at crucial junctures during the late sixties played vital roles in transforming societal awareness and public policy. Yet it was the primacy of working-class self-assertion that distinguished this campaign and that goes furthest toward explaining its efficacy. While recognition of occupational disease has always depended on cross-class coalitions, what stood out as most remarkable in this case was a confrontational style of mass mobilization that drew on the traditional militance of mine workers and the organizational resources of their local unions.[87]

Events since 1969 underscore the centrality of the miners' organization to improvements in working conditions and social provision in the coal industry. With the UMW actively facilitating the filing of claims and fighting for more open eligibility rules, by the late 1970s approximately half a million miners, widows, and other beneficiaries were receiving federal black lung benefits. (Nixon's estimate was right.) With continued union vigilance over both mine operators and federal regulators, the prevalence of dust disease has declined markedly over the past quarter century, as has the incidence of new cases. Though hardly eradicated, black lung exacts a smaller human cost than it did prior to the passage of the Federal Coal Mine Health and Safety Act.[88]

ENDNOTES

Preface

1. *Charleston Gazette* (W.Va.), Dec. 19, 1969, p. 1; *New York Times,* Dec. 18, 1969, pp. 1, 28; Sara Kaznoski, interview with author, June 6, 1994, Fairmont, W.Va. (tape in author's possession); *Congressional Record,* 91st Cong., 1st sess., 1969, 115, pt. 29: 39707–19, 39997–99.

2. *New York Times,* Dec. 30, 1969, pp. 12, 1, Dec. 31, 1969, p. 8; *Charleston Gazette,* Dec. 30, 1969, pp. 1, 13; *Sunday Gazette-Mail* (Charleston, W.Va.), Dec. 28, 1969, p. 1A; Kaznoski, interview; Ken Hechler, interview with author, July 25, 1991, Charleston, W.Va. (tape in author's possession); Ken Hechler, "Behind the Scenes on the Mine Safety Bill," Jan. 5, 1970, Ken Hechler personal papers.

3. Lorin E. Kerr, "The UMWA Looks at Coal Workers' Pneumoconiosis," *Journal of Occupational Medicine* 12 (1970): 360.

4. U.S. Department of Labor, *OWCP* [Office of Workers' Compensation Programs] *Annual Report to Congress, Fiscal Year 1995* (Washington, D.C., 1996), p. 49; U.S. Department of Labor, *OWCP Annual Report to Congress, Fiscal Year 1994* (Washington, D.C., 1995), p. 41; U.S. Department of Labor, *Black Lung Benefits Act: Annual Report on Administration of the Act during Calendar Year 1984* (Washington, D.C., 1986), p. 23; U.S. Social Security Administration, *Social Security Bulletin: Annual Statistical Supplement, 1995* (Washington, D.C., 1995), p. 351. See also Peter S. Barth, *The Tragedy of Black Lung: Federal Compensation for Occupational Disease* (Kalamazoo, Mich., 1987); Allen R. Prunty and Mark E. Solomons, "The Federal Black Lung Program: Its Evolution and Current Issues," *West Virginia Law Review* 91 (1989): 665–735; John R. Nelson, Jr., *Black Lung: A Study of Disability Compensation Policy Formation* (Chicago, 1985).

1. They Spit a Black Substance

1. H. A. Lemen, "A Case of So-Called Phthisis Pulmonalis Nigra," *Colorado Medical Journal* 1 (1882): 20. For a subtle analysis of a more restrained rhetorical strategy, see Steven M. Stowe, "Seeing Themselves at Work: Physicians and the Case Narra-

tive in the Mid-Nineteenth-Century American South," *American Historical Review* 101 (1996): 41–79.

2. Anthony F. C. Wallace, *St. Clair: A Nineteenth-Century Coal Town's Experience with a Disaster-Prone Industry* (New York, 1987), pp. 296–99; U.S. Bureau of the Census, *Historical Statistics of the United States, Colonial Times to 1970*, 2 vols. (Washington, D.C., 1975), vol. 1, pp. 606–7.

3. A number of studies have acknowledged the existence of miners' respiratory ailments in the United States prior to 1900. However, these works have given the topic only brief attention, and often no more than passing notice. See James Whiteside, *Regulating Danger: The Struggle for Mine Safety in the Rocky Mountain Coal Industry* (Lincoln, Nebr., 1990), p. 46; Jacqueline K. Corn, *Environment and Health in Nineteenth Century America* (New York, 1989), pp. 87–93; Barbara Ellen Smith, *Digging Our Own Graves: Coal Miners and the Struggle over Black Lung Disease* (Philadelphia, 1987), pp. 4–9, 37–38; Priscilla Long, *Where the Sun Never Shines: A History of America's Bloody Coal Industry* (New York, 1989), p. 50; Wallace, *St. Clair*, pp. 256–57, 279; Donald L. Miller and Richard E. Sharpless, *The Kingdom of Coal: Work, Enterprise, and Ethnic Communities in the Mine Fields* (Philadelphia, 1985), p. 106. A second group of scholars simply ignores miners' diseases in the United States, either by focusing exclusively on traumatic injuries or by treating early recognition of pneumoconiosis as an exclusively European phenomenon. See Keith Dix, *Work Relations in the Coal Industry: The Hand Loading Era* (Morgantown, W.Va., 1977), pp. 25, 67–104; Eugene P. Pendergrass, et al., "Historical Perspectives on Coal Workers' Pneumoconiosis in the United States," *Annals of the New York Academy of Sciences* 200 (1972): 835.

4. Carey P. McCord, "Occupational Health Publications in the United States Prior to 1900," *Industrial Medicine and Surgery* 24 (1955): 363–68; compare Robert T. Legge, "Progress of American Industrial Medicine in the First Half of the Twentieth Century," *American Journal of Public Health* 42 (1952): 907; Jacqueline K. Corn, "Historical Aspects of Industrial Hygiene—I: Changing Attitudes toward Occupational Health," *American Industrial Hygiene Association Journal* 39 (1978): 695. On lead intoxication, see Carey P. McCord, "Lead and Lead Poisoning in Early America," *Industrial Medicine and Surgery* 22 (1953): 393–99, 534–39, 573–77, and 23 (1954): 75–80, 120–25, 169–74. For an exceptional effort to pursue major hazards back into the nineteenth century, see Allard E. Dembe, *Occupation and Disease: How Social Factors Affect the Conception of Work-Related Disorders* (New Haven, 1996).

5. For studies of specific diseases, see, among others, David Rosner and Gerald Markowitz, *Deadly Dust: Silicosis and the Politics of Occupational Disease in Twentieth-Century America* (Princeton, 1991); David Rosner and Gerald Markowitz, eds., *Dying for Work: Workers' Safety and Health in Twentieth-Century America* (Bloomington, Ind., 1987); Martin Cherniack, *The Hawk's Nest Incident: America's Worst Industrial Disaster* (New Haven, 1986); Mark Aldrich, "Mortality from Byssinosis among New England Cotton Mill Workers, 1905–1912," *Journal of Occupational Medicine* 24 (1982): 177–80; Edward H. Beardsley, *A History of Neglect: Health Care for Blacks and Mill Workers in the Twentieth-Century South* (Knoxville, Tenn., 1987), chaps. 3, 9, 10; Claudia Clark, "Physicians, Reformers, and Occupational Disease: The Discovery of Radium Poisoning," *Women and Health* 12 (1987): 147–67; Howard Ball, *Cancer Factories: America's Tragic Quest for Uranium Self-Sufficiency* (Westport, Conn., 1993); David E. Lilienfeld, "The Silence: The Asbestos Industry and Early Occupational Cancer Research—A Case Study," *American Journal of Public Health* 81 (1991): 791–800; Ronald Bayer, ed., *The Health and Safety of Workers: Case Studies in the Politics of Professional Responsibility* (New York, 1988); Alan Derickson, "Federal Intervention in the Joplin Silicosis Epidemic,

1911–1916," *Bulletin of the History of Medicine* 62 (1988): 236–51; Wendy Richardson, "The Curse of Our Trade: Occupational Disease in a Vermont Granite Town," *Vermont History* 60 (1992): 5–28.

6. Howard N. Eavenson, *The First Century and a Quarter of American Coal Industry* (Pittsburgh, 1942), esp. pp. 29–43; Ronald L. Lewis, *Coal, Iron, and Slaves: Industrial Slavery in Maryland and Virginia, 1715–1865* (Westport, Conn., 1979), pp. 6–7, 455–80; U.S. Census, *Historical Statistics*, vol. 1, pp. 588–93, 580; Pennsylvania Bureau of Mines, *Report, 1898* ([Harrisburg], 1899), p. vii.

7. Dix, *Work Relations in Coal*; Miller and Sharpless, *Kingdom of Coal*, pp. 84–134, esp. 85–86; Cadwallader Evans, Jr., et al., "Seventy-Five Years of Progress in the Anthracite Industry," and Howard N. Eavenson, "Seventy-Five Years of Progress in Bituminous Coal Mining," both in *Seventy-Five Years of Progress in the Mineral Industry*, ed. A. E. Parsons (New York, 1947), pp. 250–51, 225–26, 229–31; U.S. Census, *Historical Statistics*, vol. 1, pp. 589–90.

8. Henry C. Sheafer, "Hygiene of Coal-Mines," in *Cyclopaedia of the Practice of Medicine*, ed. Hugo von Ziemssen, vol. 19: *On Hygiene and Public Health*, ed. Albert H. Buck (New York, 1879), pp. 232, 245, 229–32, 245–46; Dix, *Work Relations in Coal*, pp. 8–9, 25; Pennsylvania Department of Internal Affairs, *Reports of the Inspectors of Coal Mines, 1896* ([Harrisburg], 1897), p. 367; Katherine A. Harvey, *The Best-Dressed Miners: Life and Labor in the Maryland Coal Region, 1835–1910* (Ithaca, 1969), pp. 35–37; Whiteside, *Regulating Danger*, pp. 35–40.

9. John Brophy, *A Miner's Life*, ed. John O. P. Hall (Madison, 1964), pp. 39, 38–39; *United Mine Workers Journal* (hereafter cited as *UMWJ*), March 16, 1893, p. 3, Oct. 26, 1893, p. 8, Nov. 9, 1893, pp. 4, 8, Sept. 21, 1899, p. 2; Sheafer, "Hygiene of Coal-Mines," p. 245; Miller and Sharpless, *Kingdom of Coal*, pp. 102–6; Harvey, *Best-Dressed Miners*, pp. 34–35; Steve Sewell, "Amongst the Damp: The Dangerous Profession of Coal Mining in Oklahoma, 1870–1935," *Chronicles of Oklahoma* 70 (1992): 71.

10. Andrew Meiklejohn, "History of Lung Diseases of Coal Miners in Great Britain: Part I, 1800–1875," *British Journal of Industrial Medicine* 8 (1951): 127; George Rosen, *The History of Miners' Diseases: A Medical and Social Interpretation* (New York, 1943), p. 190; Russell C. Maulitz, *Morbid Appearances: The Anatomy of Pathology in the Early Nineteenth Century* (Cambridge, Eng., 1987); W. F. Bynum, *Science and the Practice of Medicine in the Nineteenth Century* (Cambridge, Eng., 1994), pp. 31–51; John S. Haller, Jr., *American Medicine in Transition, 1840–1910* (Urbana, 1981), pp. 192–233; Esmond R. Long, *A History of Pathology*, rev. ed. (New York, 1965), pp. 76–101; Oliver Wendell Holmes, et al., "Report of the Committee on Medical Literature," *Transactions of the American Medical Association*, vol. 1 (1848), rpt. in *Medical America in the Nineteenth Century: Readings from the Literature*, ed. Gert H. Brieger (Baltimore, 1972), pp. 53, 54.

11. James C. Gregory, "Case of Peculiar Black Infiltration of the Whole Lung, Resembling Melanosis," *Edinburgh Medical and Surgical Journal* 36 (1831): 389–94.

12. Thomas Stratton, "Case of Anthracosis or Black Infiltration of the Whole Lungs," *Edinburgh Medical and Surgical Journal* 49 (1838): 490–91; Edward Greenhow, "Specimen of Collier's Lung," *Transactions of the Pathological Society of London* 17 (1866): 34–36; J. W. Begbie, "On Anthracosis, or Coal Miners' Phthisis, the Spurious Melanosis of Carswell," *Glasgow Medical Journal* n.s., 1 (1866): 13–20, 169–81.

13. James A. Merchant, Geoffrey Taylor, and Thomas K. Hodous, "Coal Workers' Pneumoconiosis and Exposure to Other Carbonaceous Dusts," in U.S. National Institute for Occupational Safety and Health, *Occupational Respiratory Diseases*, ed. James A. Merchant, et al. (Washington, D.C., 1986), pp. 329–84, esp. 366–72. For other valuable overviews of the medical literature, see Michael Attfield and Gregory Wagner, "Re-

spiratory Disease in Coal Miners," in *Environmental and Occupational Medicine*, 2d ed., ed. William N. Rom (Boston, 1992), pp. 325–44; Edward L. Petsonk and Michael D. Attfield, "Coal Workers' Pneumoconiosis and Other Coal-Related Lung Disease," in *Textbook of Clinical Occupational and Environmental Medicine*, ed. Linda Rosenstock and Mark R. Cullen (Philadelphia, 1994), pp. 274–87; James L. Weeks and Gregory R. Wagner, "Compensation for Occupational Disease with Multiple Causes: The Case of Miners' Respiratory Diseases," *American Journal of Public Health* 76 (1986): 58–61. For a discussion of pathological anatomy that overlooks melanoptysis as the key link between clinical observation and pathological studies, see Smith, *Digging Our Own Graves*, pp. 8–9.

14. E. H. Greenhow, "Black Lungs from a Case of Colliers' Phthisis," *Transactions of the Pathological Society of London* 20 (1869): 42; Begbie, "On Anthracosis," pp. 17, 18, 172–73; William Thomson, "On Black Expectoration and the Deposition of Black Matter in the Lungs," *Transactions of the Medical and Chirurgical Society of London* 20 (1837): 235–36.

15. John T. Carpenter, untitled paper in "Report of the Schuylkill County Medical Society," *Transactions of the Medical Society of the State of Pennsylvania* 5th ser., pt. 2 (1869): 488, 489. For passing comments on anthracite respiratory disease that predate Carpenter's paper, see George W. Brown, "Report of the Schuylkill County Medical Society, 1856: Report on General Medicine," and Horace Ladd, "Sanitary Report of Carbon County Medical Society," *Transactions of the Medical Society of the State of Pennsylvania*, n.s., pt. 1 (1856): 202–3, and pt. 3 (1858): 51–52. For a general application of the miasmatic hypothesis to the workplace, see Charles H. Brigham, "The Influence of Occupations upon Health," Michigan Board of Health, *Third Annual Report, 1875*, rpt. in *Journal of Occupational Medicine* 18 (1976): 236–37. For the persistence of the miasma concept generally, see Phyllis Allen Richmond, "American Attitudes toward the Germ Theory of Disease (1860–1880)," *Journal of the History of Medicine and Allied Sciences* 9 (1954): 428–30.

16. Carpenter, "Schuylkill Medical Society," pp. 489, 490. The use of the terms "miner's asthma" and "miners' asthma" by Carpenter and by a host of other lay and professional observers throughout the late nineteenth century to denote a potentially serious disease refutes Barbara Ellen Smith's claim that company doctors made up "miners' asthma" as a benign condition after the turn of the century; see Smith, *Digging Our Own Graves*, pp. 16–17, 25, 222.

17. Carpenter, "Schuylkill Medical Society," pp. 490, 491. On Victorian individualism, see Thomas R. Cole, *The Journey of Life: A Cultural History of Aging in America* (Cambridge, Eng., 1992), pp. 139–52, esp. 146–47.

18. Lemen, "Phthisis Pulmonalis Nigra," p. 21; D. J. Miller, "Anthracosis," *Proceedings of the Pathological Society of Philadelphia* 16 (1891–93): 246–48; Edward Pinkowski, *John Siney, the Miners' Martyr* (Philadelphia, 1963), pp. 242, 244. Daniel Weaver of Illinois was another pioneering unionist who died of miners' asthma; see Edward A. Wieck, *The American Miners' Association: A Record of the Origin of Coal Miners' Unions in the United States* (New York, 1940), p. 190. On the broad definition of consumption in the late nineteenth century, see Katherine Ott, *Fevered Lives: Tuberculosis in American Culture since 1870* (Cambridge, Mass., 1996).

19. Gottlieb Merkel, "The Diseases Caused by the Inhalation of Those Kinds of Dust Whose Presence in the Pulmonary Tissue May Be Demonstrated," *Medical Record* (New York) 9 (1874): 670, 669–72; Frederick Peterson, "Pneumonokoniosis," *Medical News* (Philadelphia) 47 (1885): 121–22.

20. J. W. Exline, "The Sanitation of Mines," in Colorado State Medical Society, *Transactions of the Twenty-Sixth Annual Convention, 1896* (Denver, 1896), pp. 238–39.

On subsequent specialization, see Christopher C. Sellers, *Hazards of the Job: From Industrial Disease to Environmental Health Science* (Chapel Hill, 1997).

21. Austin Flint, *A Treatise on the Principles and Practice of Medicine*, 4th ed. (Philadelphia, 1873), pp. 198–200; Lemen, "Phthisis Pulmonalis Nigra," p. 22. On the importance of Flint's work, see Paul J. Edelson, "Adopting Osler's *Principles*: Medical Textbooks in American Medical Schools, 1891–1906," *Bulletin of the History of Medicine* 68 (1994): 72, 74.

22. Flint, *Treatise*, p. 200; R. Virchow, "The Pathology of Miners' Lung," *Edinburgh Medical Journal* 4 (1858): 204–13. For a critique of Virchow's approach, see Rosen, *History of Miners' Diseases*, pp. 312–13, 318–24. On the rising importance of microscopy at this time, see Russell C. Maulitz, "Pathology," in *The Education of American Physicians: Historical Essays*, ed. Ronald L. Numbers (Berkeley, 1980), pp. 123, 131–35.

23. Alfred L. Loomis, *A Text-Book of Practical Medicine* (New York, 1884), p. 182; Edward T. Bruen, "Pneumonokoniosis," in *A System of Practical Medicine*, ed. William Pepper, 5 vols. (Philadelphia, 1885), vol. 3, pp. 454–59; Adolf Strumpell, *A Text-Book of Medicine for Students and Practitioners*, trans. Herman F. Vickery and Philip C. Knapp (New York, 1887), pp. 227–28; James T. Anders, *A Text-Book of the Practice of Medicine* (Philadelphia, 1897), pp. 533–35. For other limitations of late-nineteenth-century texts, see Sellers, *Hazards of the Job*, pp. 32–33.

24. Flint, *Treatise*, pp. 198–200; Bruen, "Pneumonokoniosis," p. 459.

25. William Osler, *The Principles and Practice of Medicine* (New York, 1892), pp. 553–56; Osler, *The Principles and Practice of Medicine*, 3d ed. (New York, 1899), pp. 652–54. On the preeminence of Osler's textbook by the turn of the century, see Edelson, "Adopting Osler's *Principles*," pp. 68, 77; Kenneth M. Ludmerer, *Learning to Heal: The Development of American Medical Education* (New York, 1985), pp. 88–89. For Osler's own studies of pneumoconiosis in Canada, see William Osler, "On the Pathology of Miner's Lung," *Canada Medical and Surgical Journal* 4 (1875–76): 145–68; George Rosen, "Osler and Miners Phthisis," *Journal of the History of Medicine and Allied Sciences* 4 (1949): 259–66.

26. Osler, *Principles and Practice*, 1st ed., p. 556; *UMWJ*, Aug. 18, 1892, p. 2, Sept. 22, 1892, p. 2, Nov. 10, 1892, p. 3, Aug. 15, 1901, p. 3; *Miners' Journal* (Pottsville, Pa.), April 29, 1843, Jan. 10, 1846; George Korson, *Black Rock: Mining Folklore of the Pennsylvania Dutch* (Baltimore, 1960), p. 258. On the primacy of and possibilities for therapy, see Charles E. Rosenberg, "The Therapeutic Revolution: Medicine, Meaning, and Social Change in Nineteenth-Century America," in *The Therapeutic Revolution: Essays in the Social History of American Medicine*, ed. Morris J. Vogel and Charles E. Rosenberg (Philadelphia, 1979), pp. 3–25, esp. 15–21; William G. Rothstein, *American Physicians in the Nineteenth Century: From Sects to Science* (Baltimore, 1992), pp. 177–97; John Harley Warner, *The Therapeutic Perspective: Medical Practice, Knowledge, and Identity in America, 1820–1885* (Cambridge, Mass., 1986).

27. Roberts Bartholow, *A Treatise on the Practice of Medicine*, 7th ed. (New York, 1890), p. 407; Exline, "Sanitation of Mines," p. 241.

28. To contrast the disregard for miners' disease with the immersion of investigators in other social problems in the late nineteenth century, see Ellen Fitzpatrick, *Endless Crusade: Women Social Scientists and Progressive Reform* (New York, 1990), pp. 3–79; Kathryn Kish Sklar, *Florence Kelley and the Nation's Work: The Rise of Women's Political Culture, 1830–1900* (New Haven, 1995); Dorothy Ross, *The Origins of American Social Science* (Cambridge, Eng., 1991), pp. 53–140; Thomas L. Haskell, *The Emergence of Professional Social Science: The American Social Science Association and the Nineteenth-Century Crisis of Authority* (Urbana, 1977); Mary O. Furner, *Advocacy and Objectivity: A Crisis in the Professionalization of American Social Science, 1865–1905* (Lexington, Ky.,

1975); John Duffy, *The Sanitarians: A History of American Public Health* (Urbana, 1990), pp. 126–37; Judith Walzer Leavitt, *The Healthiest City: Milwaukee and the Politics of Health Reform* (Princeton, 1982), pp. 190–204; Alexandra Oleson and John Voss, eds., *The Organization of Knowledge in Modern America, 1860–1920* (Baltimore, 1979). For a skeptical view of the potential for civil society to remedy contemporary ills, see Adam B. Seligman, *The Idea of Civil Society* (Princeton, 1995).

29. William R. Brock, *Investigation and Responsibility: Public Responsibility in the United States, 1865–1900* (Cambridge, Eng., 1984), pp. 36, 54; Steven Kelman, "The Statistical Foundations of American Statistical Policy," in *The Politics of Numbers*, ed. William Alonzo and Paul Starr (New York, 1987), pp. 280–86. For a helpful introduction to the relationship of numerical data to public policy, see Paul Starr, "The Sociology of Official Statistics," in *The Politics of Numbers*, ed. Alonzo and Starr, pp. 7–57.

30. For the general course of state development and underdevelopment, see Brock, *Investigation and Responsibility*; Stephen Skowronek, *Building a New American State: The Expansion of National Administrative Capacities, 1877–1920* (Cambridge, Eng., 1982), pt. 2; Morton Keller, *Affairs of State: Public Life in Late Nineteenth-Century America* (Cambridge, Mass., 1977); William J. Novak, *The People's Welfare: Law and Regulation in Nineteenth-Century America* (Chapel Hill, 1996).

31. Michael J. Lacey and Mary O. Furner, eds., *The State and Social Investigation in Britain and the United States* (Cambridge, Eng., 1993); Mary O. Furner and Barry Supple, eds., *The State and Economic Knowledge: The American and British Experience* (Cambridge, Eng., 1990); Martin Bulmer, Kevin Bales, and Kathryn Kish Sklar, eds., *The Social Survey in Historical Perspective, 1880–1940* (Cambridge, Eng., 1991); Dietrich Rueschemeyer and Theda Skocpol, eds., *States, Social Knowledge, and the Origins of Modern Social Policies* (Princeton, 1996).

32. Ohio Mining Commission, *Report, 1871* (Columbus, 1872), p. 153.

33. Ohio Mining Commission, *Report, 1871*, pp. 22, 80, 155, 40, 74, 155–56, 169.

34. Pennsylvania Second Geological Survey, *Report on the Mining Methods and Appliances Used in the Anthracite Coal Fields*, by Henry M. Chance (Harrisburg, 1883), pp. 423–39. This survey avoided any systematic consideration of the distribution of the disease across the hard-coal workforce, but remarked that "the disease is most common (among coal miners) in persons over forty years of age," implying that this condition was prevalent across the hard-coal region (p. 438).

35. U.S. Industrial Commission, *Report*, vol. 12: *The Relations and Conditions of Capital and Labor Employed in the Mining Industry* (Washington, D.C., 1901), pp. 130, cxliii.

36. Margo J. Anderson, *The American Census: A Social History* (New Haven, 1988), pp. 83–115, esp. 85–86; U.S. Census Office, *Report on the Mortality and Vital Statistics of the United States as Returned at the Tenth Census (June 1, 1880)*, by John S. Billings, 2 pts. (Washington, D.C., 1885, 1886); U.S. Census Office, *Report on the Statistics of Agriculture in the United States at the Eleventh Census: 1890* (Washington, D.C., 1895), pp. 237–73; James H. Cassedy, "The Registration Area and American Vital Statistics: Development of a Health Research Resource, 1885–1915," *Bulletin of the History of Medicine* 39 (1965): 221–31; Duffy, *The Sanitarians*, 157–92; William Graebner, *Coal-Mining Safety in the Progressive Period: The Political Economy of Reform* (Lexington, Ky., 1976), pp. 23–24.

37. Duffy, *The Sanitarians*, pp. 126–56; Brock, *Investigation and Responsibility*, pp. 116–47; Charles V. Chapin, "History of State and Municipal Control of Disease," in *A Half Century of Public Health*, ed. Mazyck P. Ravenel (New York, 1921), pp. 133–60, esp. 155.

38. Pennsylvania State Board of Health and Vital Statistics, *First Annual Report, 1885* (Harrisburg, 1886), p. 9.

39. Pennsylvania Board of Health, *Report, 1885*, p. 13; Pennsylvania, *Laws, 1885*

(Harrisburg, 1885), pp. 56–59. On the weakness of the health boards, see Duffy, *The Sanitarians*, pp. 126–56, esp. 153–54.

40. Pennsylvania Board of Health, *Report, 1885*, pp. 29–30; Pennsylvania State Board of Health and Vital Statistics, *Fourth Annual Report, 1888* (Harrisburg, 1891), pp. 62, 81, 367–73; Spencer M. Free, "Sanitation in Mining Towns," *Annals of Hygiene* 3 (1888): 303–8; Illinois State Board of Health, *Eighth Annual Report, 1885* (Springfield, 1886), pp. 85–282; Illinois State Board of Health, *Ninth Annual Report, 1886* (Springfield, 1889), pp. 5–159; Harvey, *Best-Dressed Miners*, pp. 86–87. On the policy implications of the deep institutionalization of individualistic ideology in U.S. health data systems, see Nancy Krieger, "The Making of Public Health Data: Paradigms, Politics, and Policy," *Journal of Public Health Policy* 13 (1992): 412–27.

41. Pennsylvania Board of Health, *Report, 1888*, pp. 371–73. On the state's dependence on and deference to local health authorities, see Barbara Gutmann Rosenkrantz, *Public Health and the State: Changing Views in Massachusetts, 1842–1936* (Cambridge, Mass., 1972), pp. 52–73, esp. 70. On localism generally, see Keller, *Affairs of State*, pp. 112–21, 130, 319–22.

42. Pennsylvania State Board of Health and Vital Statistics, *Seventeenth Annual Report, 1901*, 2 vols. ([Harrisburg], 1902), vol. 1, pp. 323, 323–25. The relationship between alcohol consumption and miners' health may not have been what Fulton imagined. In the anthracite fields, work-induced disabilities forced many miners and their families into the tavern business, and many of their former co-workers felt obliged to patronize their establishments. See *Miners' Journal*, July 3, 1869.

43. Pennsylvania State Board of Health and Vital Statistics, *Second Annual Report, 1886* (Harrisburg, 1887), pp. 506, 507. For a class analysis of changing conceptions of consumption, see Rosner and Markowitz, *Deadly Dust*, pp. 13–20.

44. Pennsylvania State Board of Health and Vital Statistics, *Fifth Annual Report, 1889* (Harrisburg, 1891), p. 374. On the initial phase of vital statistics, see James H. Cassedy, *American Medicine and Statistical Thinking, 1800–1860* (Cambridge, Mass., 1984), pp. 178–206.

45. Pennsylvania State Board of Health and Vital Statistics, *Fifth Annual Report, 1889*, p. 188; Kentucky State Board of Health, *Biennial Report, 1898–99* (Louisville, 1899), pp. 26, 19–20; Luzerne County, Pennsylvania, "Register of Deaths," 1893–99, 3 vols., Luzerne County Records (Luzerne County Courthouse Annex, Wilkes-Barre); Lackawanna County, Pennsylvania, "Return of All Deaths," 1893–97, Lackawanna County Records (Lackawanna County Courthouse, Scranton); Brock, *Investigation and Responsibility*, pp. 127–28; Arthur Koenig, "The Defective Vital Statistics of the United States," *Pennsylvania Medical Journal* 7 (1904): 208.

46. Ohio State Mine Inspector, *Third Annual Report, 1876* (Columbus, 1876), pp. 92, 86–94. On mining regulations in Ohio, see K. Austin Kerr, "The Movement for Coal Mine Safety in Nineteenth-Century Ohio," *Ohio History* 86 (1977): 3–18. On "bad air," see Sheafer, "Hygiene of Coal-Mines," pp. 229–50, esp. 230, 246, 248; R. W. Raymond, "The Hygiene of Mines," *Transactions of the American Institute of Mining Engineers* 8 (1880): 98–108; Brophy, *Miner's Life*, p. 39.

47. Andrew Roy, "Miners' Hospitals," *Ohio Mining Journal* 7 (1889): 24.

48. Pennsylvania Department of Internal Affairs, *Reports of the Inspectors of Mines of the Anthracite Coal Regions, 1881* (Harrisburg, 1882), pp. 10–11; Pennsylvania, *Laws, 1885*, pp. 238–39; Alexander Trachtenberg, *The History of Legislation for the Protection of Coal Miners in Pennsylvania, 1824–1915* (New York, 1942), p. 119; Pennsylvania Department of Internal Affairs, *Reports of the Inspectors of Mines of the Anthracite and Bituminous Coal Regions, 1892* (Harrisburg, 1893), p. 112; Pennsylvania Department of Internal Affairs, *Reports of the Inspectors of Mines, 1886–1900* (titles vary slightly) (Har-

risburg, 1887–1901). On the first laws safeguarding Pennsylvania miners, see Trachtenberg, *History of Legislation*, chaps. 3–4, 6–7. For a national overview, see Jacqueline Corn, "Protective Legislation for Coal Miners, 1870–1900: Response to Safety and Health Hazards," in *Dying for Work*, ed. Rosner and Markowitz, pp. 67–82.

49. Pennsylvania Bureau of Mines, *Report, 1899* ([Harrisburg], 1900), pp. 812–13, 908–9; West Virginia State Inspector/s of Mines, *Annual Report* series for 1888–1900 (Charleston, 1889–1901); Kentucky Inspector of Mines, *Annual Report* series for 1893–1900 (Frankfort/Louisville, 1894–1901); Iowa State Mine Inspector/s, *Biennial Report* series for 1880–1901 (Des Moines, 1882–1901). Andrew Roy's successors also turned a blind eye to the hazard of respirable dust. See Ohio Chief Inspector of Mines, *Annual Report* series for 1884–1900 (Columbus/Norwalk, 1885–1902).

50. James Leiby, *Carroll Wright and Labor Reform: The Origin of Labor Statistics* (Cambridge, Mass., 1960); Kenneth Fones-Wolf, "Class, Professionalism and the Early Bureaus of Labor Statistics," *Insurgent Sociologist* 10 (1980): 38–45; Wendell D. MacDonald, "The Early History of Labor Statistics in the United States," *Labor History* 13 (1972): 267–78.

51. On the paucity of statistical data on occupational disease, see Jacqueline Corn, "Historical Aspects of Industrial Hygiene—I: Changing Attitudes toward Occupational Health," *American Industrial Hygiene Association Journal* 39 (1978): 695.

52. On the distinction between clinical entity and disease entity, see Lester S. King, *Medical Thinking: A Historical Preface* (Princeton, 1982), 146–64, esp. 151.

2. Twice a Boy

1. William Keating, "Down, Down, Down," in George Korson, *Minstrels of the Mine Patch: Songs and Stories of the Anthracite Industry* (Philadelphia, 1938), pp. 48, 38–41, 48–53. This keenly observant folklorist reported that pneumoconiotic singers frequently interrupted their performances to catch their breath. See George Korson, *Black Rock: Mining Folklore of the Pennsylvania Dutch* (Baltimore, 1960), p. 351.

2. Korson, *Black Rock*, p. 258; Donald L. Miller and Richard E. Sharpless, *The Kingdom of Coal: Work, Enterprise, and Ethnic Communities in the Mine Fields* (Philadelphia, 1985), p. 210; *Frostburg Mining Journal* (Maryland), April 20, 1872. On the self-care tradition, see *Medicine without Doctors: Home Health Care in American History*, ed. Guenter B. Risse, Ronald L. Numbers, and Judith Walzer Leavitt (New York, 1977).

3. *United Mine Workers Journal* (hereafter *UMWJ*), Aug. 15, 1901, p. 3, Aug. 18, 1892, p. 2, Nov. 10, 1892, p. 3; *Frostburg Mining Journal*, Dec. 9, 1871, Jan. 4, 1873, April 6, 1878; Miller and Sharpless, *Kingdom of Coal*, p. 210; *Miners' Journal* (Pottsville, Penn.), June 8, 1844, Jan. 10, 1846; *Anthracite Monitor* (Tamaqua, Penn.), Dec. 9, 1871. On the enormous nineteenth-century patent medicine industry, see James Harvey Young, *The Toadstool Millionaires: A Social History of Patent Medicines in America before Federal Regulation* (Princeton, 1961).

4. *Frostburg Mining Journal*, April 25, 1874, Dec. 16, 1871, June 1, 1872.

5. Anthony F. C. Wallace, *St. Clair: A Nineteenth-Century Coal Town's Experience with a Disaster-Prone Industry* (New York, 1987); Miller and Sharpless, *Kingdom of Coal*, pp. 1–134, esp. 85–87.

6. George O. Virtue, "The Anthracite Mine Laborers," *Bulletin of the Department of Labor* 13 (1897): 730; Homer Greene, *Coal and the Coal Mines* (Boston, 1889), p. 227.

7. U.S. Bureau of the Census, *Historical Statistics of the United States, Colonial Times to 1970*, 2 vols. (Washington, D.C., 1975), vol. 1, pp. 592–93, 590; Edgar A. Haine, *An-*

thracite Coal (Chicago, 1987), after p. 66; Alfred D. Chandler, Jr., "Anthracite Coal and the Beginnings of the Industrial Revolution in the United States," *Business History Review* 46 (1972): 141–81; Miller and Sharpless, *Kingdom of Coal*, pp. 51–82.

8. Wallace, *St. Clair*, p. 33; Robert Allison, "Early History of Coal Mining and Mining Machinery in Schuylkill County," *Publications of the Historical Society of Schuylkill County* 4 (1914): 137. For similar developments in other industries, see William H. Sewell, Jr., "Uneven Development, the Autonomy of Politics, and the Dockworkers of Nineteenth-Century Marseille," *American Historical Review* 93 (1988): 605; Raphael Samuel, "Workshop of the World: Steam Power and Hand Technology in Mid-Victorian Britain," *History Workshop* 3 (1977): 6–72.

9. *Miners' Journal*, March 2, May 25, 1844; Wallace, *St. Clair*, pp. 15–17, 33–36; Allison, "Early History," pp. 140–41; Miller and Sharpless, *Kingdom of Coal*, p. 121; *Scranton Republican*, Aug. 8, 1872, rpt. in *Saward's Coal Trade Circular*, Aug. 14, 1872, p. 1.

10. Wallace, *St. Clair*, p. 36; Rowland Berthoff, "The Social Order of the Anthracite Region, 1825–1902," *Pennsylvania Magazine of History and Biography* 89 (1965): 278; John F. Crowell, "The Employment of Children," *Andover Review* 4 (1885): 43, 52; Pennsylvania, *Laws, 1885* (Harrisburg, 1885), p. 233; Henry George, "Labor in Pennsylvania—II," *North American Review*, Sept. 1886, p. 269; Pennsylvania Bureau of Mines, *Report, 1902* ([Harrisburg], 1903), p. 5; U.S. Census Office, *Report on Mineral Industries in the United States at the Eleventh Census: 1890* (Washington, D.C., 1892), p. 402. On the expansion of child labor across the economy in the late nineteenth century, see Walter I. Trattner, *Crusade for the Children: A History of the National Child Labor Committee and Child Labor Reform in America* (Chicago, 1970), pp. 22–23, 41–42.

11. U.S. Anthracite Coal Strike Commission [hereafter cited as ACSC], "Proceedings," vol. 12, p. 1472, Michael J. Kosik Collection, box 1, Historical Collections and Labor Archives, Pattee Library, Pennsylvania State University, University Park; Phoebe E. Gibbons, "The Miners of Scranton," *Harper's New Monthly Magazine*, Nov. 18,99, p. 921; Perry K. Blatz, *Democratic Miners: Work and Labor Relations in the Anthracite Coal Industry, 1875–1925* (Albany, N.Y., 1994), p. 67; Crowell, "Employment of Children," p. 52; Joseph M. Speakman, "Unwillingly to School: Child Labor and Its Reform in Pennsylvania in the Progressive Era" (Ph.D. diss., Temple University, 1976), p. 135.

12. Greene, *Coal and the Coal Mines*, pp. 230, 218; George, "Labor in Pennsylvania," p. 271; U.S. Industrial Commission, *Report*, vol. 12: *On the Relations of Capital and Labor Employed in the Mining Industry* (Washington, D.C., 1901), p. 149; Berthoff, "Social Order of Anthracite," p. 278; ACSC, "Proceedings," vol. 12, p. 1558, vol. 14, pp. 1846–49, Kosik Collection, box 1; ACSC, "Proceedings," vol. 20, pp. 2869–71, Kosik Collection, box 2. On family economic theory and its application to the allocation of children's time, see Patrick M. Horan and Peggy G. Hargis, "Children's Work and Schooling in the Late Nineteenth-Century Family Economy," *American Sociological Review* 56 (1991): 583–96.

13. Peter Roberts, *The Anthracite Coal Industry* (New York, 1901), p. 217; Wallace, *St. Clair*, pp. 15–17; *Saward's Coal Trade Circular*, April 3, 1872, p. 3, Aug. 14, 1872, p. 1; H. Benjamin Powell, "The Pennsylvania Anthracite Industry, 1769–1976," *Pennsylvania History* 47 (1980): 15; *Coal Trade Journal*, Nov. 5, 1902, p. 710.

14. Henry C. Sheafer, "Hygiene of Coal-Mines," in *Cyclopaedia of the Practice of Medicine*, ed. Hugo von Ziemssen, vol. 19: *On Hygiene and Public Health*, ed. Albert H. Buck (New York, 1879), p. 245; Kellogg Durland, "Child Labor in Pennsylvania," *Outlook*, May 9, 1903, p. 126.

15. Greene, *Coal and the Coal Mines*, p. 215; Stephen Crane, "In the Depths of a Coal Mine," *McClure's Magazine*, Aug. 1894, pp. 195–96; Robert L. Reid, "Drove Headings for Thirty Years," p. 2, n.d. [ca. 1939], RG-13, Pennsylvania Historical Commission,

Records of the WPA Pennsylvania Historical Survey, box 12, folder: Job 54, FN 305–49, Pennsylvania State Archives, Harrisburg; Pennsylvania Second Geological Survey, *Report on the Mining Methods and Appliances Used in the Anthracite Coal Fields,* by Henry M. Chance (Harrisburg, 1883), p. 439.

16. Greene, *Coal and the Coal Mines,* pp. 217, 216–17; ACSC, "Proceedings," vol. 37, p. 6053, Kosik Collection, box 3; ACSC, "Proceedings," vol. 6, p. 777, Kosik Collection, box 1; Korson, *Black Rock,* p. 315.

17. Pennsylvania Department of Internal Affairs, *Reports of the Inspectors of Mines of the Anthracite Coal Regions, 1881* (Harrisburg, 1882), pp. 11, 10–11; ACSC, "Proceedings," vol. 16, pp. 2061–62, 2068, 2106, 2109, vol. 17, p. 2313, Kosik Collection, box 2; Greene, *Coal and the Coal Mines,* p. 227.

18. [no first name] Raymond, "Boys' Lot Dreary in Coal Breakers," *Chicago Daily Tribune,* Aug. 7, 1906, p. 1; Plymouth No. 3 Colliery, Hudson Coal Company, Payroll, April 1901, Hudson Coal Company Payroll Records, roll 3, frame 1657, Historical Collections and Labor Archives, Pattee Library, Pennsylvania State University, University Park.

19. Gibbons, "Miners of Scranton," p. 921; Francis H. Nichols, "Children of the Coal Shadow," *McClure's Magazine,* Feb. 1903, p. 444; George, "Labor in Pennsylvania—II," p. 270; John Mitchell, "The Mine Worker's Life and Aims," *Cosmopolitan,* Oct. 1901, p. 629.

20. Korson, *Minstrels of the Mine Patch,* p. 94; Wallace, *St. Clair,* p. 20; Mitchell, "Mine Worker's Life," p. 629; Pennsylvania, *Laws, 1885,* p. 233; Miller and Sharpless, *Kingdom of Coal,* pp. 98–102; Perry Blatz, "Ever-Shifting Ground: Work and Labor Relations in the Anthracite Coal Industry, 1868–1903" (Ph.D. diss., Princeton University, 1987), pp. 30–32.

21. Joseph Reardon, "Memories of an Old Coal Miner," Jan. 1, 1939, RG-13, Pennsylvania Historical Commission, Records of the WPA Pennsylvania Historical Survey, box 11, folder: Job 54, Field Notes 122–30, Pennsylvania State Archives, Harrisburg; Miller and Sharpless, *Kingdom of Coal,* pp. 94–96; Sheafer, "Hygiene of Coal-Mines," p. 245; Korson, *Minstrels of the Mine Patch,* pp. 51, 52.

22. Mitchell, "Mine Worker's Life," p. 629; U.S. Census Office, *Mineral Industries: 1890,* p. 402; Harold W. Aurand, "Social Motivation of the Anthracite Mine Workers: 1901–1920," *Labor History* 18 (1977): 363–65; Greene, *Coal and the Coal Mines,* p. 227; Virtue, "Anthracite Mine Laborers," p. 730.

23. Mitchell, "Mine Worker's Life," p. 629; U.S. Census Office, *Report on Vital and Social Statistics at the Eleventh Census: 1890* (Washington, D.C., 1896), vol. 1, p. 172; ACSC, "Proceedings," vol. 7, pp. 911, 916–18, 967–68, Kosik Collection, box 1; George, "Labor in Pennsylvania—II," p. 271.

24. Pennsylvania Second Geological Survey, *Mining Methods and Appliances,* pp. 436–38; U.S. Industrial Commission, *Report,* vol. 12, p. 130; Blatz, "Ever-Shifting Ground," pp. 8, 10, 22; ACSC, "Proceedings," vol. 7, pp. 911–14, 949, Kosik Collection, box 1; ACSC, "Proceedings," vol. 18, p. 2403, Kosik Collection, box 2.

25. Mitchell, "Mine Worker's Life," p. 629; Pennsylvania Second Geological Survey, *Mining Methods and Appliances,* p. 472; Frank J. Warne, "The Effect of Unionism upon the Mine Worker," *Annals of the American Academy of Political and Social Science* 21 (1903): 21; Berthoff, "Social Order of Anthracite," p. 290; ACSC, "Proceedings," vol. 19, pp. 2626–27, Kosik Collection, box 2.

26. Blatz, "Ever-Shifting Ground," pp. 155–75; Ray Ginger, "Company-Sponsored Welfare Plans in the Anthracite Industry before 1900," *Bulletin of the Business History Society* 27 (1953): 112–20; Virtue, "Anthracite Mine Laborers," pp. 770–73. On the emotional burdens borne by the wives of pneumoconiosis victims a century later, see

Carol A. B. Giesen, *Coal Miners' Wives: Portraits of Endurance* (Lexington, Ky., 1995), pp. 56–60.

27. Jack Johnson, "The Miner's Life," in Korson, *Minstrels of the Mine Patch*, p. 276; ACSC, "Proceedings," vol. 19, pp. 2626–27, Kosik Collection, box 2; Miller and Sharpless, *Kingdom of Coal*, p. 104; Blatz, "Ever-Shifting Ground," pp. 33, 340–41, 477; John Bodnar, *Workers' World: Kinship, Community, and Protest in an Industrial Society, 1900–1940* (Baltimore, 1982), pp. 79, 84; Mitchell, "Mine Worker's Life," pp. 627, 629.

28. Charles B. Spahr, "The Coal Miners of Pennsylvania," *Outlook*, Aug. 5, 1899, p. 807; Caroline Golab, "The Impact of the Industrial Experience on the Immigrant Family: The Huddled Masses Reconsidered," in *Immigrants in Industrial America, 1850–1920*, ed. Richard L. Ehrlich (Charlottesville, Va., 1977), pp. 5, 8, 12–14, 19; Michael R. Haines, "Industrial Work and the Family Life Cycle, 1889–1890," *Research in Economic History* 4 (1979): 289–356, esp. 290, 298; Michael R. Haines, "Fertility, Marriage, and Occupation in the Pennsylvania Anthracite Region, 1850–1880," *Journal of Family History* 2 (1977): 28–55; John Modell, "Patterns of Consumption, Acculturation, and Family Income Strategies in Late Nineteenth-Century America," in *Family and Population in Nineteenth-Century America*, ed. Tamara K. Hareven and Maris A. Vinovskis (Princeton, 1978), pp. 234, 235.

29. George, "Labor in Pennsylvania—II," p. 271; Spahr, "Miners of Pennsylvania," p. 807; U.S. Industrial Commission, *Report*, vol. 12, p. 149; William Keating, "Down, Down, Down," in Korson, *Minstrels of the Mine Patch*, pp. 39–41, 48–53. Textile firms in the region apparently obtained labor with comparable ease. Francis Nichols met a girl who had gone to work in a knitting mill at age eleven after her father died of miners' dust disease; see Nichols, "Coal Shadow," p. 440.

30. Virtue, "Anthracite Mine Laborers," pp. 770–73; Pennsylvania Department of Internal Affairs, *Reports of the Inspectors of Mines of the Anthracite Coal Regions, 1883* (Harrisburg, 1884), pp. 244–47; Murray W. Latimer, *Industrial Pension Systems in the United States and Canada*, 2 vols. (New York, 1932), vol. 1, p. 55; Pennsylvania Commission on Old Age Pensions, *Report, 1919* (Harrisburg, 1919), pp. 116–18, 137. On the family as the main welfare institution for the aging in this period, see Daniel S. Smith, "Life Course, Norms, and the Family System of Older Americans in 1900," *Journal of Family History* 4 (1979): 285–98. Besides loss of income, it seems reasonable to infer that many pneumoconiotic ex-miners burdened their families with demands for long-term health care, though I have not found positive evidence on this dimension of the problem. On this unpaid, onerous job of wives, daughters, and other female family members, see Debbie Ward, "Women and the Work of Caring," *Second Opinion* 19 (1993): 11–25; Giesen, *Coal Miners' Wives*, p. 59.

31. Anonymous, "The Old Miner's Refrain," in Korson, *Minstrels*, p. 273; Pennsylvania, *Laws, 1879* (Harrisburg, 1879), pp. 157–58; Pennsylvania, *Laws, 1887* (Harrisburg, 1887), pp. 399–401; Harold W. Aurand, *From the Molly Maguires to the United Mine Workers: The Social Ecology of an Industrial Union, 1869–1897* (Philadelphia, 1971), pp. 156–57; [Anonymous], "A Miner's Story," *Independent*, June 12, 1902, p. 1409; Warne, "Effect of Unionism," p. 21; Berthoff, "Social Order of Anthracite," p. 282. On institutionalization as threat and reality for aging workers, see Carole Haber and Brian Gratton, *Old Age and the Search for Security: An American History* (Bloomington, Ind., 1994), pp. 116–42.

32. Crane, "In Depths," pp. 209, 198–200; George Korson, *Songs and Ballads of the Anthracite Miners* (New York, 1927), pp. 90, 90–91; Luzerne County, "Register of Deaths," 1893–1902, 5 vols., Luzerne County Records, Luzerne County Courthouse Annex, Wilkes-Barre, Penn.; *Wilkes-Barre Record* (Penn.), July 13, 1896, p. 12; Pennsylvania Board of Health, *Report, 1901*, vol. 1, p. 323; [Anonymous], "Miner's Story," p. 1407.

33. Craig Phelan, *Divided Loyalties: The Public and Private Life of Labor Leader John Mitchell* (Albany, N.Y., 1994), pp. 108, 93–122, esp. 107–8; Miller and Sharpless, *Kingdom of Coal,* pp. 220–55; Aurand, *From the Molly Maguires,* pp. 135–42; Edward J. Davies II, *The Anthracite Aristocracy: Leadership and Social Change in the Hard Coal Region of Northeastern Pennsylvania, 1800–1930* (DeKalb, Ill., 1985).

34. Robert J. Cornell, *The Anthracite Coal Strike of 1902* (Washington, D.C., 1957); Miller and Sharpless, *Kingdom of Coal,* pp. 255–76.

35. Phelan, *Divided Loyalties,* pp. 183–87; Blatz, *Democratic Miners,* pp. 137–40. For the importance (and the limitations) of this affair for the evolution of federal policy on labor-management relations, see Melvyn Dubofsky, *The State and Labor in Modern America* (Chapel Hill, 1994), pp. 39–42; Jonathan Grossman, "The Coal Strike of 1902— Turning Point in U.S. Policy," *Monthly Labor Review* 98 (Oct. 1975): 21–28.

36. UMW, *Minutes of Special Convention, 1902* (Indianapolis, 1902), pp. 49, 48–51; Mitchell, "Mine Worker's Life," pp. 623–30; ACSC, "Proceedings," vols. 55–56, pp. 9,841–10,046, esp. 9,843, 9,853, 10,043–46, Kosik Collection, box 5; Miller and Sharpless, *Kingdom of Coal,* pp. 256–79, esp. 260; Phelan, *Divided Loyalties,* pp. 159–97; Lincoln Steffens, "A Labor Leader of Today: John Mitchell and What He Stands For," *McClures,* Aug. 1902, pp. 355–57.

37. Mother Jones, *The Autobiography of Mother Jones,* 3d ed., ed. Mary Field Parton (Chicago, 1976), p. 61; Frederick L. Hoffman, "Problems of Life and Labor in Anthracite Mining," *Engineering and Mining Journal,* Nov. 29, 1902, p. 710. On the widespread fears that child labor would subvert national vitality, see Alan Derickson, "Making Human Junk: Child Labor as a Health Issue in the Progressive Era," *American Journal of Public Health* 82 (1992): 1280–90.

38. John Harris Jones to Whom It May Concern, Nov. 3, 1902, John Mitchell Papers, microfilm ed. (Glen Rock, N.J., 1974), reel 5. The UMW's relatively passive approach to obtaining health information contrasts with the aggressive field investigations of sweatshop conditions by women unionists, working in alliance with middle-class activists. See Sklar, *Florence Kelley,* pp. 209–14; Ralph Scharnau, "Elizabeth Morgan, Crusader for Labor Reform," *Labor History* 14 (1973): 342–47.

39. ACSC, "Proceedings," vol. 2, pp. 13, 13–14, 45–46, Kosik Collection, box 1; ACSC, "Proceedings," vol. 55, pp. 9883, 9878, 9882–83, vol. 56, p. 9941, Kosik Collection, box 5.

40. ACSC, "Proceedings," vol. 7, p. 911, 912, 911–14, 925, 942, 952, vol. 8, pp. 987–88, vol. 10, p. 1172, Kosik Collection, box 1.

41. ACSC, "Proceedings," vol. 7, pp. 949, 911–12, 944, vol. 8, pp. 966, 988, 962–67, 993, Kosik Collection, box 1; ACSC, "Proceedings," vol. 18, pp. 2398, 2403, Kosik Collection, box 2.

42. ACSC, "Proceedings," vol. 7, pp. 915, 911–15, 921, 949, 952, vol. 8, pp. 993, 965–67, Kosik Collection, box 1; ACSC, "Proceedings," vol. 18, p. 2403, vol. 19, pp. 2626–27, Kosik Collection, box 2. On the development of veterans' pensions, see Theda Skocpol, *Protecting Soldiers and Mothers: The Political Origins of Social Policy in the United States* (Cambridge, Mass., 1992), pp. 102–51.

43. ACSC, "Proceedings," vol. 8, p. 984, vol. 7, pp. 944–45, 921, vol. 6, pp. 765–66, vol. 11, p. 1306, Kosik Collection, box 1.

44. ACSC, "Proceedings," vol. 7, pp. 913, 920, 911, 920–21, vol. 8, pp. 989, 996, vol. 2, p. 13, vol. 10, p. 1172, vol. 11, p. 1264, Kosik Collection, box 1; S. L. Fleishman to Walter E. Weyl, Nov. 28, 1902, Mitchell Papers, reel 5. I have yet to find any strong substantiation for Miller and Sharpless's contention that three-fourths of aging anthracite miners had disabling pneumoconiosis; see Miller and Sharpless, *Kingdom of Coal,* p. 106.

45. *Pittsburgh Press*, Nov. 21, 1902, p. 1, Nov. 14, 1902, p. 3; *New York Times*, Nov. 15, 1902, p. 3, Nov. 21, 1902, p. 5; *Chicago Tribune*, Nov. 21, 1902, p. 16; *Great Falls Daily Tribune* (Mont.), Nov. 30, 1902, p. 2.

46. ACSC, "Proceedings," vol. 22, p. 3313, vol. 30, p. 4713, Kosik Collection, box 2; ACSC, "Proceedings," vol. 32, pp. 5146–48, 5171–74, vol. 37, pp. 6217–19, Kosik Collection, box 3.

47. ACSC, "Proceedings," vol. 32, pp. 5154, 5166, 5152–55, 5197–98, 5207–9, vol. 34, pp. 5476, 5544, 5551, 5559–60, 5581, 5594–95, vol. 35, pp. 5704–6, 5715, Kosik Collection, box 3; ACSC, "Proceedings," vol. 7, p. 952, vol. 8, p. 997, Kosik Collection, box 1; ACSC, "Proceedings," vol. 53, p. 9440, Kosik Collection, box 5.

48. ACSC, *Report to the President* (Washington, D.C., 1903), p. 51; Phelan, *Divided Loyalties*, pp. 197–99.

49. Owen R. Lovejoy, "Child Labor in the Coal Mines," *Annals of the American Academy of Political and Social Science* 27 (1906): 293–94; Owen R. Lovejoy, "The Extent of Child Labor in the Anthracite Industry," *Annals of the American Academy of Political and Social Science* 29 (1907): 35–41.

3. The Atmosphere of the Mine Is Now Vindicated

1. Ronald D. Eller, *Miners, Millhands, and Mountaineers: Industrialization of the Appalachian South, 1880–1930* (Knoxville, Tenn., 1982), pp. 228–29, 234–35; Olivier Zunz, *Making America Corporate, 1870–1920* (Chicago, 1990); Robert H. Wiebe, *The Search for Order, 1877–1920* (New York, 1967); John Ettling, *The Germ of Laziness: Rockefeller Philanthropy and Public Health in the New South* (Cambridge, Mass., 1981); John C. Burnham, "Medical Specialists and Movements toward Social Control in the Progressive Era: Three Examples," in *Building the Organizational Society: Essays on Associational Activities in Modern America*, ed. Jerry Israel (New York, 1972), pp. 19–30. On the changing social composition, class location, and ideology of the medical profession in the Progressive Era, see Paul Starr, *The Social Transformation of American Medicine* (New York, 1982), pp. 116–27, 142–44; E. Richard Brown, *Rockefeller Medicine Men: Medicine and Capitalism in America* (Berkeley, 1979).

2. R. S. Trotter, "The So-Called Anthracosis and Phthisis in Coal Miners," *British Medical Journal* 1 (May 23, 1903): 1197–98, rpt. in *Coal Trade Journal*, July 15, 1903, pp. 516–17; Thomas Oliver, "Pneumoconiosis," in *A System of Medicine*, 2d ed., ed. Clifford Allbutt and Humphry D. Rolleston, 8 vols. (London, 1909), vol. 5, pp. 449, 465; *Coal Age*, Sept. 25, 1915, p. 513, Aug. 31, 1912, p. 303.

3. Samuel R. Haythorn, "Some Histological Evidences of the Disease Importance of Pulmonary Anthracosis," *Journal of Medical Research* 29 (1913): 277, 259–79; Oskar Klotz, "Pulmonary Anthracosis—A Community Disease," *American Journal of Public Health* 4 (1914): 887–916, esp. 890; Henry S. Willis, "Spontaneous Pneumonokoniosis in the Guinea Pig," *American Review of Tuberculosis* 5 (1921): 197–215; J. A. Myers, "Studies on the Respiratory Organs in Health and Disease: Effects of Bituminous Coal Mining on Vital Capacity of Lungs," *American Review of Tuberculosis* 9 (1924): 50.

4. Thomas Oliver, "Dust Diseases of the Lungs," in *Industrial Health*, ed. George M. Kober and Emery R. Hayhurst (Philadelphia, 1924), p. 703; Henry K. Pancoast and Eugene P. Pendergrass, "A Review of Our Present Knowledge of Pneumoconiosis, Based upon Roentgenologic Studies, with Notes on the Pathology of the Condition," *American Journal of Roentgenology and Radium Therapy* 14 (1925): 390.

5. On tuberculosis in industrializing America, see U.S. Bureau of the Census, *Histo-*

rical Statistics of the United States, Colonial Times to 1970, 2 vols. (Washington, D.C., 1975), vol. 1, pp. 58, 63; Barbara Bates, *Bargaining for Life: A Social History of Tuberculosis, 1876–1938* (Philadelphia, 1992); Sheila M. Rothman, *Living in the Shadow of Death: Tuberculosis and the Social Experience of Illness in American History* (New York, 1994); Michael E. Teller, *The Tuberculosis Movement: A Public Health Campaign in the Progressive Era* (Westport, Conn., 1988); Georgina D. Feldberg, *Disease and Class: Tuberculosis and the Shaping of Modern North American Society* (New Brunswick, 1995); Katherine Ott, *Fevered Lives: Tuberculosis in American Culture since 1870* (Cambridge, Mass., 1996).

6. T. Mitchell Prudden, *Dust and Its Dangers*, 2d ed. (New York, 1910), pp. 58–73; Frederick L. Hoffman, "The Mortality from Consumption in the Dusty Trades," *Bulletin of the Bureau of Labor* 79 (1908): 633–875; Frederick L. Hoffman, "Dust as a Factor in Occupation [sic] Mortality," *Medical Examiner and General Practitioner* 17 (1907): 360–75; Teller, *Tuberculosis Movement*, pp. 104–8; Ohio State Board of Health, *Consumption and Preventable Deaths in American Occupations*, by Emery R. Hayhurst (Columbus, 1914), p. 7.

7. Andrew Smart, "Note on Anthracosis," *British Medical Journal* 2 (Sept. 5, 1885): 439; John Tatham, "Dust-Producing Occupations," in *Dangerous Trades*, ed. Thomas Oliver (New York, 1902), p. 158; Trotter, "So-Called Anthracosis," p. 1198; ACSC, "Proceedings," vol. 32, p. 5150, Michael J. Kosik Collection, box 3, Historical Collections and Labor Archives, Pattee Library, Pennsylvania State University, University Park.

8. Jonathan M. Wainwright and Harry J. Nichols, "The Relation between Anthracosis and Pulmonary Tuberculosis," *American Journal of the Medical Sciences* n.s., 130 (1905): 403, 409–10.

9. Ibid., pp. 411–13.

10. Ibid., pp. 411–12, 403–4.

11. Dr. Miner et al., "Discussion" [of Jonathan M. Wainwright and H. T. Nichols, "Two Phases of Anthracite Mine Hygiene"], *Transactions of the Luzerne County Medical Society* 13 (1905): 116, 116–17; William Osler, *The Principles and Practice of Medicine*, 7th ed. (New York, 1911), p. 632; Henry R. M. Landis, "Diseases of the Lungs," in George W. Norris, Henry R. M. Landis, and Edward B. Krumbhaar, *Diseases of the Chest and the Principles of Physical Diagnosis* (Philadelphia, 1917), p. 438; H. R. M. Landis, "The Pathological and Clinical Manifestations Following the Inhalation of Dust," *Journal of Industrial Hygiene* 1 (1919): 123–24; Myers, "Studies on Respiratory Organs," pp. 50–51.

12. M. C. Carr to Editor, Nov. 21, 1905, *Journal of the American Medical Association* 45 (1905): 1892; Samuel Mengel, "Some Medical and Surgical Problems and Their Solutions from the Point of View of the Mining Surgeon," *Pennsylvania Medical Journal* 21 (1918): 348; Pancoast and Pendergrass, "Review of Present Knowledge," pp. 412–13.

13. *Coal Age*, May 11, 1912, pp. 1015–16, March 16, 1912, p. 750, Aug. 3, 1912, pp. 163–64, Aug. 24, 1912, pp. 269–70, Aug. 31, 1912, pp. 293–94, 303–4; *Coal Trade Journal*, Sept. 7, 1904, p. 651.

14. *Coal Age*, June 26, 1915, p. 1089, Aug. 19, 1916, p. 310, March 25, 1920, pp. 598–99, Dec. 11, 1924, p. 821.

15. Wainwright and Nichols, "Anthracosis and Tuberculosis," p. 405; George Rosen, *The History of Miners' Diseases: A Medical and Social Interpretation* (New York, 1943), esp. pp. 285–401.

16. Landis, "Diseases of the Lungs," pp. 442–43.

17. Edgar L. Collis, "Industrial Pneumonoconioses, with Special Reference to Dust-Phthisis," *Public Health* 28 (1915): 252–64, 295–96; Irving J. Selikoff, "Widening Perspectives of Occupational Lung Disease," *Preventive Medicine* 2 (1973): 412.

18. Edgar L. Collis, "Industrial Pneumonoconioses, with Special Reference to Dust-Phthisis," *Public Health* 29 (1915): 16, 43, 11–20, 38–40; Collis, "Industrial Pneumono-conioses," *Public Health* 28 (1915): 295.

19. Collis, "Industrial Pneumonoconioses," *Public Health* 29 (1915): following 38, 39, following 40.

20. Edgar L. Collis, "Physiological Effects of Mine Dusts," *Transactions of the American Institute of Mining and Metallurgical Engineers* 75 (1927): 97–103; "Discussion [of "Physiological Effects of Mine Dusts"]," *Transactions of the American Institute of Mining and Metallurgical Engineers* 75 (1927): 104–6; V. C. V., "The Inhalation of Coal Dust, Anthracosis," *Hygiea* 1 (1923): 183; Henry K. Pancoast, "Roentgenologic Studies of Pneumoconiosis and Other Fibrosing Conditions of Lungs," *Annals of Clinical Medicine* 2 (1923): 11, 11–12, 16.

21. Pancoast and Pendergrass, "Review of Our Present Knowledge," pp. 382, 390–92, 411; Eugene P. Pendergrass, "Memoir of Henry Khunrath Pancoast, M.D.," *Transactions and Studies of the College of Physicians of Philadelphia* 4th ser., 8 (1940): 48, 50–51; Lynne A. Leopold, *Radiology at the University of Pennsylvania, 1890–1975* (Philadelphia, 1981), pp. 21–71, esp. 36–38, 40, 52–53, 64. On the problems and promise of X-rays and other "objective" tests in diagnosis, see Stanley Joel Reiser, *Medicine and the Reign of Technology* (Cambridge, Eng., 1978), pp. 58–68, 158–73, esp. 67; Hughes Evans, "Losing Touch: The Controversy over the Introduction of Blood Pressure Instruments into Medicine," *Technology and Culture* 34 (1993): 784–807; Barron H. Lerner, "The Perils of 'X-Ray Vision': How Radiographic Images Have Historically Influenced Perception," *Perspectives in Biology and Medicine* 35 (1992): 382–97. On technology shaping disease definition, see Keith Wailoo, *Drawing Blood: Technology and Disease Identity in Twentieth-Century America* (Baltimore, 1997).

22. Henry K. Pancoast and Eugene P. Pendergrass, *Pneumoconiosis [Silicosis]: A Roentgenological Study with Notes on Pathology* (New York, 1926), pp. 6, 11, 123.

23. Pancoast and Pendergrass, *Pneumoconiosis [Silicosis]*, pp. 49, 123, 129.

24. Pancoast and Pendergrass, *Pneumoconiosis [Silicosis]*, pp. x, ix, 12, 38, 49, 51, 74, 84; Reiser, *Reign of Technology*, pp. 166–71.

25. Landis, "Pathological and Clinical Manifestations," p. 138; Pancoast and Pendergrass, *Pneumoconiosis [Silicosis]*, pp. 71–73; Henry K. Pancoast, T. G. Miller, and Henry R. M. Landis, "A Roentgenologic Study of the Effects of Dust Inhalation upon the Lungs," *American Journal of Roentgenology* 5 (1918): 138. For an even earlier comment on the diffusely mottled chest X-ray of a coal worker, see W. W. Boardman, "Pneumonoconiosis," *American Journal of Roentgenology* 4 (1917): 296.

26. Thomas Oliver, *Diseases of Occupation from the Legislative, Social, Medical Points of View* (London, 1908), pp. 267, 272; Thomas Oliver, "Phthisis and Occupation," *Journal of Industrial Hygiene* 2 (1920): 115; Frank Shufflebotham, "The Hygienic Aspect of the Coal-Mining Industry in the United Kingdom," *British Medical Journal* 1 (1914): 588.

27. *Coal Age*, Nov. 25, 1916, p. 894, March 25, 1920, p. 599, March 6, 1924, p. 350.

28. Wainwright and Nichols, "Anthracosis and Tuberculosis," p. 409; Mengel, "Medical and Surgical Problems," p. 348.

29. *Coal Age*, Feb. 24, 1927, p. 291, March 25, 1920, p. 599, May 11, 1912, p. 1015.

30. *Coal Age*, June 26, 1915, p. 1089, Sept. 25, 1915, p. 513.

31. *Coal Age*, Aug. 19, 1916, pp. 310, 310–11; July 24, 1919, p. 133.

32. Owen R. Lovejoy, "School-House or Coal-Breaker," *Outlook*, Aug. 26, 1905, pp. 1013, 1013–15; Lewis W. Hine, "Report: Photographic Investigation of Child Labor Conditions in the Mines of Eastern Pennsylvania," Jan. 1911, pt. 1, p. 2, National Child Labor Committee Papers, box 4, folder: "Penn.—Coal Mines—1911," Manuscript Division, Library of Congress, Washington; Edward F. Brown, "Child Labor in the Anthracite Coal Fields of Eastern Pennsylvania," April 1, 1912, pp. 1, 6, NCLC Papers,

box 4, folder: "Penn.—Coal—1912"; *Chicago Tribune*, Aug. 6, 1906, pp. 1, 7, Aug. 7, 1906, pp. 1, 7, Aug. 8, 1906, pp. 1, 5; Edwin Markham, "The Hoe-Man in the Making: Little Slaves of the Coal Mines," *Cosmopolitan*, Nov. 1906, p. 26; John Spargo, *The Bitter Cry of the Children* (New York, 1906), pp. 164, 176; Florence L. Sanville, "Social Legislation in the Keystone State," *Survey*, Feb. 6, 1915, p. 482.

33. Wainwright and Nichols, "Anthracosis and Tuberculosis," pp. 413–14; *Engineering and Mining Journal*, April 2, 1910, p. 734.

34. U.S. Bureau of Labor Statistics, *Mortality from Respiratory Diseases in Dusty Trades (Inorganic Dusts)*, by Frederick L. Hoffman, Bulletin 231 (Washington, D.C., 1918), p. 378; Keith Dix, *Work Relations in the Coal Industry: The Hand Loading Era* (Morgantown, W. Va. 1977), pp. 14–38, esp. 25; Howard N. Eavenson, "Seventy-Five Years of Progress in Bituminous Coal Mining," and Cadwallader Evans, Jr., et al., "Seventy-Five Years of Progress in the Anthracite Industry," in *Seventy-Five Years of Progress in the Mineral Industry*, ed. A. E. Parsons (New York, 1947), pp. 226–36, 254–55; U.S. Census, *Historical Statistics*, vol. 1, pp. 580, 589–90; Henry R. O'Brien, "The Industrial Hygiene of the Buckeye Coal Company, Nemacolin, Penna.," Oct. 6, 1921, p. 3, RG 70, Records of the U.S. Bureau of Mines, Health and Safety Branch, Records of the Picher, Oklahoma, Clinic, 1927–1932, box 2, file 082, Washington National Records Center, National Archives and Records Administration, Suitland, Maryland; Harrington, "Dust Elimination," pp. 200–201.

35. Daniel Harrington, "The Engineering-Hygienic Aspects of Dust Elimination in Mines," *Journal of Industrial Hygiene* 7 (1975): 202–3; J. J. Forbes and Alden H. Emery, "Sources of Dust in Coal Mines," *Transactions of the American Institute of Mining and Metallurgical Engineers* 75 (1927): 645–58, esp. 648.

36. Frederick S. Crum, "The Mortality from Diseases of the Lungs in American Industry," *Pennsylvania Medical Journal* 20 (Oct. 1916): 37.

37. *Fuel*, n.d., rpt. in *UMWJ*, March 15, 1906, p. 3; *UMWJ*, Jan. 19, 1911, p. 12; Thomas Kennedy, "Wages, Hours and Working Conditions in the Anthracite Industry," *Annals of the American Academy of Political and Social Science* 111 (1924): 51.

38. Joseph L. Pico to Editor, Jan. 28, 1911, *UMWJ*, Feb. 16, 1911, p. 7; A. M. Schott to Editor, n.d., *Illinois Miner* (Springfield), Aug. 25, 1923, p. 3; Joseph Koleno, interview with author, May 16, 1994, Clarence, Pa. (tape in author's possession).

39. Oskar Klotz, "Pulmonary Anthracosis—A Community Disease," *American Journal of Public Health* 4 (1914): 903; H. R. M. Landis, "The Relation of Organic Dust to Pneumonokoniosis," *Journal of Industrial Hygiene* 7 (1925): 1; Edgar L. Collis, "A Study of the Mortality of Coal Miners, England and Wales," *Journal of Industrial Hygiene* 4 (1922): 264; Henry S. Willis, "Studies on Tuberculous Infection, IX: The Influence of the Inhalation of Coal Dust on Tuberculous Infection in Guinea Pigs," *American Review of Tuberculosis* 6 (1922): 810; "The Coal Mine as a Tuberculosis Sanitarium," *American Labor Legislation Review* 12 (1922): 131.

40. *UMWJ*, March 15, 1906, p. 3, March 25, 1915, pp. 4, 5; *Illinois Miner* (Springfield), July 29, 1922, p. 3.

41. *UMWJ*, Oct. 5, 1911, p. 2.

42. Wainwright and Nichols, "Anthracosis and Tuberculosis," pp. 412–13; Mengel, "Medical and Surgical Problems," p. 348; Landis, "Diseases of the Lungs," pp. 434, 442–43; John A. Koch, "Dust: Its Relation to Disease," *Illinois Medical Journal* 12 (1907): 513; W. G. Thompson, *The Occupational Diseases: Their Causation, Symptoms, Treatment and Prevention* (New York, 1914), pp. 613–14.

43. Robert T. Legge, "Miners' Silicosis: Its Pathology, Symptomatology and Prevention," *Journal of the American Medical Association* 81 (Sept. 8, 1923): 809; Boardman, "Pneumonoconiosis," pp. 292–99. Curiously, not long before his absorption in silico-

sis, Pancoast himself espoused the more inclusive view; see Pancoast, Miller, and Landis, "Roentgenologic Study," p. 130.

4. Sheep-like Acceptance of Half-Baked Statements

1. Stephen Skowronek, *Building a New American State: The Expansion of National Administrative Capacities, 1877–1920* (Cambridge, Eng., 1982), pp. 163–284; Morton Keller, *Regulating a New Society: Public Policy and Social Change in America, 1900–1933* (Cambridge, Mass., 1994); Richard Hofstadter, *The Age of Reform: From Bryan to F.D.R.* (New York, 1955), pp. 131–271; Robert M. Crunden, *Ministers of Reform: The Progressives' Achievement in American Civilization, 1889–1920* (New York, 1982); Alan Dawley, *Struggles for Justice: Social Responsibility and the Liberal State* (Cambridge, Mass., 1991), pts. 1-2.

2. David A. Moss, *Socializing Security: Progressive-Era Economists and the Origins of American Social Policy* (Cambridge, Mass., 1996), esp. pp. 10–11, 183n28; David Brian Robertson, "The Bias of American Federalism: The Limits of Welfare-State Development in the Progressive Era," *Journal of Policy History* 1 (1989): 261–91; William Graebner, "Federalism in the Progressive Era: A Structural Interpretation of Reform," *Journal of American History* 64 (1977): 331–57.

3. Alice Hamilton and Gertrude Seymour, "The New Public Health II: The Program of a State Board of Health," *Survey*, Jan. 20, 1917, pp. 456–57; Iowa State Board of Health, *Thirteenth Report, 1904–1906* (Des Moines, 1906), pp. 105–7; L. W. Hutchcroft, "The Mortality from Industrial Diseases," *American Journal of Public Hygiene* 19 (1909): 112–13; Emery R. Hayhurst, "Health Hazards of Non-Poisonous Dusts: A Resume of Some Recent Investigations," *American Journal of Public Health* 10 (1920): 62, 60 65; Emery R. Hayhurst, "The Health Hazards and Mortality Statistics of Soft Coal Mining in Illinois and Ohio," *Journal of Industrial Hygiene* 1 (1919): 362; Ohio State Board of Health, *Industrial Health-Hazards and Occupational Diseases in Ohio*, by E. R. Hayhurst (Columbus, 1915), p. 18; John Duffy, *The Sanitarians: A History of American Public Health* (Urbana, 1990), pp. 221–38; Shirley G. Schoonover, "Alabama Public Health Campaign, 1900–1919," *Alabama Review* 28 (1975): 218–33. Hutchcroft soberly reminded his colleagues in vital statistics that "in attempting to summarize what has been done in the various States to investigate the extent, nature and cause of occupational diseases, we must keep clearly in mind that, with the exception of two or three investigations which have been made of certain isolated industries, practically nothing has been done." See Hutchcroft, "Mortality from Industrial Diseases," p. 109.

4. Emery R. Hayhurst, "Health of Ohio Coal Miners," in Ohio Health and Old Age Insurance Commission, *Health, Health Insurance, Old Age Pensions: Report, Recommendations, Dissenting Opinions* (Columbus, 1919), pp. 358, 370, 361, 370–72; Emery R. Hayhurst, "Health of Illinois Coal Miners," in Illinois Health Insurance Commission, *Report* (Springfield, Ill., 1919), pp. 374, 385–86, 388–90; Pennsylvania Health Insurance Commission, *Report* (Harrisburg, 1919), pp. 176, 184, 193. Hayhurst characterized miners' asthma as a dwindling problem despite his own inspection of forty-three Ohio mines, which disclosed high levels of dust contamination in numerous jobs both under and above ground; see Hayhurst, "Health of Ohio Miners," pp. 364–66.

5. Lawrence F. Schmeckebier, *The Public Health Service: Its History, Activities, and Organization* (Baltimore, 1923); Fred W. Powell, *The Bureau of Mines: Its History, Ac-*

tivities, and Organization (New York, 1922); William Graebner, *Coal-Mining Safety in the Progressive Period: The Political Economy of Reform* (Lexington, Ky., 1976); James Harvey Young, "The Pig That Fell into the Privy: Upton Sinclair's *The Jungle* and the Meat Inspection Amendments of 1906," *Bulletin of the History of Medicine* 59 (1985): 467–80; Ilyse D. Barkan, "Industry Invites Regulation: The Passage of the Pure Food and Drug Act of 1906," *American Journal of Public Health* 75 (1985): 18–26; Elizabeth W. Etheridge, *The Butterfly Caste: A Social History of Pellagra in the South* (Westport, Conn., 1972); D. J. Soviero, "The Nationalization of a Disease: A Paradigm?," *Public Health Reports* 101 (1986): 399–404; J. Stanley Lemons, "The Sheppard-Towner Act: Progressivism in the 1920s," *Journal of American History* 55 (1969): 776–86; R. Alton Lee, "The Eradication of Phossy Jaw: A Unique Development of Federal Police Power," *Historian* 29 (1966): 1–21; Moss, *Socializing Security*, pp. 77–96; Manfred Waserman, "The Quest for a National Health Department in the Progressive Era," *Bulletin of the History of Medicine* 49 (1975): 353–80, esp. 370; Victoria A. Harden, *Inventing the NIH: Federal Biomedical Research Policy, 1887–1937* (Baltimore, 1986), pp. 27–68.

6. John Lombardi, *Labor's Voice in the Cabinet: A History of the Department of Labor from Its Origins to 1921* (New York, 1942), esp. pp. 68–70, 75–89; Melvyn Dubofsky, "Abortive Reform: The Wilson Administration and Organized Labor, 1913–1920," in *Work, Community, and Power: The Experience of Labor in Europe and America, 1900–1925,* ed. James E. Cronin and Carmen Sirianni (Philadelphia, 1983), pp. 197–220, esp. 204–5; Nancy DiTomaso, "Class Politics and Public Bureaucracy: The U.S. Department of Labor," in *Classes, Class Conflict, and the State: Empirical Studies in Class Analysis,* ed. Maurice Zeitlin (Cambridge, Mass., 1980), pp. 135–52, esp. 140–41. On the lead project, see Alice Hamilton, *Exploring the Dangerous Trades: The Autobiography of Alice Hamilton, M.D.* (Boston, 1943), pp. 127–38.

7. U.S. Bureau of Labor Statistics, *Mortality from Respiratory Diseases in Dusty Trades,* by Frederick L. Hoffman, Bulletin 231 (Washington, D.C., 1918), pp. 398, 344, 380–81, 399–400, 403.

8. Ibid., pp. 388, 397–98, 403–6.

9. Ibid., pp. 408–9. For a contemporaneous study that emphasized tuberculosis and glossed over the occupational respiratory disease byssinosis, see U.S. Bureau of Labor Statistics, *Preventable Death in Cotton Manufacturing Industries,* by Arthur R. Perry, Bulletin 251 (Washington, D.C., 1919).

10. U.S. Bureau of Labor Statistics, *Occupation Hazards and Diagnostic Signs: A Guide to Impairments to Be Looked for in Hazardous Occupations,* by Louis I. Dublin and Philip Leiboff, Bulletin 306 (Washington, D.C., 1922), pp. 14, 14–15; U.S. Bureau of Labor Statistics, *Occupation Hazards and Diagnostic Signs: A Guide to Impairments to Be Looked for in Hazardous Occupations,* by Louis I. Dublin and Robert J. Vane, Bulletin 582 (Washington, D.C., 1933), p. 19; U.S. Bureau of Labor Statistics, *Causes of Death, by Occupation: Occupational Mortality Experience of the Metropolitan Life Insurance Company, Industrial Department, 1922–1924,* by Louis I. Dublin and Robert J. Vane, Bulletin 507 (Washington, D.C., 1930), pp. 33, 124.

11. James P. Johnson, *The Politics of Soft Coal: The Bituminous Industry from World War I through the New Deal* (Urbana, 1979), pp. 102–7; Maier B. Fox, *United We Stand: The United Mine Workers of America, 1890–1990* (Washington, D.C., 1990), pp. 187–90; UMW, *Proceedings of the Twenty-Seventh Consecutive and Fourth Biennial Convention, 1919,* 3 vols. (Indianapolis, 1919), vol. 3, pp. 102–3, 409; S. A. Traylor to Editor, n.d., *UMWJ,* March 1, 1920, p. 16.

12. U.S. Bituminous Coal Commission, Proceedings, vol. 1, pp. 110, 67, 80, UMW Archive, UMW International Office, Washington, D.C., or Historical Collections and Labor Archives, Pattee Library, Pennsylvania State University, University Park. (In

1994, the UMW agreed to transfer its records to Pennsylvania State University. By mid-1997, the union had sent most of its historical material to Penn State and had plans to move additional material there. Thus far, however, records at Penn State have undergone only preliminary archival processing, or no processing at all.)

13. U.S. Bituminous Coal Commission, Proceedings, vol. 1, pp. 315, 316, vol. 2, p. 1232, UMW Archive.

14. U.S. Bituminous Coal Commission, Proceedings, vol. 1, p. 718, vol. 2, pp. 1012–15, 1191–92, 1194–96, 1205–7, UMW Archive; UMW, *The Case of the Bituminous Coal Mine Workers . . . as Presented to the President's Coal Commission* (Washington, D.C., 1920), p. 54; Roger W. Babson, *W. B. Wilson and the Department of Labor* (New York, 1919), p. 19; *UMWJ*, March 15, 1906, p. 3, March 1, 1963, pp. 6, 18–20.

15. U.S. Bituminous Coal Commission, *Award and Recommendations* (Washington, D.C., 1920), pp. 46, 86–87.

16. Districts 1, 7, and 9, UMW, *Proceedings of the Tri-District Convention, 1919* (Scranton, n.d.), pp. 33, 73, 123, 151, 170; Joint Conference of Anthracite Operators and Mine Workers, "Minutes, 1920," p. 7, UMW Archive, Anthracite Tri-Distri~t General Scale Committee Files, folder: Anthracite Wage Conference, 1920; Fox, *United We Stand*, pp. 193–94; Harold K. Kanarek, "Progressivism in Crisis: The United Mine Workers and the Anthracite Coal Industry during the 1920s" (Ph.D. diss., University of Virginia, 1972), pp. 34, 41, 44.

17. Kanarek, "Progressivism in Crisis," pp. 41–43, 49–51; District 9, UMW, *Report of Proceedings of the Nineteenth Successive Constitutional and Second Biennial Convention, 1920* (Mount Carmel, Pa., n.d.), pp. 141–42; *Coal Age*, July 8, 1920, p. 82; UMW, *Occupation Hazard of Anthracite Miners* (Washington, D.C., 1920), esp. pp. 5, 7, 22–24; Philip Murray, *The Case of the Anthracite Coal Mine Workers* (n.p., 1920), pp. 29–30; U.S. Anthracite Coal Commission, "Proceedings," vol. 2, pp. 507–12, UMW Archive; U.S. Anthracite Coal Commission, *Report, Findings, and Award* (Washington, D.C., 1920), pp. 10–18.

18. Anthracite Coal Commission, "Proceedings," vol. 5, pp. 1596, 1594–629, UMW Archive; Anthracite Operators, *Before the United States Anthracite Coal Commission: Exhibits of the Anthracite Operators in Reply to Exhibits Presented by the Anthracite Mine Workers* (Scranton, 1920), pp. 13, 3, 5, 7, 20–23; Frederick L. Hoffman to Forrest F. Dryden, July 12, 1920, Frederick L. Hoffman Papers, box 8, item 25, Rare Book and Manuscript Library, Butler Library, Columbia University, New York; Hoffman to Dryden, July 15, 1920, Hoffman Papers, box 8.

19. Anthracite Coal Commission, *Report, Findings, and Award*, pp. 22–33; Kanarek, "Progressivism in Crisis," pp. 67–74; *UMWJ*, Sept. 15, 1920, p. 6; Fox, *United We Stand*, pp. 194–95.

20. Robert H. Zieger, *Republicans and Labor, 1919–1929* (Lexington, Ky., 1969), pp. 218–27; Fox, *United We Stand*, pp. 239–44.

21. U.S. Coal Commission, *Report*, 5 vols. (Washington, D.C., 1925), vol. 1, pp. 32, 149, vol. 2, pp. 603–25, vol. 3, pp. 1441–50, 1603–46, 1662, 1687; Robert Olesen et al., Sanitary Surveys, 1923, RG 68, Records of the U.S. Coal Commission, Records of the Office of Commissioner George Otis Smith, entry 13: Public Health Service Sanitary Surveys of Coal Communities, boxes 7–8, Washington National Records Center, National Archives and Records Administration, Suitland, Md. For another campaign to use germ theory and class biases in early-twentieth-century epidemiology, see Naomi Rogers, *Dirt and Disease: Polio before FDR* (New Brunswick, N.J., 1992), pp. 138–64.

22. Joseph A. Holmes, "The Work of the United States Bureau of Mines," *American Labor Legislation Review* 2 (1912): 125–30; U.S. Surgeon General, *Annual Report . . . for the Fiscal Year 1911* (Washington, D.C., 1912), p. 65. On the establishment and early de-

velopment of the BOM, see William Graebner, *Coal-Mining Safety in the Progressive Period: The Political Economy of Reform* (Lexington, Ky., 1976).

23. S. C. Hotchkiss, "Occupational Diseases in the Mining Industry," *American Labor Legislation Review* 2 (1912): 132; Alan Derickson, "Federal Intervention in the Joplin Silicosis Epidemic, 1911–1916," *Bulletin of the History of Medicine* 62 (1988): 236–51; W. A. Lynott, "Fatalities and Diseases in Coal Mining Districts," in National Safety Council, *Proceedings of the Fourth Annual Safety Congress, 1915* (n.p., n.d.), pp. 239–40; *Coal Age*, April 8, 1916, p. 629, April 15, 1916, p. 664.

24. L. R. Thompson to Surgeon General, June 1925, RG 90, Files of Domestic Stations, Washington, D. C., Office of Industrial Hygiene and Sanitation, box 61, file 0135–58; M. J. White to Secretary of the Treasury, April 10, 1924, Files of Domestic Stations, Washington, D.C., Office of Industrial Hygiene and Sanitation, box 61, file 0245–184; W. G. Platt to James F. Rogers, Feb. 14, 1923, RG 90, General Correspondence, 1897–1923, box 195, file 2048-K; Platt to Thomas J. O'Brien, Feb. 14, 1923, RG 90, General Correspondence, 1897–1923, box 195, file 2048-K; A. M. Stimson to Surgeon General, Sept. 27, 1923, RG 90, General Correspondence, 1897–1923, box 188, file 2048; all in Records of the Public Health Service, National Archives, Washington, D.C.

25. U.S. Surgeon General, *Annual Report . . . for the Fiscal Year 1923* (Washington, D.C., 1923), p. 22; L. R. Thompson to Surgeon General, July 25, 1925, RG 90, Files of Domestic Stations, Washington, D.C., Office of Industrial Hygiene and Sanitation, box 62, file 1975–85; U.S. Public Health Service, *The Health of Workers in Dusty Trades: III. Exposure to Dust in Coal Mining*, by Dean K. Brundage and Elizabeth S. Frasier, Public Health Bulletin 208 (Washington, D.C., 1933), pp. iv, 2, 7–8.

26. PHS, *Health in Dusty Trades*, pp. 4, 9–11.

27. M. J. White to Secretary of the Treasury, April 19, 1924, RG 90, Records of the PHS, Files of Domestic Stations, Washington, D.C., Office of Industrial Hygiene and Sanitation, box 61, file 0115–42; PHS, *Health in Dusty Trades*, pp. 3, 8–9.

28. PHS, *Health in Dusty Trades*, pp. 10–11, 4–5.

29. Ibid., pp. 12–15.

30. Ibid., pp. 15–16; L. R. Thompson to Surgeon General, Aug. 6, 1923, RG 90, General Correspondence, 1897–1923, box 195, file 2048-K; U.S. Surgeon General, *Annual Report . . . for the Fiscal Year 1926* (Washington, D.C., 1926), p. 45; Leroy U. Gardner, Donald E. Cummings, and Gerald R. Dowd, "Experimental Inhalation of Bituminous Coal Dust and Its Effects upon Primary Tuberculosis Infection in Guinea Pigs," *Journal of Industrial Hygiene* 15 (1933): 457.

31. Gardner, Cummings, and Dowd, "Bituminous Dust and Tuberculosis," pp. 464, 456–65; L. R. Thompson to Surgeon General, Nov. 6, 1925, box 62, file 1910; C. C. Pierce to Secretary of the Treasury, April 7, 1927, box 62, file 1515–17; both in RG 90, Files of Domestic Stations, Office of Industrial Hygiene and Sanitation.

32. F. V. Meriwether, "Report . . . , November 1922," Dec. 14, 1922, RG 70, Records of the Bureau of Mines, Health and Safety Branch, Records of the Picher, Oklahoma, Clinic, 1927–1932, box 3, file 087, Washington National Records Center, National Archives and Records Administration, Suitland, Maryland; F. V. Meriwether to Daniel Harrington, Aug. 2, 1923, box 8, file 104. On the destruction of the UMW in Alabama after the First World War, see Daniel Letwin, *The Challenge of Interracial Unionism: Alabama Coal Miners, 1878–1921* (Chapel Hill, 1998).

33. Daniel Harrington and J. J. Forbes to A. C. Fieldner, Oct. 11, 1923, box 3, file 087; F. V. Meriwether, "Report . . . , October 1923," Oct. 31, 1923, box 3, file 087; Meriwether to Sara Davenport, Nov. 23, 1923, box 8, file 104; all in RG 70, Records of the Bureau of Mines, Health and Safety Branch, Records of the Picher, Oklahoma, Clinic, 1927–1932; R. R. Sayers to Surgeon General, Aug. 6, 1924, RG 70, Federal Agencies Files, box 13, file 1850–15.

34. F. V. Meriwether to F. Flinn, Feb. 13, 1924, box 3, file 087; J. J. Forbes to Alden H. Emery, May 14, 1924, box 8, file 104; both in RG 70, Health and Safety Branch, Records of the Picher, Oklahoma, Clinic, 1927–1932.

35. D. A. Lyon to L. E. Geohegan, June 26, 1924, box 8, file 104; George S. Rice to Dr. Sayers and Mr. van Siclen, July 3, 1924; both in RG 70, Health and Safety Branch, Records of the Picher, Oklahoma, Clinic, 1927–1932. Russell M. Cunningham, "The Relation of Coal Mines to Health and Disease as Applied to the Convict Labor System of Alabama," *Alabama Medical and Surgical Age* 5 (1893): 537, 480–81, 536ff. The most infamous racist research venture of the PHS commenced a decade later in Alabama; see James H. Jones, *Bad Blood: The Tuskegee Syphilis Experiment* (New York, 1981).

36. C. A. Herbert to J. J. Forbes, Jan. 3, 1925, box 197, file 437.1; M. van Siclen to J. J. Forbes, Aug. 5, 1924; F. V. Meriwether to R. R. Sayers, Jan. 31, 1925; all in RG 70, General Correspondence, 1910–50. Meriwether, Report, February 1925, Feb. 28, 1925, RG 70, Health and Safety Branch, Records of the Picher, Oklahoma, Clinic, 1927–1932, box 3, file 087.

37. H. Foster Bain to Milton H. Fies, July 24, 1924, box 3, file 087; J. J. Forbes and F. V. Meriwether to M. van Siclen, July 10, 1924; D. A. Lyon to James Nicol, Jr., July 11, 1925; all in RG 70, Health and Safety Branch, Records of the Picher, Oklahoma, Clinic, 1927–1932. Lyon to Fies, Nov. 8, 1924, RG 70, General Correspondence, 1910–50, box 1061, file 432.1.

38. J. J. Forbes and F. V. Meriwether to M. van Siclen, June 16, 1924, RG 70, Health and Safety Branch, Records of the Picher, Oklahoma, Clinic, 1927–1932, box 8, file 104; J. J. Forbes and Alden H. Emery, "Sources of Dust in Coal Mines," *Transactions of the American Institute of Mining and Metallurgical Engineers* 75 (1927): 645–63.

39. U.S. Surgeon General, *Annual Report . . . for Fiscal Year 1924* (Washington, D.C., 1924), p. 31; R. R. Sayers to Surgeon General, Aug. 6, 1924, RG 90, Federal Agencies Files, box 13, file 1850–15; F. V. Meriwether, "Report . . . , May 1926," June 2, 1926, RG 70, Health and Safety Branch, Records of the Picher, Oklahoma, Clinic, 1927–1932, box 3, file 087.

40. M. van Siclen to J. J. Forbes and F. V. Meriwether, July 13, 1925, RG 70, Health and Safety Branch, Records of the Picher, Oklahoma, Clinic, 1927–1932, box 3, file 087.

41. D. Harrington, "Even Coal and Non-Siliceous Dusts Harmful to Health," *Coal Age*, March 20, 1924, pp. 417, 418; F. V. Meriwether to Harrington, Aug. 13, 1926, RG 70, General Correspondence, 1910–50, box 457, file 437.1. For Harrington's view of the engineer's key role in improving working conditions, see U.S. BOM, *Review of Literature on Effects of Breathing Dusts with Special Reference to Silicosis*, by Daniel Harrington and Sara J. Davenport, Bulletin 400 (Washington, D.C., 1937), p. 145. For one source of Harrington's vision, see George C. Whipple, "Human Health and the American Engineer," *Journal of Industrial Hygiene* 1 (1919): 75–84, esp. 81–82.

42. D. Harrington, "Is Coal Industry Blind to Health Hazards of Mine?" *Coal Age*, Nov. 27, 1924, p. 759; D. Harrington, "Dust and the Health of Miners," *Mining and Metallurgy*, Jan. 1925, pp. 29–31.

43. Harrington, "Is Coal Industry Blind," pp. 757–61.

44. Daniel Harrington, "The Engineering-Hygienic Aspects of Dust Elimination in Mines," *Journal of Industrial Hygiene* 7 (1925): 212, 199–214; *Coal Age*, Aug. 14, 1924, p. 228; *Coal Age*, Nov. 27, 1924, pp. 743–44.

45. F. W. Meriwether, "The Effects of Mine Dust on Health," in National Safety Council, *Transactions of the . . . Sixteenth Annual Safety Congress, 1927*, 3 vols. ([Chicago], 1928), vol. 2, pp. 248, 250.

46. Ibid., pp. 249, 250–51.

47. Ibid., pp. 249–51.

48. Ibid., pp. 251–55. For a more recent case in which a demolition contractor pro-

fessed ignorance of the hazards of asbestos while making sure that his own son worked out of harm's way, see Don J. Lofgren, *Dangerous Premises: An Insider's View of OSHA Enforcement* (Ithaca, 1989), pp. 13–41, esp. 23.

49. Daniel Harrington, "Miner's Health," *National Safety News*, Oct. 1933; *Coal Age*, March 1930, p. 158; D. Harrington to S. H. Ash, April 14, 1930, RG 70, Health and Safety Branch, Records of the Picher, Oklahoma, Clinic, 1927–1932, box 15, file 440. On Meriwether's work with metal miners, see Alan Derickson, "'On the Dump Heap': Employee Medical Screening in the Tri-State Zinc-Lead Industry, 1924–1932," *Business History Review* 62 (1988): 667–76.

50. F. V. Meriwether, "Pneumonoconiosis Due to Coal Dust," n.d. [ca. Aug. 27, 1927], esp. pp. 14–18, box 4, file 087; Meriwether to R. R. Sayers, Aug. 27, 1927; both in RG 70, Health and Safety Branch, Records of the Picher, Oklahoma, Clinic, 1927–1932. Alden H. Emery, "Concentration and Composition of Atmospheric Dusts from the Sipsey, Alabama, Mines," Sept. 24, 1924, Table II, RG 70, Records of the Office of the Chief Surgeon, 1916–33, box 84, folder: Dust Ventilation—Alabama. For one of the occasions on which the Alabama Mining Institute passed by an opportunity to take notice of the Meriwether project, see James L. Davidson, "Safety Practices in and about Alabama Coal Mines," in National Safety Council, *Transactions of the Fifteenth Annual Safety Congress, 1926*, 3 vols. ([Chicago], 1926), vol. 2, pp. 194–206. On the institute's goal of preserving the health of mine employees and, to that end, on its close working relationship with the BOM, see Alabama Mining Institute, "Constitution," Article III, Oct. 11, 1921; James L. Davidson, "Annual Report, 1923–24," n.d. [ca. Oct. 1924]; Davidson, "Annual Report, 1924–25," Oct. 6, 1925; Board of Governors, Alabama Mining Institute, "Minutes," Nov. 10, 1925; all in Alabama Coal Operators Association Records, box 1, Department of Archives and Manuscripts, Birmingham Public Library, Birmingham, Ala. The Alabama-Kentucky study also is historiographically invisible; see, for example, Barbara Ellen Smith, *Digging Our Own Graves: Coal Miners and the Struggle over Black Lung Disease* (Philadelphia, 1987), esp. pp. 19–20, 222.

51. D. Harrington to John F. Knudsen, Sept. 29, 1943, box 4274, file 437.4; O. P. Hood to H. G. Hensel, July 2, 1931, box 1393, file 437.4; both in RG 70, General Correspondence, 1910–50. David Rosner and Gerald Markowitz, "A 'Gift of God'?: The Public Health Controversy over Leaded Gasoline during the 1920s," *American Journal of Public Health* 75 (1985): 344–52; Graebner, *Coal-Mining Safety*, pp. 25–27, 43–71; Daniel J. Curran, *Dead Laws for Dead Men: The Politics of Federal Coal Mine Health and Safety Legislation* (Pittsburgh, 1993), pp. 66–68.

52. U.S. Bureau of Mines, *Health Hazards in the Mining Industry*, by R. R. Sayers, Report of Investigaton 2660 ([Washington, D.C.], 1924), pp. 5–8; *Coal Age*, Dec. 11, 1924, p. 821.

53. Fox, *United We Stand*, pp. 212–305; Robert H. Zieger, *John L. Lewis: Labor Leader* (Boston, 1988), pp. 26–61.

54. Pennsylvania, *Laws, 1903* (Harrisburg, 1903), pp. 249, 248–50; Pennsylvania, *Laws, 1904* ([Harrisburg], 1905), pp. 542–43; *UMWJ*, Oct. 5, 1905, p. 5; UMW, *Minutes of the Fifteenth Annual Convention, 1904* (Indianapolis, 1904), p. 140. Anthony F. C. Wallace contends that mid-nineteenth-century plans for an anthracite asylum specifically aimed to deal with victims of miners' asthma; see *St. Clair: A Nineteenth-Century Coal Town's Experience with a Disaster-Prone Industry* (New York, 1987), pp. 279–80. However, I have found corroboration for this claim neither in the sources cited by Wallace nor in other sources from the period.

55. *UMWJ*, Dec. 21, 1905, pp. 1, 4; UMW, *Proceedings of the Twentieth Annual Convention, 1909*, 2 vols. (Indianapolis, 1909), vol. 1, p. 373; William B. Wilson to Executive Council, AFL, June 11, 1909, William B. Papers, Chronological File, 1880–1913, Historical Society of Pennsylvania, Philadelphia; UMW, *Proceedings of the Twenty-First An-*

nual Convention, 1910 (Indianapolis, 1910), pp. 436, 529–31; District 1, UMW, *Proceedings of the Fourteenth Annual Convention, 1912* (Scranton, n.d.), p. 75; John Brophy, *A Miner's Life*, ed. John O. P. Hall (Madison, 1964), pp. 117–18; *Coal Age*, Feb. 10, 1921, p. 281; *Illinois Miner* (Springfield), May 5, 1923, p. 1, May 26, 1923, p. 3, May 17, 1924, p. 4; Christopher Anglim and Brian Gratton, "Organized Labor and Old Age Pensions," *International Journal of Aging and Human Development* 25 (1987): 91–107, esp. pp. 96–98; Jill Quadagno and Madonna Harrington Meyer, "Organized Labor, State Structures, and Social Policy Development: A Case Study of Old Age Assistance in Ohio, 1916–1940," *Social Problems* 36 (1989): 184–86.

56. *UMWJ*, Sept. 11, 1913, p. 1, July 3, 1913, p. 2; American Association for Labor Legislation, *Standards for Workmen's Compensation Laws* (New York, 1914), p. 8; John B. Andrews, "Occupational Diseases and Legislative Remedies," *American Journal of Public Health* 4 (1914): 179–84; Roy Lubove, *The Struggle for Social Security, 1900–1935*, 2d ed. (Pittsburgh, 1986), pp. 45–65; Moss, *Socializing Security*, pp. 59–76, 117–31.

57. Van Bittner, "General Discussion," *American Labor Legislation Review* 5 (1915): 30; John Mitchell, "General Discussion," *American Labor Legislation Review* 5 (1915): 22; *UMWJ*, Jan. 7, 1915, p. 6. British miners faced a similar dilemma with regard to compensation for nystagmus; see Karl Figlio, "How Does Illness Mediate Social Relations? Workmen's Compensation and Medico-Legal Practices, 1890–1940," in *The Problem of Medical Knowledge: Examining the Social Construction of Medicine*, ed. Peter Wright and Andrew Treacher (Edinburgh, 1982), pp. 187, 189.

58. District 1, UMW, *Proceedings of the Sixteenth Consecutive and First Biennial Convention, 1915* (Scranton, n.d.), pp. 79, 79–80; *UMWJ*, Oct. 5, 1916, p. 7; District 9, UMW, *Proceedings of the Seventeenth Annual Convention, 1916* (Shenandoah, Penn., n.d.), pp. 64, 248.

59. District 1, UMW, *Report of the Proceedings of the Twentieth Successive and Fifth Biennial Convention, 1923* (Scranton, n.d.), p. 111; District 1, UMW, *Report of the Proceedings of the Twenty-First Successive and Sixth Biennial Convention, 1925* (Scranton, n.d.), pp. 122, 255; *UMWJ*, Oct. 15, 1924, p. 5, Nov. 1, 1926, p. 8; District 9, UMW, *Report of Proceedings of the Twenty-Third Successive Constitutional and Sixth Biennial Convention, 1928* (Mahanoy City, Pa., n.d.), p. 129; District 7, UMW, *Report of Proceedings of the Twenty-Fifth Consecutive and Ninth Biennial Convention, 1930* (Hazleton, Pa., n.d.), pp. 40, 183, 215, 251.

60. [John Walker] to John Steele, Jan. 5, 1926 [1927], folder 234; [Walker] to Subcommittee . . . Working Out Agreed Amendments to the Workmen's Compensation Act, Jan. 14, 1929, folder 775; both in John H. Walker Papers, Illinois Historical Survey Library, University of Illinois, Urbana. *Illinois Miner*, Aug. 23, 1924, pp. 3, 5; *Illinois State Federation of Labor Weekly News Letter* (Chicago), Sept. 27, 1924, p. 5, Jan. 8, 1927, pp. 1–2, Jan. 29, 1927, p. 1; John H. Keiser, "John H. Walker: Labor Leader from Illinois," in *Essays in Illinois History*, ed. Keiser (Carbondale, Ill., 1968), pp. 75–100.

61. UMW, *Proceedings of the Twenty-Ninth Consecutive and Sixth Biennial Convention, 1924*, 3 vols. (Indianapolis, 1924), vol. 2, p. 568; District 1, UMW, *Report of Proceedings of the Twenty-Fourth Consecutive and Ninth Biennial Convention, 1931* (n.p., n.d.), pp. 209, 274; District 7, UMW, *Report of the Proceedings of the Twenty-Sixth Consecutive and Tenth Biennial Convention, 1932*, 2 vols. (Hazleton, n.d.), vol. 1, pp. 41, 172; American Association for Labor Legislation, *Standards for Workmen's Compensation Laws, Revised to January 1, 1929* (New York, n.d.), p. 8. For an endorsement of the scheduling approach that acknowledges its British inspiration, see National Conference of Commissioners on Uniform State Laws, *Draft of Uniform Occupational Diseases Act* (n.p., n.d. [ca. 1916]). On the British policy, see Thomas M. Legge, "Industrial Diseases under the Workmen's Compensation Act," *Journal of Industrial Hygiene* 2 (1920): 25–32.

62. Pennsylvania Department of Mines, *Report, Part II: Bituminous, 1909* (Harris-

burg, 1910), pp. lviii, lx; John A. Garcia, "State Coal Mining Laws Concerning Venti-lation," *Transactions of the American Institute of Mining and Metallurgical Engineers* 74 (1927): 409–16; E. A. Holbrook, "Importance of Uniformity in Mine Safety Legisla-tion," *American Labor Legislation Review* 14 (1924): 54–59; Graebner, *Coal-Mining Safety*, pp. 72–111; Alexander Trachtenberg, *The History of Legislation for the Protection of Coal Miners in Pennsylvania, 1824–1915* (New York, 1942), pp. 173–77; James Whiteside, *Regulating Danger: The Struggle for Mine Safety in the Rocky Mountain Coal Industry* (Lin-coln, Neb., 1990), pp. 84–114, 145–54; Price V. Fishback, *Soft Coal, Hard Choices: The Economic Welfare of Bituminous Coal Miners, 1890–1930* (New York, 1992), pp. 112–18.

63. Linda Gordon, "The New Feminist Scholarship on the Welfare State," in *Women, the State, and Welfare*, ed. Gordon (Madison, 1990), pp. 9–35; Linda Gordon, "Social Insurance and Public Assistance: The Influence of Gender in Welfare Thought in the United States, 1890–1935," *American Historical Review* 97 (1992): 19–54; Theda Skoc-pol, *Protecting Soldiers and Mothers: The Political Origins of Social Policy in the United States* (Cambridge, Mass., 1992); Barbara J. Nelson, "The Gender, Race, and Class Ori-gins of Early Welfare Policy and the Welfare State: A Comparison of Workmen's Com-pensation and Mothers' Aid," in *Women, Politics, and Change*, ed. Louise A. Tilly and Patricia Gurin (New York, 1990), pp. 413–35; Seth Koven and Sonya Michel, "Wom-anly Duties: Maternalist Policies and the Origins of Welfare States in France, Germany, Great Britain, and the United States, 1880–1920," *American Historical Review* 95 (1990): 1076–108; Ann Shola Orloff, "Gender in Early U.S. Social Policy," *Journal of Policy History* 3 (1991): 249–81; Kathryn Kish Sklar, "The Historical Foundations of Women's Power in the Creation of the American Welfare State, 1830–1930," in *Mothers of a New World: Maternalist Politics and the Origins of Welfare States*, ed. Seth Koven and Sonya Michel (New York, 1993), pp. 43–93.

64. On social empiricist investigation in this period, see Mary O. Furner, "Knowing Capitalism: Public Investigation and the Labor Question in the Long Progressive Era," in *The State and Economic Knowledge: The American and British Experiences*, ed. Furner and Barry Supple (Cambridge, Eng., 1990), pp. 241–86; Libby Schweber, "Progressive Reformers, Unemployment, and the Transformation of Social Inquiry in Britain and the United States, 1880s-1920s," and John R. Sutton, "Social Knowledge and the Gen-eration of Child Welfare Policy," both in *States, Social Knowledge, and the Origins of Modern Social Policies*, ed. Dietrich Rueschemeyer and Theda Skocpol (Princeton, 1996), pp. 163–200, 201–30; Martin Bulmer, "The Decline of the Social Survey Move-ment and the Rise of American Empirical Sociology," in *The Social Survey in Historical Perspective, 1880–1940*, ed. Bulmer, Kevin Bales, and Kathryn Kish Sklar (Cambridge, Eng., 1991), pp. 291–315.

5. To Bits

1. U.S. Bureau of the Census, *Historical Statistics of the United States, Colonial Times to 1970*, 2 vols. (Washington, D.C., 1975), vol. 1, pp. 589, 592; Curtis Seltzer, *Fire in the Hole: Miners and Managers in the American Coal Industry* (Lexington, Ky., 1985), pp. 34–41; Donald L. Miller and Richard E. Sharpless, *The Kingdom of Coal: Work, Enterprise, and Ethnic Communities in the Mine Fields* (Philadelphia, 1985), pp. 287–91; Irving Bernstein, *The Lean Years: A History of the American Worker, 1920–1933* (Boston, 1960), pp. 127–29.

2. U.S. Census, *Historical Statistics*, vol. 1, pp. 591–92; U.S. Bureau of Labor Statis-tics, *Technological Change and Productivity in the Bituminous Coal Industry, 1920–60*, Bulletin 1305 (Washington, D.C., 1961), p. 15; Keith Dix, *What's a Miner to Do?: The Mechanization of Coal Mining* (Pittsburgh, 1988), esp. pp. 17, 83–88, 218; Miller and

Sharpless, *Kingdom of Coal*, pp. 288–305; Bernstein, *Lean Years*, pp. 130–32, 381–82; Robert H. Zieger, *Republicans and Labor, 1919–1929* (Lexington, Ken., 1969), pp. 216–47.

3. *Coal Age*, Dec. 1933, p. 427; U.S. Census, *Historical Statistics*, vol. 1, p. 170; Harold W. Aurand, "Self-Employment: Last Resort of the Unemployed," *International Social Science Review* 58 (1983): 8; Michael Kozura, "We Stood Our Ground: Anthracite Miners and the Expropriation of Corporate Property, 1930–41," in *"We Are All Leaders": The Alternative Unionism of the Early 1930s*, ed. Staughton Lynd (Urbana, 1996), pp. 199–237; Bernstein, *Lean Years*, pp. 360–64; Marlene Rikard, "An Experiment in Welfare Capitalism: The Health Care Services of the Tennessee Coal, Iron and Railroad Company" (Ph.D. diss., University of Alabama, 1983), pp. 269, 278–79; Malcolm Ross, *Machine Age in the Hills* (New York, 1933), pp. 109–24; John F. Bauman and Thomas F. Coode, *In the Eye of the Great Depression: New Deal Reporters and the Agony of the American People* (DeKalb, Ill., 1988), pp. 94–115, 216, 227–28; Richard C. Keller, "Pennsylvania's Little New Deal" (Ph.D. diss., Columbia University, 1960), pp. 66–100, esp. 70–71; Homer L. Morris, *The Plight of the Bituminous Coal Miner* (Philadelphia, 1934), pp. 105–14; Sonya Jason, *Icon of Spring* (Pittsburgh, 1993), pp. 13, 33–34, 76, 83, 118, 144. For an especially insightful study of the inability of ethnic and religious welfare institutions to meet the needs of workers during the depression, see Lizabeth Cohen, *Making a New Deal: Industrial Workers in Chicago, 1919–1939* (Cambridge, Eng., 1990), pp. 218–38.

4. Morris, *Plight of Bituminous Miner*, pp. 41–42, 39–42, 179–80; Carl D. Oblinger, *Divided Kingdom: Work, Community, and the Mining Wars in the Central Illinois Coal Fields during the Great Depression* (Springfield, Ill., 1991), pp. 120–22; Alan Derickson, "Part of the Yellow Dog: U.S. Coal Miners' Opposition to the Company Doctor System, 1936–1946," *International Journal of Health Services* 19 (1989): 711–13.

5. David Rosner and Gerald Markowitz, *Deadly Dust: Silicosis and the Politics of Occupational Disease in Twentieth-Century America* (Princeton, 1991), pp. 78–82; District 1, UMW, *Report of Proceedings of the Nineteenth Successive and Fourth Biennial Convention, 1921* (Scranton, n.d.), pp. 62, 289, 293; District 1, UMW, *Report of Proceedings of the Twenty-Sixth Consecutive and Eleventh Biennial Convention, 1935* (n.p., n.d.), pp. 51–52; Steve Nelson, James R. Barrett, and Rob Ruck, *Steve Nelson: American Radical* (Pittsburgh, 1981), pp. 94–124, 153–82; Miller and Sharpless, *Kingdom of Coal*, pp. 315–19.

6. Charlotte E. Carr to P. S. Stahlnecker, Aug. 19, 1931, Gifford Pinchot Papers, box 2264, folder: Labor and Industry, Department of, Carr, Charlotte, Correspondence, AS 1932, Manuscript Division, Library of Congress; "Eastern Interstate Conference on Labor Legislation," *Monthly Labor Review* 33 (1931): 302–3; M. Nelson McGeary, *Gifford Pinchot: Forester-Politician* (Princeton, 1960), pp. 358–86.

7. Gifford Pinchot, "Address of Governor Pinchot at Banquet of Pennsylvania Safety Conference," May 12, 1932, Pinchot Papers, box 823, folder: 5–13–32, Penna. Safety Conference; John Campbell, "The Conference Discussion of Industrial Disease," *Labor and Industry*, June 1932, pp. 24–28.

8. Pennsylvania Commission on Compensation for Occupational Disease, *Occupational Disease Compensation: A Report* (Harrisburg, 1933), pp. 5, 7–8.

9. T. Henry Walnut to John B. Andrews, Oct. 20, 1932, American Association for Labor Legislation Papers, reel 48, Labor-Management Documentation Center, Catherwood Library, Cornell University, Ithaca.

10. Pennsylvania Commission on Compensation, *Occupational Disease Compensation*, p. 32; *UMWJ*, March 1, 1958, p. 15. On changing definitions of disability, see Deborah A. Stone, *The Disabled State* (Philadelphia, 1984); Edward D. Berkowitz, *Disabled Policy: America's Programs for the Handicapped* (Cambridge, Eng., 1987).

11. A. J. Lanza to Daniel Harrington, Dec. 12, 1932; Lanza to R. R. Sayers, Dec. 12,

1932; both in RG 70, Records of the U.S. Bureau of Mines, General Correspondence, 1910–50, box 1584, file 437.4, Washington National Records Center, National Archives and Records Administration, Suitland, Maryland.

12. A. J. Lanza to Daniel Harrington, Dec. 12, 1932; Harrington to Lanza, Dec. 29, 1932; both in RG 70, Records of the U.S. Bureau of Mines, General Correspondence, 1910–50, box 1584, file 437.4. T. Henry Walnut to Gifford Pinchot, Dec. 13, 1932, Pinchot Papers, box 2266, folder: Labor and Industry, Department of, Committees— Occupational Diseases, AS 1932; Walnut to John B. Andrews, Nov. 2, 1932, AALL Papers, reel 48.

13. T. Henry Walnut to John B. Andrews, Oct. 20, 1932; Andrews to Thomas Kennedy, Oct. 10, 1932; Elizabeth B. Bricker to Andrews, Oct. 28, 1932; Andrews to Charlotte E. Carr, Nov. 1, 1932; Andrews to A. Estelle Lauder, Nov. 1, 1932; all in AALL Papers, reel 48. A. J. Lanza, "Occupational Diseases: Their Prevalence and Relative Importance," *Safety Engineering*, May 1934, p. 210.

14. T. Henry Walnut to Gifford Pinchot, March 2, 1933, Pinchot Papers, box 2266, folder: Labor and Industry, Department of, Committees[,] Occupational Diseases, Members, AS 1932.

15. Pennsylvania Commission on Compensation, *Occupational Disease Compensation*, pp. 5–6, 10, 20–27, 31, 39, 46–47, 61–62, 81–88.

16. Ibid., pp. 23, 26, 31–33, 66.

17. Ibid., pp. 59, 7.

18. Ibid., pp. 26–27, 7, 36; T. Henry Walnut to Gifford Pinchot, May 19, 1933, Pinchot Papers, box 2266, folder: Labor and Industry[,] Department of, Committee—Occupational Diseases, Members, AS 1932. On the use of expert commissions to put off reform, see Robert R. Alford, *Health Care Politics: Ideological and Interest Group Barriers to Reform* (Chicago, 1975).

19. Governor's Office, "Statement," April 21, 1933, Pinchot Papers, box 2266, folder: Labor and Industry[,] Department of, Committee—Occupational Disease, AS 1933; Governor's Office, "Statement," July 5, 1933, Pinchot Papers, box 852, folder: July 5, 1933, U.S. Public Health Service Survey of Miners' Asthma, SN.

20. H. S. Cumming to Gifford Pinchot, April 22, 1933, Pinchot Papers, box 2266, folder: Labor and Industry[,] Department of, Committee—Occupational Disease, AS 1933; Charlotte E. Carr to Pinchot, May 17, 1933, Pinchot Papers, box 2266, folder: Labor and Industry, Department of, Committee–Occupational Disease, AS 1933; R. R. Sayers, "Memorandum," May 15, 1933, RG 70, General Correspondence, 1910–50, box 1779, file 437.4; Pennsylvania, Department of Labor and Industry, *Anthraco-Silicosis (Miners' Asthma): A Preliminary Report of a Study Made in the Anthracite Region of Pennsylvania by United States Public Health Service*, Special Bulletin 41 (Harrisburg, 1934), p. 8.

21. Pennsylvania, *Anthraco-Silicosis (Miners' Asthma)*, pp. 17–20, 48–50.

22. Ibid., pp. 20–23, 51, 69.

23. Ibid., pp. 23–25, 31–32.

24. Ibid., pp. 12, 21, 23.

25. Ibid., p. 10.

26. Ibid., pp. 12, 27–28, 42–43, 53, 62–66.

27. Ibid., pp. 10, 20, 36–39, 50.

28. Ibid., *passim*, esp. p. 12.

29. Charlotte E. Carr, "Foreword," p. 3; A. M. Boyd, et al. to Gifford Pinchot, "Letter of Transmittal," Nov. 28, 1934, p. 5; both in Pennsylvania, *Anthraco-Silicosis (Miners' Asthma)*. R. R. Sayers to Surgeon General, Sept. 15, 1934, and Oct. 1, 1934, RG 90, Records of the U.S. Public Health Service, General Files, 1924–1935, box 97, file 0875–96, National Archives, Washington; *UMWJ*, July 1, 1935, p. 15.

30. U.S. PHS, *Anthraco-Silicosis among Hard Coal Miners*, by J. J. Bloomfield et al., Public Health Bulletin 221 (Washington, D.C., 1936), pp. 51–69.

31. Ibid., *passim*, esp. pp. 2, 5, 73–83. For squeamishness on the hazard of coal dust in the preliminary report, see Pennsylvania, *Anthraco-Silicosis (Miners' Asthma)*, pp. 12–13.

32. U.S. Department of Labor, Division of Labor Standards, *Anthraco-Silicosis (Miners' Asthma in Anthracite Mines): Its Cause and Prevention* (Washington, D.C., 1935), pp. 2, 3. For the liberal stance of DOL on silicosis at this time, see Rosner and Markowitz, *Deadly Dust*, pp. 101–65.

33. R. R. Sayers to Surgeon General, Aug. 16, 1932; Sayers to Surgeon General, Oct. 14, 1932; Sayers to Surgeon General, Nov. 30, 1932; Albert E. Russell to Surgeon General, March 23, 1933; Russell to Surgeon General, May 17, 1933; all in RG 90, Federal Agencies Files, box 13, file 1850. Sayers to L. R. Thompson, March 25, 1933, RG 90, Files of Domestic Stations, Washington, D.C., Office of Industrial Hygiene and Sanitation, box 62, file 1850.

34. D. Harrington to L. E. Young, March 2, 1936, RG 70, General Correspondence, 1910–50, box 2429, file 437.4; Harrington to Walter A. Jones, April 5, 1933, RG 70, General Correspondence, 1910–50, box 1779, file 437.4; R. R. Sayers to Surgeon General, Feb. 7, 1936, RG 90, General Correspondence, 1936–44, box 88, file 0875-96-49. Dependent on Public Health Service expertise, the U.S. Department of Labor was also held back by PHS's failure to publish the report on Powellton. See Division of Labor Standards, *Anthraco-Silicosis*, p. 4: "When further studies [beyond anthracite] are completed, another booklet will be issued with special reference to the bituminous-coal-dust hazard."

35. *Fayette Journal* (Fayetteville, W. Va.), Jan. 13, 1933, p. 3; Albert E. Russell to E. R. Hayhurst, June 21, 1933, box 2428, file 437.4; Russell to Hayhurst, June 24, 1933, box 2428, file 437.4; C. E. Mahan to Bureau of Mines, June 16, 1937, box 2638, file 437.4; all in RG 70, General Correspondence, 1910–50. Martin Cherniack, *The Hawk's Nest Incident: America's Worst Industrial Disaster* (New Haven, 1986); Martin Cherniack, "Pancoast and the Image of Silicosis," *American Journal of Industrial Medicine* 18 (1990): 599–612.

36. BOM, *Review of Literature on Effects of Breathing Dusts with Special Reference to Silicosis*, by D. Harrington and Sara J. Davenport, Bulletin 400 (Washington, D.C., 1937), esp. pp. 22–25, 34–35, 74, 115, 159–69. On the preceding circulars, see for example, BOM, *Review of Literature on Effects of Breathing Dusts with Special Reference to Silicosis, Part II-B*, by D. Harrington and Sara J. Davenport, Information Circular 6848 ([Washington, D.C.], 1935).

37. Keller, "Pennsylvania's Little New Deal"; *Labor News* (Wilkes-Barre, Pa.), March 31, 1934, p. 1, June 22, 1935, p. 1; *Anthracite Tri-District News* (Hazleton, Pa.), Jan. 18, 1935, pp. 1, 8.

38. *Anthracite Tri-District News*, March 26, 1937, p. 1, June 11, 1937, p. 1; Keller, "Pennsylvania's Little New Deal," pp. 263, 271; Pennsylvania, *Laws, 1937*, 2 vols. (Harrisburg, 1937), vol. 2, pp. 2714–19. For cost containment through similar discriminatory restrictions on compensation benefits for silicosis victims in New York, see Rosner and Markowitz, *Deadly Dust*, pp. 93–95.

39. Pennsylvania, *Laws, 1937*, vol. 2, pp. 2715, 2714–15; District 9, UMW, *Report of Proceedings of the Twenty-Sixth Successive Constitutional and Ninth Biennial Convention, 1934* (Tremont, Pa., n.d.), pp. 42, 177–78; District 1, UMW, *Report of Proceedings of the Twenty-Sixth Consecutive and Eleventh Biennial Convention, 1935* (n.p., n.d.), pp. 51–52, 96, 267–68, 290, 323.

40. D. Harrington to L. E. Young, Oct. 26, 1938; Young to Harrington, Oct. 13, 1938;

Harrington to Young, Oct. 19, 1938; Young to Harrington, Oct. 21, 1938; Young to Harrington, Feb. 25, 1939; all in RG 70, General Correspondence, 1910–50, box 2851, file 437.1.

41. UMW, *Proceedings of the Thirty-Fifth Constitutional Convention, 1938*, 2 vols. (n.p., n.d.), vol. 1, p. 437; UMW, *Proceedings of the Thirty-Seventh Constitutional Convention, 1942*, 2 vols. (n.p., n.d.), vol. 1, p. 89. On the misuses of employee medical examinations, see Derickson, "Yellow Dog," pp. 711–13.

42. Pennsylvania, *Laws, 1939* (Harrisburg, 1939), pp. 568–602, esp. 571, 587; compare Pennsylvania, *Laws, 1937*, vol. 2, pp. 2717–18. On the changing concerns of pathology, see Pennsylvania, *Anthraco-Silicosis*, pp. 13, 33–34.

43. Pennsylvania, *Laws, 1939*, p. 569.

44. Districts 1, 7, and 9, UMW, *Proceedings of the Tri-District Convention, 1941* (Washington, D.C., n.d.), pp. 69, 45. Mary Lawler to R. R. Sayers, n.d. [April 13, 1942]; Sayers to Lawler, April 22, 1942; both in RG 70, General Correspondence, 1910–50, box 3926, file 437.4. *UMWJ*, Oct. 15, 1939, p. 15, Jan. 15, 1941, p. 16; *Anthracite Tri-District News*, July 4, 1941, p. 1; Districts 1, 7, and 9, UMW, *Proceedings of the Tri-District Scale Convention, 1943* (Hazleton, n.d.), p. 64; Moses Behrend, "Workmen's Compensation and Occupational Disease Laws in the Commonwealth of Pennsylvania," *Pennsylvania Medical Journal* 43 (1939): 20; International Executive Board, UMW, "Proceedings," Dec. 14, 1939, pp. 119–24, UMW Archive; John W. Stephenson, "Report of the Accomplishments of the Compensation Department of District No. 2," n.d. [ca. 1944], District 2, UMW, Collection, box 63, folder 6, Special Collections, Stapleton Library, Indiana University of Pennsylvania, Indiana, Pa.

45. *Anthracite Tri-District News*, April 3, 1942, p. 7.

46. *Anthracite Tri-District News*, Sept. 20, 1940, p. 4, March 7, 1941, p. 4, May 8, 1942, p. 9; Carl A. Peterson, notebook, entries of Feb. 22, 1940, March 24, 1941; Peterson, "Diary, 1940"; Peterson, "Diary, 1941"; Peterson, "Diary, 1942"; all in Carl A. Peterson Papers, box 2, folder 1, Historical Collections and Labor Archives, Pattee Library, Pennsylvania State University, University Park.

47. Walter F. Dodd to D. Harrington, Feb. 12, 1934, RG 70, General Correspondence, 1910–50, box 1962, file 437.4; Illinois, *Laws, 1936, Third Special Session* (Springfield, Ill., n.d.), pp. 40–74; Albert T. Helbing, "Occupational Disease Legislation in Illinois," *Social Service Review* 12 (1938): 105–22; Joseph D. Cronin to John B. Andrews, Sept. 25, 1937, AALL Papers, reel 56; Indiana, *Laws, 1937* (Fort Wayne, 1937), pp. 334–71; *UMWJ*, April 15, 1937, p. 5, Sept. 15, 1937, p. 17.

48. Kentucky, *Acts, 1944* (Frankfort, Ky., n.d.), pp. 144–55; A. C. Hirth to Albert E. Russell, March 10, 1933, RG 70, General Correspondence, 1910–50, box 1779, file 437.4; West Virginia, *Acts and Resolutions, 1935* (n.p., n.d.), pp. 345–58; A. G. Mathews to John B. Andrews, May 17, 1937, AALL Papers, reel 56. At Inland Steel Company's mining operations in Wheelwright, Kentucky, management dealt with threats of litigation and compensation by an elaborate medical program and vigorous controversion of claims. See E. R. Price to H. M. Wilkinson, Jan. 24, 1936, box 80, folder 2; Price to Clarence B. Randall, March 31, 1938, box 80, folder 2; A. G. Kammer to W. J. [J. W.] Bailey, March 28, 1941, box 82, folder 2; [Bailey] to John S. Harter, March 19, 1951, box 82, folder 3; all in Wheelwright Collection, Department of Special Collections and Archives, King Library, University of Kentucky, Lexington.

49. *UMWJ*, Nov. 15, 1944, p. 5; Maryland Medical Board for Occupational Diseases, *First Annual Report, 1940* (n.p., n.d.); Ohio, *Legislative Acts, 1937–38* (Columbus, 1938), pp. 268–72; Utah, *Laws, 1941* (Kaysville, Utah, 1941), pp. 79–87; Emery R. Hayhurst to John B. Andrews, Sept. 27, 1937, AALL Papers, reel 56. Like Pennsylvania, Ohio

placed a lower limit on the benefits payable in silicosis cases. At least one employers' attorney found this unjust; see Theodore Waters, "Critical Review," *Mining Congress Journal*, Dec. 1939, p. 35.

50. District 22, UMW, *Proceedings, Twelfth Biennial Convention, 1939* (Cheyenne, Wyo., n.d.), pp. 136, 136–40, 154; PHS, *Soft Coal Miners: Health and Working Environment*, by Robert H. Flinn, et al., Public Health Bulletin 270 (Washington, D.C., 1941).

51. PHS, *Soft Coal Miners*, pp. 48, 1, 8, 59; B. G. Clarke and C. E. Moffet, "Silicosis in Soft Coal Miners," *Journal of Industrial Hygiene and Toxicology* 23 (1941): 176–86. Inland Steel, site of the Clarke-Moffet study, found its findings favorable enough to send to the Kentucky State Department of Health. See E. H. Carleton to Wayne L. Ritter, Feb. 22, 1945, Wheelwright Collection, box 82, folder 2. For another reductionist study at this time, see R. Harold Jones, "Pneumonoconiosis Encountered in Bituminous Coal Miners," *Journal of the American Medical Association* 119 (1942): 611–15.

52. Robert H. Flinn, Harry E. Seifert, and Hugh P. Brinton, "Anthraco-Silicosis among Bituminous Coal Miners," *Industrial Medicine* 11 (1942): 470, 470–73; compare PHS, *The Health of Workers in Dusty Trades: III. Exposure to Dust in Coal Mining*, by Dean K. Brundage and Elizabeth S. Frasier, Public Health Bulletin 208 (Washington, D.C., 1933), pp. 15–16.

53. Districts 17 and 29, UMW, *Special Joint Convention, 1943* (Charleston, W.Va., n.d.), pp. 123–24, 122–24.

54. UMW, *Proceedings of the Thirty-Eighth Constitutional Convention, 1944*, 2 vols. (n.p., n.d.), vol. 1, pp. 340, 340–41; James P. Johnson, *The Politics of Soft Coal: The Bituminous Industry from World War I through the New Deal* (Urbana, 1979), pp. 135–245; John R. Bowman, *Capitalist Collective Action: Competition, Cooperation, and Conflict in the Coal Industry* (Cambridge, Eng., 1989), pp. 178–210; Karl Figlio, "How Does Illness Mediate Social Relations? Workmen's Compensation and Medico-Legal Practices, 1890–1940," in *The Problem of Medical Knowledge: Examining the Social Construction of Medicine*, ed. Peter Wright and Andrew Treacher (Edinburgh, 1982), pp. 174–224, esp. 185; Rosner and Markowitz, *Deadly Dust*, pp. 82–133.

55. Bernard Feder, "The Collective Bargaining and the Legislative Policies of the United Mine Workers of America, 1933–1947" (Ph.D. diss., New York University, 1957), pp. 291–93; Maier B. Fox, *United We Stand: The United Mine Workers of America, 1890–1990* (Washington, D.C., 1990), pp. 362–63.

56. U.S. Senate, Committee on Mines and Mining, *Inspections and Investigations in Coal Mines: Hearings . . . on S. 2420, 1939* (Washington, D.C., 1939), pp. 85, 84–85, 14–15; U.S. House of Representatives, Committee on Mines and Mining, *Inspections and Investigations in Coal Mines: Hearings . . . on S. 2420, 1940* (Washington, D.C., 1940), pp. 78, 77, 89–90; James J. Davis, "Statement," Jan. 19, 1940, AALL Papers, reel 64; *UMWJ*, June 1, 1939, p. 10, Aug. 1, 1939, p. 9; UMW, *Proceedings of the Thirty-Sixth Constitutional Convention, 1940*, 2 vols. (n.p., n.d.), vol. 1, pp. 55–56, 112, 113, vol. 2, pp. 115–16; Feder, "Bargaining and Legislative Policies," pp. 293–302.

57. House, *Inspections and Investigations*, pp. 546, 546–47; Senate, *Inspections and Investigations*, pp. 151, 59.

58. U.S., *Statutes at Large*, vol. 55, pt. 1 (Washington, D.C., 1942), pp. 177, 177–80; Daniel J. Curran, *Dead Laws for Dead Men: The Politics of Federal Coal Mine Health and Safety Legislation* (Pittsburgh, 1993), pp. 91–93.

59. D. Harrington to H. H. Schrenk, Dec. 2, 1943, box 4274, file 437.1; C. W. Owings, "Report on Atmospheric Dust Study, Mine No. 1 . . . April 30 to May 4, 1945," n.d., box 4274, file 437.1; Harrington to Henry C. Rose, May 1, 1946, box 4274, file 437.1; Schrenk, "Industrial Hygiene Activities of the Bureau of Mines," March 20, 1945,

box 4995, file 937–30795; Harrington to G. W. Grove, Oct. 18, 1946, box 5199, file 437.1; Harrington to Richard Maize, Nov. 20, 1946; all in RG 70, General Correspondence, 1910–50.

60. J. J. Forbes to Edward Griffith, Oct. 2, 1943, box 4274, file 437.4; D. Harrington to Supervising Engineers, Sept. 18, 1943, box 4274, file 437.4; G. P. Hevenor to Forbes, July 31, 1944, box 2428, file 437.1; H. H. Schrenk, "Industrial Hygiene Activities of the Bureau of Mines," March 20, 1945, box 4995, file 937–30795; Harrington to R. Dawson Hall, Aug. 16, 1946, box 5294, file 937–43069; all in RG 70, General Correspondence, 1910–50. BOM, *Health Hazards from Inadequate Coal-Mine Ventilation*, by R. R. Sayers, Information Circular 7221 ([Washington, D.C.], 1942), esp. pp. 12–13.

61. Irving Bernstein, *A Caring Society: The New Deal Confronts the Great Depression* (Boston, 1985); Daniel Nelson, *Unemployment Insurance: The American Experience, 1915–1935* (Madison, 1969), pp. 192–222; Ann Shola Orloff, "The Political Origins of America's Belated Welfare State," in *The Politics of Social Policy in the United States*, ed. Margaret Weir, Orloff, and Theda Skocpol (Princeton, 1988), pp. 65–80. On the limits and failures of New Deal initiatives to provide for workers, see, among many others, Ellis W. Hawley, *The New Deal and the Problem of Monopoly* (Princeton, 1966); Theda Skocpol and Kenneth Finegold, "State Capacity and Economic Intervention in the Early New Deal," *Political Science Quarterly* 97 (1982): 255–78; Colin Gordon, *New Deals: Business, Labor, and Politics, 1920–1935* (Cambridge, Eng., 1994); Alan Brinkley, *The End of Reform: New Deal Liberalism in Recession and War* (New York, 1996).

6. Frightening Figures

1. Eugene P. Pendergrass, "Some Considerations Concerning the Roentgen Diagnosis of Pneumoconiosis and Silicosis," *American Journal of Roentgenology and Radium Therapy* 48 (1942): 571–94; William S. McCann, "Pneumonoconiosis," in *A Textbook of Medicine*, 7th ed., ed. Russell L. Cecil (Philadelphia, 1947), pp. 963–64; William Osler and Henry A. Christian, *The Principles and Practice of Medicine*, 15th ed. (New York, 1944), pp. 836–40; B. G. Clarke and C. E. Moffet, "Silicosis in Soft Coal Miners," *Journal of Industrial Hygiene and Toxicology* 23 (1941): 176–86; Leroy U. Gardner, "The Pathology and Roentgenographic Manifestations of Pneumoconiosis," *Journal of the American Medical Association (JAMA)* 114 (1940): 535–45; R. Harold Jones, "Pneumonoconiosis Encountered in Bituminous Coal Miners," *JAMA* 119 (1942): 611–15; Eugene P. Pendergrass and Simon S. Leopold, "Benign Pneumonoconiosis," *JAMA* 127 (1945): 701; George W. Wright, "Disability Evaluation in Industrial Pulmonary Disease," *JAMA* 141 (1949): 1218–22; BOM, *Review of Literature on Dusts*, by J. J. Forbes, Sara J. Davenport, and Genevieve G. Morgis, Bulletin 478 (Washington, D.C., 1950).

2. Paul Starr, *The Social Transformation of American Medicine* (New York, 1982), pp. 338–47; John Duffy, *The Sanitarians: A History of American Public Health* (Urbana, 1990), pp. 273–93; Elizabeth W. Etheridge, *Sentinel for Health: A History of the Centers for Disease Control* (Berkeley, 1992). For a similar disregard for, and even hostility to, research into occupational cancer within the burgeoning federal cancer bureaucracy, see Robert N. Proctor, *Cancer Wars: How Politics Shapes What We Know and Don't Know about Cancer* (New York, 1995), pp. 36–48.

3. UMW, *Proceedings of the Thirty-Sixth Constitutional Convention, 1940*, 2 vols. (n.p., n.d.), vol. 2, p. 65; UMW, *Proceedings of the Thirty-Fifth Constitutional Convention, 1938*, 2 vols. (n.p., n.d.), vol. 2, pp. 9, 31, 43, 113; UMW, *Proceedings of the Thirty-Seventh Constitutional Convention, 1942*, 2 vols. (n.p., n.d.), vol. 2, pp. 3, 58; District 7, UMW, *Pro-*

ceedings of the Twenty-Ninth Consecutive and Thirteenth Biennial Convention, 1938 (Hazleton, n.d.), pp. 36–37; Districts 1, 7, and 9, UMW, *Proceedings of the Tri-District Convention, 1939* (n.p., n.d.), pp. 39–40.

4. *United Mine Workers Journal*, May 15, 1947, p. 22, May 15, 1946, p. 16, May 1, 1946, p. 20, Aug. 15, 1947, p. 14; William Green, *Labor and Democracy* (Princeton, 1939), pp. 30–31; UMW, *Proceedings, 1940*, vol. 2, p. 68.

5. Melvyn Dubofsky and Warren Van Tine, *John L. Lewis: A Biography* (New York, 1977), pp. 450–54; Alan Derickson, "Part of the Yellow Dog: U.S. Coal Miners' Opposition to the Company Doctor System, 1936–1946," *International Journal of Health Services* 19 (1989): 709–20. On the general drift to employment-based benefits, see Nelson Lichtenstein, "Labor in the Truman Era: Origins of the 'Private Welfare State,'" in *The Truman Presidency*, ed. Michael J. Lacey (Cambridge, Eng., 1989), pp. 128–55; Nelson Lichtenstein, "From Corporatism to Collective Bargaining: Organized Labor and the Eclipse of Social Democracy in the Postwar Era," in *The Rise and Fall of the New Deal Order, 1930–1980*, ed. Steve Fraser and Gary Gerstle (Princeton, 1989), pp. 122–52; Beth Stevens, "Labor Unions, Employee Benefits, and the Privatization of the American Welfare State," *Journal of Policy History* 2 (1990): 233–60.

6. *UMWJ*, March 15, 1945, p. 18, May 15, 1945, pp. 8–9; Dubofsky and Van Tine, *Lewis*, pp. 454–55.

7. UMW, *Proceedings of the Thirty-Ninth Convention, 1946*, 2 vols. (n.p., n.d.), vol. 1, p. 148; Allen Croyle to Harold L. Ickes, n.d., rpt. in *UMWJ*, May 1, 1946, p. 20; *UMWJ*, April 15, 1946, p. 17, March 15, 1946, pp. 5, 23.

8. UMW and U.S. Coal Mines Administrator, *National Bituminous Wage Agreement, Effective May 29, 1946* (n.p., [1946]), pp. 2, 2–3; UMW and Operators, *National Bituminous Wage Agreement of 1947* (n.p., [1947]), pp. 3–5; UMW and Operators, *National Bituminous Wage Agreement of 1950* (n.p., [1950]), pp. 3–5; Dubofsky and Van Tine, *Lewis*, pp. 459–61. For background on the fund, see Richard P. Mulcahy, "Serving the Union: The United Mine Workers of America Welfare and Retirement Fund, 1946–1978" (Ph.D. diss., West Virginia University, 1988).

9. UMW and Mines Administrator, *Bituminous Agreement, 1946*, p. 3; Joel T. Boone, "New Horizons in Industrial Health and Welfare: Progress in Industrial Health," *JAMA* 132 (1946): 756, 756–57; Coal Mines Administration, Medical Survey Group, "Survey Outline: Avenue #2 Mine, Allegheny Coal and Coke Company," July 24, 1946, RG 245, Records of the U.S. Solid Fuels Administration for War, Coal Mines Administration—Navy, 1946–1948, Medical Survey Group, box 2678, file 2, National Archives, Archives II, College Park, Maryland; *UMWJ*, Jan. 1, 1947, p. 10.

10. U.S. Department of the Interior, Coal Mines Administration, *A Medical Survey of the Bituminous-Coal Industry: A Report of the Coal Mines Administration*, by Joel T. Boone (Washington, D.C., 1947), pp. 92, 113–14, 225, 226.

11. Coal Mines Administration, *Medical Survey*, p. ix; N. H. Collisson to J. A. Krug, May 2, 1947, RG 48, Records of the Office of the Secretary of the Interior, Office Records of Oscar Chapman, 1933–53, box 4, folder: Coal Mines Administration, National Archives, Washington, D.C.

12. Districts 1, 7, and 9, UMW, *Resolutions Submitted to the Tri-District Convention, 1946* (Washington, D.C., n.d.), pp. 45, 17, 31; *UMWJ*, June 15, 1946, pp. 20, 3–4, May 15, 1946, pp. 5, 16, 18; Districts 1, 7, and 9, UMW, *Proceedings of Tri-District Convention, 1946* (Washington, D.C., n.d.), pp. 10, 26–28, 32, 48–49; Maier B. Fox, *United We Stand: The United Mine Workers of America, 1890–1990* (Washington, D.C., 1990), pp. 406–7. On the customary death watch in one bituminous region, see James K. Crissman, *Death and Dying in Central Appalachia: Changing Attitudes and Practices* (Urbana, 1994), pp. 16–21.

13. President, Board of Trustees, Jefferson Medical College to Thomas Kennedy, April 1, 1947, United Mine Workers of America Health and Retirement Funds Archives (hereafter HRFA), ser. III, UMWA Correspondence, box 2, folder: JLL—Anthracite Health and Welfare Fund, Silicosis—Barton Mem[orial Division], West Virginia and Regional Collection, West Virginia University Library, Morgantown; *UMWJ*, June 15, 1947, p. 7, Jan. 15, 1948, p. 5, Oct. 1, 1948, pp. 6–7, Oct. 15, 1954, p. 11; UMW, *Proceedings of the Forty-First Consecutive Constitutional Convention, 1952*, 2 vols. (n.p., n.d.), vol. 1, pp. 259–63; UMW, *Proceedings of the Forty-Fifth Consecutive Constitutional Convention, 1968*, 2 vols. (n.p., n.d.), vol. 1, p. 177; Steven M. Spencer, "Their Lungs Don't Have to Be Ravaged," *Saturday Evening Post*, Sept. 8, 1951, pp. 26–27, 48, 51–52, 56.

14. UMW, *Proceedings, 1952*, vol. 1, pp. 279, 325; UMW, *Proceedings of the Fortieth Consecutive Convention, 1948*, 2 vols. (n.p., n.d.), vol. 1, pp. 198, 259–60; *UMWJ*, Feb. 15, 1948, p. 5; Burgess Gordon et al., "Anthracosilicosis and Its Symptomatic Treatment," *West Virginia Medical Journal* 45 (1949): 125–32; Burgess Gordon, "The Silicosis Problem," *West Virginia Medical Journal* 47 (1951): 1–8; Richard T. Cathcart, Peter A. Theodos, and William Fraimow, "Anthracosilicosis: Selected Aspects Related to the Evaluation of Disability, Cavitation, and the Unusual X-Ray," *Archives of Internal Medicine* 106 (1960): 368–77; Dr. Kerr to Dr. Draper, Nov. 5, 1954, HRFA, ser. III, Health Care Delivery, box 13, folder: Pneumoconiosis Publications. On Kennedy's self-diagnosis of miners' asthma, see Spencer, "Their Lungs," p. 48.

15. Lorin E. Kerr, interview with author, June 26, 1989, Chevy Chase, Md. (tape in author's possession); Leslie A. Falk, interview with author, July 12, 1991, Montpelier, Vt. (tape in author's possession); Michael R. Grey, "Dustbowls, Disease, and the New Deal: The Farm Security Administration Migrant Health Programs, 1935–1947," *Journal of the History of Medicine and Allied Sciences* (*JHMAS*) 48 (1993): 3–39; Michael R. Grey, "Poverty, Politics, and Health: The Farm Security Administration Medical Care Program, 1935–1945," *JHMAS* 44 (1989): 320–50; Monte M. Poen, *Harry S. Truman versus the Medical Lobby: The Genesis of Medicare* (Columbia, Missouri, 1979), pp. 49–50. For the international movement, see Iago Galdston, ed., *Social Medicine: Its Derivations and Objectives* (New York, 1949); Rene Sand, *The Advance to Social Medicine* (London, 1952), esp. pp. 295–343; Henry E. Sigerist, "The Place of the Physician in Modern Society," *Proceedings of the American Philosophical Society* 90 (1946): 275–79.

16. Kerr, interview, 1989; Allen N. Koplin to Warren F. Draper, Aug. 16, 1949, HRFA, ser. III, Medical, Hospital and Health Services Correspondence, box 1, folder: 1947 Fund—Area Reports.

17. Allen N. Koplin, interview with author, Sept. 29, 1990, New York (tape in author's possession); John Winebrenner, interview with author, Aug. 14, 1992, Knoxville, Tenn. (tape in author's possession); Falk, interview; Kerr, interview, 1989.

18. Michael Micklow, interview with author, May 17, 1994, Russellton, Pa. (tape in author's possession); Theodore Venesky, interview with author, May 17, 1994, Russellton, Pa. (tape in author's possession); Daniel Fine, interview with author, Feb. 18, 1992, New Kensington, Pennsylvania (tape in author's possession); Murray Hunter, interview with author, Feb. 15, 1992, Ann Arbor, Mich. (tape in author's possession); Winebrenner, interview; Koplin, interview; Janet E. Ploss, "A History of the Medical Care Program of the United Mine Workers of America Welfare and Retirement Fund" (master's thesis, Johns Hopkins University, 1981); Ivana Krajcinovic, *From Company Doctors to Managed Care: The United Mine Workers' Noble Experiment* (Ithaca, 1997); Richard Mulcahy, "A New Deal for Coal Miners: The UMWA Welfare and Retirement Fund and the Reorganization of Health Care in Appalachia," *Journal of Appalachian Studies* 2 (1996): 29–52; "Discussion," in National Conference on Labor Health Services, *Papers and Proceedings, 1958* (Washington, D.C., 1958), pp. 78–79; T. A. Ferrier to

Leslie A. Falk, April 13, 1953, HRFA, ser. III, Health Care Delivery, box 13, folder: Pneumoconiosis—Public Health Service; Milton D. Levine and Murray B. Hunter, "Clinical Study of Pneumoconiosis of Coal Workers in Ohio River Valley," *JAMA* 163 (1957): 1–4; R. E. Hyatt, A. D. Kistin, and T. K. Mahan, "Respiratory Disease in Southern West Virginia Coal Miners," *American Review of Respiratory Diseases* 89 (1964): 387–401.

19. S. L. Cummins, "The Pneumonoconioses in South Wales," *Journal of Hygiene* 36 (1936): 547, 547–58; Edgar L. Collis and J. C. Gilchrist, "Effects of Dust upon Coal Trimmers," *Journal of Industrial Hygiene* 10 (1928): 101–10; S. W. Fisher, "Medico-Legal Aspects of Coal-Mining," *Medico-Legal and Criminological Review* 6 (1938): 250–51; Andrew Meiklejohn, "History of Lung Diseases of Coal Miners in Great Britain: Part III, 1920–1952," *British Journal of Industrial Medicine* 9 (1952): 213–15; A. G. Heppleston, "Coal Workers' Pneumoconiosis: A Historical Perspective on Its Pathogenesis," *American Journal of Industrial Medicine* 22 (1992): 905–23, esp. 911–13.

20. Jethro Gough, "Pneumonoconiosis in Coal Trimmers," *Journal of Pathology and Bacteriology* 51 (1940): 277–85; Great Britain, Medical Research Council, *Chronic Pulmonary Disease in South Wales Coalminers: I. Medical Studies*, Special Report Series, No. 243 (London, 1942); Great Britain, Medical Research Council, *Chronic Pulmonary Disease in South Wales Coalminers: II. Environmental Studies*, Special Report Series, No. 244 (London, 1943); Meiklejohn, "Lung Diseases: Part III," pp. 215–16; Andrew Meiklejohn, "The Development of Compensation for Occupational Diseases of the Lungs in Great Britain," *British Journal of Industrial Medicine* 11 (1954): 209.

21. Jethro Gough, "Pneumonoconiosis in Coal Workers in Wales," *Occupational Medicine* 4 (1947): 86–97; A. G. Heppleston, "The Essential Lesion of Pneumokoniosis in Welsh Coal Workers," *Journal of Pathology and Bacteriology* 59 (1947): 453–60; A. G. Heppleston, "Coal Workers' Pneumoconiosis: Pathological and Etiological Considerations," *Archives of Industrial Hygiene and Occupational Medicine* 4 (1951): 270–88, esp. 273, 288; C. M. Fletcher, "Pneumoconiosis of Coal-Miners," *British Medical Journal* 1 (1948): 1015–22, 1065–74; C. M. Fletcher, et al., "The Classification of Radiographic Appearances in Coal-Miners' Pneumoconiosis," *Journal of the Faculty of Radiologists* 1 (1949): 40–60; International Labor Office, "Suggested International Scheme for the Classification of Radiographs in Some of the Pneumoconioses," in Third International Conference of Experts on Pneumoconiosis, *Record of Proceedings, 1950*, 2 vols. (Geneva, 1953), vol. 1, pp. 130–33; Meiklejohn, "Lung Diseases: Part III," pp. 217–20.

22. Compare Barbara Ellen Smith, *Digging Our Own Graves: Coal Miners and the Struggle over Black Lung Disease* (Philadelphia, 1987), pp. 21, 25. Smith erroneously contends that the battle began with the publication of Joseph Martin's article in 1954.

23. William E. Mitch to author, Nov. 1, 1989 (letter in author's possession); Koplin, interview; Lloyd Noland, "The Organization and Operation of an Industrial Health Department," *Transactions of the Southern Surgical Association* 38 (1926): 275–84, esp. 281; Marlene H. Rikard, "An Experiment in Welfare Capitalism: The Health Care Services of the Tennessee Coal, Iron and Railroad Company" (Ph.D. diss., University of Alabama, 1983), p. 329. [Phil] Woods, "Cost of Contract Medical Service to Miners in Alabama Based on Check-off for September and October 1947," n.d. [ca. Nov. 1947], Health Care Delivery, box 3, folder: Hospital Facilities and Services in Mining Areas in Alabama; Allen N. Koplin to Warren F. Draper, Aug. 16, 1949, Medical, Hospital and Health Service Correspondence, box 1, folder: 1947 Fund—Area Reports; Koplin to Draper, June 13, 1952, Regional Office Files, box 14, folder: Health and Medical Services, District 20; all in HRFA, ser. III. James L. Jarvis to John L. Lewis, Aug. 22, 1949, UMW Archive, President-District Correspondence, folder: District 20 Correspondence, 1949, Aug.-Sept.

24. Louis L. Friedman, "Pneumoconiosis in Soft-Coal Workers (Miner's Asthma,

Anthracosilicosis)," n.d. [ca. 1951], Louis L. Friedman personal papers (in Friedman's possession, Las Vegas, Nev.); Louis L. Friedman, "Significant Case of Pneumoconiosis in a Soft-Coal Worker," *Archives of Internal Medicine* 95 (1955): 328–32; Koplin, interview; William Mitch to Earl E. Houck, Feb. 16, 1956, UMW Archive, Legal Department Files, folder: District 20 Correspondence, 1947–63.

25. H. Ellsworth Steele, "Negro and White Miners under Alabama's Pneumoconiosis Law," *Industrial Medicine and Surgery* 31 (1962): 383; Mitch to author, Nov. 1, 1989; Koplin, interview; U.S. House of Representatives, Committee on Mines and Mining, *Inspections and Investigations in Coal Mines: Hearings before a Subcommittee . . . on S. 2420*, 77th Cong., 3d sess., 1940 (Washington, D.C., 1940), pp. 89–90; UMW, *Proceedings of the Thirty-Eighth Constitutional Convention, 1944*, 2 vols. (n.p., n.d.), vol. 2, p. 90.

26. Mitch to author, Nov. 1, 1989; Koplin interview; J. J. Forbes to J. L. Shores, Aug. 11, 1949, RG 70, Records of the Bureau of Mines, General Correspondence, 1910–50, box 6182, file 937, Washington National Records Center, National Archives and Records Administration, Suitland, Md.

27. Friedman, "Pneumoconiosis in Soft-Coal Workers"; Koplin, interview.

28. William E. Mitch, untitled address at Knoxville pneumoconiosis conference, May 6, 1953, William E. Mitch personal papers (in Mitch's possession, Birmingham, Ala.); Mitch to author, Nov. 1, 1989; Koplin interview; Legislative Committee, Alabama Mining Institute, "Report, 1949," March 31, 1950, Alabama Coal Operators Association Records, box 1, Department of Archives and Manuscripts, Birmingham Public Library, Birmingham, Ala.

29. Alabama, *Laws, 1951, Regular Session*, 2 vols. (Montgomery, 1951), vol. 1, pp. 427–28, 427–33.

30. Fox, *United We Stand*, p. 420; Dubofsky and Van Tine, *Lewis*, pp. 484–89, 510–13; Mulcahy, "Serving the Union," pp. 62–63; Falk, interview; Koplin, interview; [Josephine Roche] to Mr. Lewis, Oct. 31, 1957, HRFA, ser. II, UMW Correspondence, box 3, folder: John L. Lewis, Southern Coal Producers' Association.

31. Lorin E. Kerr, interview with author, Sept. 6, 1990 (tape in author's possession); Kerr, interview, 1989; Koplin, interview; Falk, interview; Winebrenner, interview. There was a loophole in the research policy. Although the fund per se did not subsidize research, the Miners Memorial Hospital Association did finance some clinical research. See Mulcahy, "Serving the Union," p. 178.

32. International Executive Board, UMW, "Proceedings," Oct. 26, 1951, pp. 320, 320–21, 305, 313–14, 318–21, UMW Archive; Koplin, interview.

33. William Mitch to Josephine Roche and Warren F. Draper, Nov. 2, 1951, UMW Archive, President-District Correspondence, folder: District 20 Correspondence, 1951. For evidence of improved dust suppression in Alabama in the wake of pneumoconiosis compensation, see *Coal Age*, July 1956, pp. 57–59.

34. Kerr, interview, 1989.

35. Warren F. Draper to Area Medical Administrators, May 28, 1954, box 13, folder: Pneumoconiosis Memos (distributing Joseph E. Martin, Jr., "Coal Miners' Pneumoconiosis," *American Journal of Public Health* 44 [1954]: 581–91); Draper to All Area Administrators, Dec. 14, 1955, box 13, folder: Pneumoconiosis Memos; Draper to Asa Barnes, Dec. 17, 1957, box 13, folder: Charles M. Fletcher's Visit; Lorin E. Kerr to Philip Hugh-Jones, Aug. 3, 1954, box 13, folder: Pneumoconiosis—Dr. Kerr's Proposed Report; Kerr to Charles M. Fletcher, Feb. 15, 1955, box 13, folder: Pneumoconiosis Publications; Kerr to Allen N. Koplin, Nov. 24, 1954, box 13, folder: Pneumoconiosis Publications; A. G. Heppleston to Kerr, box 14, folder: Pneumoconiosis Standard Films; J. C. Gilson to Kerr, March 16, 1961, box 14, folder: Pneumoconiosis Standard Films; all in HRFA, ser. III, Health Care Delivery. Lorin E. Kerr, "Coal Work-

ers' Pneumoconiosis," *Industrial Medicine and Surgery* 28 (1956): 355–62; Koplin, interview; Kerr, interview, 1989.

36. Thompson A. Ferrier, "Office Session on Coal Workers' Pneumoconiosis by Jethro Gough, M.D.," Feb. 10, 1958, box 11, folder: Pneumoconiosis Conferences; Lorin E. Kerr to William A. Dorsey, Oct. 7 and Oct. 14, 1952, box 12, folder: Pneumoconiosis Consultants; both in HRFA, ser. III, Health Care Delivery. *UMWJ*, Oct. 1, 1955, p. 10, Oct. 15, 1955, p. 12, Dec. 1, 1957, p. 11; Koplin, interview; Kerr, interview, 1989.

37. John Rogan to Lorin E. Kerr, Sept. 30, 1955, box 12, folder: Pneumoconiosis— General; Kerr to A. G. Heppleston, June 10, June 21, and July 14, 1954, box 13, folder: Pneumoconiosis Publications; Heppleston to Kerr, June 24 and July 6, 1954, box 13, folder: Pneumoconiosis Publications; all in HRFA, ser. III, Health Care Delivery. For the contention that a substantial proportion of the disability suffered by pneumoconiotic miners was psychogenic, see W. Donald Ross, et al., "Emotional Aspects of Respiratory Disorders among Coal Miners," *Journal of the American Medical Association* 156 (1954): 484–87.

38. Rutherford T. Johnstone and Seward E. Miller, *Occupational Diseases and Industrial Medicine* (Philadelphia, 1960), pp. 239, 200–49; Adolph G. Kammer, "Occupational Health Problems of the Bituminous Coal Miner," *Archives of Industrial Health* 15 (1957): 466–67; Koplin, interview; Warren F. Draper to Area Medical Administrators, Aug. 28, 1959, HRFA, ser. III, Health Care Delivery, box 13, folder: Pneumoconiosis— Memos to All Area Offices.

39. Warren F. Draper to C. M. Fletcher, Aug. 22, 1952, folder: Pneumoconiosis— General; Ian McCallum to Lorin E. Kerr, May 28, 1953, folder: Pneumoconiosis Consultants; Kerr to McCallum, June 23, 1953, folder: Pneumoconiosis Consultants; all in HRFA, ser. III, Health Care Delivery, box 12. C. M. Fletcher, "Epidemiological Studies of Coal Miners' Pneumoconiosis in Great Britain," *Archives of Industrial Health* 11 (1955): 29–41; Kerr, interview, 1989; Warren F. Draper, "Health Programs of the United Mine Workers," in *The House of Labor: Internal Operations of American Unions*, ed. J. B. S. Hardman and Maurice F. Neufeld (New York, 1951), pp. 302–3. For other instances in which epidemiology figured prominently in disease recognition and health policy, see David Michaels, "Waiting for the Body Count: Corporate Decision Making and Bladder Cancer in the U.S. Dye Industry," *Medical Anthropology Quarterly*, n.s., 2 (1988): 215–32; Angela Nugent, "The Power to Define a New Disease: Epidemiological Politics and Radium Poisoning," in *Dying for Work: Workers' Safety and Health in Twentieth-Century America*, ed. David Rosner and Gerald Markowitz (Bloomington, Ind., 1987), pp. 177–91; Barbara Berney, "Round and Round It Goes: The Epidemiology of Childhood Lead Poisoning, 1950–1990," *Milbank Quarterly* 71 (1993): 3–39; Gerald M. Oppenheimer, "In the Eye of the Storm: The Epidemiological Construction of AIDS," in *AIDS: The Burdens of History*, ed. Elizabeth Fee and Daniel M. Fox (Berkeley, 1988), pp. 267–300.

40. Warren F. Draper to Leonard A. Scheele, Oct. 27, 1952; Lorin E. Kerr to Leslie A. Falk, April 27, 1952; both in HRFA, ser. III, Health Care Delivery, box 13, folder: Pneumoconiosis—PHS.

41. John D. Winebrenner to Warren F. Draper, Aug. 15, 1949, John Winebrenner Papers, box 1, folder: Correspondence, 1948–55, West Virginia and Regional Collection, West Virginia University Library, Morgantown; Winebrenner, interview. Draper to Leonard A. Scheele, Oct. 27, 1952; Scheele to Draper, Nov. 7, 1952, both in HRFA, ser. III, Health Care Delivery, box 13, folder Pneumoconiosis—Public Health Service.

42. Allen N. Koplin to Warren F. Draper, May 14, 1953, HRFA, ser. III, Health Care Delivery, box 14, folder: Pneumoconiosis, Knoxville Chest Group (Chest Disability); Winebrenner, interview; Koplin, interview.

43. Henry N. Doyle to Lorin E. Kerr, Sept. 18, 1953; Seward E. Miller to Warren F.

Draper, Sept. 23, 1953; Henry N. Doyle and Tracy Levy, "A Preliminary Survey of Chest Disability in American Bituminous Coal Miners," Sept. 1953; all in HRFA, ser. III, Health Care Delivery, box 13, folder: Pneumoconiosis—Public Health Service. Harold J. Magnuson to William G. Reidy, Aug. 21, 1957, RG 90, Records of the Public Health Service, Occupational Health Program, Subject Files, 1955–1957, box 45, folder: Diseases 9—Studies and Surveys, Washington National Records Center, National Archives and Records Administration, Suitland, Maryland. In retrospect, Doyle saw this moment as a missed opportunity: "By 1953 there was ample evidence to indicate an increasing incidence of pneumoconiosis among bituminous coal miners. However, action was not taken by management, labor, or government." See Henry N. Doyle, "The Impact of Changing Technology on Health Problems in the Coal Mining Industry," in National Conference on Medicine and the Federal Coal Mine Health and Safety Act of 1969, *Papers and Proceedings, 1970* (n.p., 1970), pp. 195–96.

44. Leslie A. Falk to Warren F. Draper, Dec. 14, 1953, Health Care Delivery, box 12, folder: Pneumoconiosis Consultants; Falk to Draper, July 14, 1955, Subject Files, box 21, folder: Informational Reports, 1954; both in HRFA, ser. III. Falk, interview; Kerr, interview, 1989. On the ongoing distribution of the ILO radiographs to practitioners and researchers far and wide, see Draper to Area Medical Administrators, June 11, 1954; F. D. Mott to Lorin E. Kerr, June 25, 1954; both in HRFA, ser. III, Health Care Delivery, box 14, folder: Pneumoconiosis Standard Films.

45. Leslie A. Falk to Warren F. Draper, July 2, 1954; Lorin E. Kerr to Draper, Sept. 27, 1954; Kerr to Draper, Oct. 1, 1954; Kerr to Draper and Staff, Oct. 8, 1954; all in HRFA, ser. III, Health Care Delivery, box 12, folder: Pneumoconiosis Consultants. Kerr, interview, 1989; Martin, "Coal Miners' Pneumoconiosis," pp. 587, 589–91.

46. International Association of Industrial Accident Boards and Commissions, "A Resolution for a Prevalence Study of Pneumoconiosis among Coal Workers in the United States," Sept. 29, 1955, Lorin E. Kerr personal papers. Lorin E. Kerr to Charles M. Fletcher, Nov. 30, 1955, box 12, folder: Pneumoconiosis—General; Warren F. Draper to Leonard A. Scheele, Nov. 4, 1955, box 13, folder: Pneumoconiosis—Public Health Service; both in HRFA, ser. III, Health Care Delivery. Kerr, interview, 1989; *UMWJ*, Oct. 1, 1955, p. 10, Oct. 15, 1955, p. 12.

47. Centerville [Medical Group], "Pneumoconiosis—Coal Miners," 1956, Russellton Miners Clinic Records, box 1, folder: Pneumoconioses Studies, Historical Collections and Labor Archives, Pattee Library, Pennsylvania State University, University Park; Centerville [Medical Group], "Coal Miners Pneumonioconiosis [sic]," Jan. 30, 1956, HRFA, ser. III, Health Care Delivery, box 14, folder: Pneumoconiosis Treatment; Falk, interview; Fine, interview.

48. Leslie A. Falk to Warren F. Draper, March 5, 1957, box 11, folder: Pneumoconiosis Conferences; Falk to Draper, June 20, 1957, box 14, folder: Pneumoconiosis Research; both in HRFA, ser. III, Health Care Delivery. Falk, interview; Kerr, interviews, 1989 and 1990; Pennsylvania, Department of Health, *Annual Report, 1959* (n.p., n.d.), p. 61; Pennsylvania, Joint State Government Commission, *Anthracosilicosis and Commonwealth Expenditures under the Occupational Disease Law* (Harrisburg, 1959); Paul K. Reed to Thomas Kennedy, Feb. 10, 1958, UMW Archive, President's Office Files, folder: Interior (U.S. Department of)—Bureau of Mines, 1958.

49. W. W. McBride, E. G. Pendergrass, and J. Lieben, "Pneumoconiosis Study of Pennsylvania Anthracite Miners," *Journal of Occupational Medicine* 8 (1966): 365–76.

50. Jan Lieben, "Pneumoconiosis in Pennsylvania," *Pennsylvania Medical Journal* 63 (Aug. 1960): 1183; Lieben to Allen Croyle, July 23, 1959; Lieben to Joseph J. Boyko, July 27, 1959; both in District 2, UMW, Collection, box 144, folder: Chest X-Rays, Special Collections, Stapleton Library, Indiana University of Pennsylvania, Indiana, Pa. David H. Kurtzman to David L. Lawrence, March 29, 1960, MG-191, David L.

Lawrence Papers, General File, box 97, folder: UMWA, 1959–62, Pennsylvania State Archives, Harrisburg; Lieben to Falk, Dec. 15, 1960, Russellton Miners' Clinic Records, box 1, folder: Pneumoconioses Studies. For Pendergrass's conversion, see Eugene P. Pendergrass, *The Pneumoconiosis Problem, with Emphasis on the Role of the Radiologist* (Springfield, Ill., 1958), pp. 105–10.

51. Jan Lieben and W. Wayne McBride, "Pneumoconiosis in Pennsylvania's Bituminous Mining Industry," *JAMA* 183 (1963): 179, 176–79; Lieben, Eugene Pendergrass, and McBride, "Pneumoconiosis Study in Central Pennsylvania Coal Mines: I. Medical Phase," *Journal of Occupational Medicine* 3 (1961): 493–506; McBride, Pendergrass, and Lieben, "Pneumoconiosis Study of Western Pennsylvania Bituminous-Coal Miners," *Journal of Occupational Medicine* 5 (1963): 376–88; John H. Vinyard and Lieben, "Pneumoconiosis Mortality in Pennsylvania," *Pennsylvania Medical Journal* 63 (1960): 1117–20, Lieben and Philip C. Hill, "Pneumoconiosis Mortality in Pennsylvania," *Pennsylvania Medical Journal* 65 (1962): 1475–78.

52. U.S. PHS, Division of Occupational Health, "Proposal for the Study of Chronic Chest Disease in Bituminous Coal Miners," Oct. 8, 1962, pp. 2, 4; Henry N. Doyle to Warren F. Draper, Oct. 12, 1962; both in HRFA, ser. III, Subject Files, box 20, folder: Reports—Chest Diseases in Bituminous Coal Miners. Kerr, interview, 1990.

53. Henry N. Doyle, "A Study of Chronic Chest Disease in Bituminous Coal Miners," in Mine Inspectors' Institute of America, *Proceedings of the Fifty-Third Convention, 1963* (n.p., n.d.), pp. 113–19; U.S. PHS, *Pneumoconiosis in Appalachian Bituminous Coal Miners*, by W. S. Lainhart, et al., PHS Publication 2000 (Cincinnati, 1969).

54. Kerr, interviews, 1990, 1989; Murray C. Brown, "Pneumoconiosis in Bituminous Coal Miners," *Mining Congress Journal*, Aug. 1965, pp. 44–48. Kerr repeated his contention that 100,000 Americans had indications of CWP in congressional hearings the following year. See U.S. Senate, Committee on Labor and Public Welfare, Subcommittee on Labor, *Occupational Safety and Health Act of 1968: Hearings . . . on S. 2864*, 90th Cong., 2d sess., 1968 (Washington, D.C., 1968), p. 503. For further criticism of suppression of data by the PHS, see *Washington Post*, Sept. 22, 1968, pp. A1, A12.

55. Ralph Nader to Stewart L. Udall, March 23, 1968, rpt. in U.S. Senate, Committee on Labor and Public Welfare, Subcommittee on Labor, *Occupational Safety and Health Act of 1968: Hearings . . . on S. 2864*, 90th Cong., 2d sess., 1968 (Washington, D.C., 1968), p. 527; W. K. C. Morgan, "The Prevalence of Coal Workers' Pneumoconiosis," *American Review of Respiratory Disease* 98 (1968): 306–10; Kerr, interview, 1990.

56. Eugene P. Pendergrass to William W. Scranton, Dec. 3, 1963; Pennsylvania, Governor's Office, news release, April 6, 1964; both in MG-208, William W. Scranton Papers, General File, 1963–66, box 49, folder: Governor's Conference on Pneumoconiosis, Pennsylvania State Archives, Harrisburg. From his long service on the board of directors of a leading coal firm, Scranton was familiar with the mounting costs of disease compensation even under the restrictive Occupational Disease Act. See Franklin B. Gelder to F. O. Case, Jan. 20, 1954, William W. Scranton Papers, box 78, folder 2, Historical Collections and Labor Archives, Pattee Library, Pennsylvania State University, University Park.

57. C. L. Wilbar, Jr., "Opening Remarks"; William W. Scranton, "Opening Remarks"; H. Beecher Charmbury, "Opening Remarks"; all in Pennsylvania Governor's Conference on Pneumoconiosis (Anthraco-Silicosis), *Proceedings, 1964* (n.p., n.d.), pp. 1, 3, 4–7.

58. Henry N. Doyle, Murray C. Brown, and George H. Dillard, "Coal Pneumoconiosis as a World-Wide Problem"; Eugene Robin, "The Spectrum of Pneumoconiotic Disease in Pennsylvania"; both in Pennsylvania Governor's Conference on Pneumoconiosis (Anthraco-Silicosis), *Proceedings, 1964*, pp. 63, 62, 61–67, 73–78.

59. Leon Cander, "Special Session on Disability Evaluation: Report of the Chair-

man," in Pennsylvania Governor's Conference on Pneumoconiosis (Anthraco-Silico-sis), *Proceedings, 1964*, pp. 247, 247–49.

60. John Curtin, Jr., "Special Session on Workmen's Compensation Legislation: Report of the Chairman," in Pennsylvania Governor's Conference on Pneumoconiosis (Anthraco-Silicosis), *Proceedings, 1964*, pp. 259, 257–59. W. A. Boyle to Presidents of All UMWA Districts in Pennsylvania, June 12, 1964, box 149, folder: Pennsylvania Governor's Conference on Pneumoconiosis; UMW representatives, minutes of meeting, Nov. 19, 1964, box 146, folder: Governor's Conference on Pneumoconiosis; both in District 2, UMW, Collection.

61. Pennsylvania, *Laws, 1965*, 2 vols. (Harrisburg, 1965), vol. 1, pp. 695, 695–704; District 1, UMW, *Proceedings of the Sixth Quadrennial Constitutional Convention, 1965* (Wilkes-Barre, n.d.), pp. 73–75, 154; Brit Hume, *Death and the Mines: Rebellion and Murder in the United Mine Workers* (New York, 1971), pp. 167–68; Walter Orzechowski to Joseph Yablonski, Nov. 20, 1965, District 5, UMW, Collection, box 10, folder 10, Special Collections, Stapleton Library, Indiana University of Pennsylvania, Indiana, Pa.

62. Virginia, *Acts and Joint Resolutions, 1952* (Richmond, 1952), p. 931; Virginia, *Acts and Joint Resolutions, 1958* (Richmond, 1958), pp. 584–85; Winebrenner, interview; William H. Anderson to Joseph Beasley, Dec. 14, 1956, RG 90, Occupational Health Program, Subject Files, 1955–1957, box 45, folder: Diseases 9—Studies and Surveys, N-Z. John D. Winebrenner to Lorin E. Kerr, May 8, 1957; William F. Schmidt to Joseph N. Cridlin, April 24, 1957; both in HRFA, ser. III, Health Care Delivery, box 12, folder: Pneumoconiosis—General.

63. Virginia, *Acts and Joint Resolutions, Regular Session, 1968* (Richmond, 1968), pp. 349, 348–49; *Roanoke Times*, Feb. 24, 1960, p. 18; *UMWJ*, March 15, 1960, p. 8, Feb. 1, 1968, p. 11, April 1, 1968, p. 8; W[arren] D[raper] to Dr. Kerr, March 29, 1960, HRFA, ser. III, Health Care Delivery, box 11, folder: Pneumoconiosis Compensation.

64. U.S. Bureau of Labor Statistics, *Technological Change and Productivity in the Bituminous Coal Industry, 1920–60*, Bulletin 1305 (Washington, D.C., 1961), pp. 13–17, 27, 89; U.S. Bureau of Mines, *Some Preliminary Data on Methods for Controlling the Dust Hazards in Mechanical Mining*, Information Circular 7151 (Washington, D.C., 1941), pp. 2–4; Keith Dix, *What's a Miner to Do?: The Mechanization of Coal Mining* (Pittsburgh, 1988), pp. 84, 93, 104–5; *Coal Age*, July 1956, pp. 56, 57; Murray Jacobson, "Respirable Dust in Bituminous Coal Mines in the U.S.," in *Inhaled Particles, III: Proceedings of an International Symposium Organized by the British Occupational Hygiene Society, 1970*, ed. W. H. Walton, 2 vols. (Old Woking, Eng., 1971), vol. 2, pp. 752–53.

65. Kerr, interview, 1990. B. I. Golden to John L. Lewis, Sept. 17, 1955; H. D. Hatfield to Lewis, Nov. 3, 1952; both in HRFA, ser. III, Health Care Delivery, box 14, folder: Pneumoconiosis Symposium at Golden Clinic. William Mitch to Josephine Roche and Warren F. Draper, Nov. 2, 1951, UMW Archive, President-District Correspondence, folder: District 20 Correspondence, 1951; compare Mulcahy, "Serving the Union," p. 311. On Lewis's financial support for Golden's research on miners' asthma in the thirties, see Benjamin I. Golden to Harrison A. Williams, March 31, 1969, rpt. in U.S. Senate, Committee on Labor and Public Welfare, Subcommittee on Labor, *Coal Mine Health and Safety: Hearings*, 1969, 5 pts. (Washington, D.C., 1969), pt. 2, p. 871. Roche did not attend Golden's conference in 1955. Three years earlier, however, Draper had informed her of the ideas under discussion at the first Golden Symposium. See Warren F. Draper to Miss Roche, Nov. 12, 1952, HRFA, ser. III, Health Care Delivery, box 14, folder: Pneumoconiosis Symposium at Golden Clinic.

66. U.S. Bureau of Mines, *Minerals Yearbook, 1960*, 3 vols. (Washington, D.C., 1961), vol. 2, pp. 4–5; Dix, *What's a Miner to Do*, pp. 126–214; Dubofsky and Van Tine, *Lewis*, pp. 494, 505; Morton S. Baratz, *The Union and the Coal Industry* (New Haven, 1955),

pp. 70–72; David Brody, *In Labor's Cause: Main Themes on the History of the American Worker* (New York, 1993), pp. 131–74, esp. 162–64; UMW, *Minutes of the Twelfth Annual Convention, 1901* (Indianapolis, n.d.), pp. 46–47; UMW, *Minutes of the Fifteenth Annual Convention, 1904* (Indianapolis, 1904), p. 32; *UMWJ*, May 1, 1949, p. 3; Peter Navarro, "Union Bargaining Power in the Coal Industry, 1945–1981," *Industrial and Labor Relations Review* 36 (1983): 214–29, esp. 218–20.

67. Koplin, interview; Kerr, interview, 1990. On belief in and problems of social quantification, see Theodore M. Porter, *Trust in Numbers: The Pursuit of Objectivity in Science and Public Life* (Princeton, 1995).

68. UMW, *Proceedings, 1968*, vol. 1, pp. 316, 320, 313–21, vol. 2, pp. 132–33; *UMWJ*, Oct. 1, 1968, pp. 10–13.

69. UMW, *Proceedings, 1968*, vol. 1, pp. 432–33, 462.

7. Extreme Solidarity

1. Clarence Y. H. Lo, "Communities of Challengers in Social Movement Theory," in *Frontiers in Social Movement Theory*, ed. Aldon D. Morris and Carol McClurg Mueller (New Haven, 1992), pp. 224–47. For other insightful criticisms of the tendency of the dominant resource-mobilization paradigm to avoid or denigrate the disruptive protest movements of the lower classes, see Frances Fox Piven and Richard A. Cloward, "Normalizing Collective Protest," in *Frontiers in Social Movement Theory*, ed. Morris and Mueller, pp. 301–25.

2. Theodore C. Waters, "Medicolegal Aspects of the Pneumoconioses," in *The Pneumoconioses*, ed. A. J. Lanza (New York, 1963), pp. 129–50; Lorin Kerr, "The Occupational Pneumoconiosis of Coal Miners as a Public Health Problem," *Virginia Medical Monthly* 96 (1969): 124.

3. UMW, *Proceedings of the Forty-Fourth Consecutive Constitutional Convention, 1964*, 2 vols. (Washington, D.C., n.d.), vol. 2, p. 63; UMW, *Proceedings of the Forty-Fifth Consecutive Constitutional Convention, 1968*, 2 vols. (n.p., n.d.), vol. 2, pp. 164, 75, 163, vol. 1, p. 432. Jess Warden to W. A. Boyle, ca. Feb. 1, 1969, folder: District 29, 1969, Jan.-Feb.; Fulton C. Wooding to Boyle, Feb. 14, 1969, folder: District 29, 1969, March; both in UMW Archive, President-District Correspondence. Davitt McAteer, interview with author, May 20, 1993, Shepherdstown, W. Va. (tape in author's possession); *New York Times*, Feb. 12, 1969, p. 36; West Virginia, *Acts, 1960–62* (Charleston, n.d.), pp. 881–82; Donald L. Rasmussen, interview with author, July 26, 1991, Beckley, W. Va. (tape in author's possession). On the political economy of West Virginia as related to miners' disease and its compensation, see J. Davitt McAteer, *Coal Mine Health and Safety: The Case of West Virginia* (New York, 1973).

4. Craig Robinson, interview with author, June 4, 1993, Scarbro, W. Va. (tape in author's possession); Rick Bank, interview with author, May 21, 1993, Washington, D.C. (tape in author's possession); K. W. Lee, "Catalyst of the Black Lung Movement," in *Appalachia in the Sixties: Decade of Reawakening*, ed. David S. Walls and John B. Stephenson (Lexington, Ky., 1972), pp. 201–9.

5. Robinson, interview; Richard P. Mulcahy, "Serving the Union: The United Mine Workers of America Welfare and Retirement Fund, 1946–1978" (Ph.D. diss., West Virginia University, 1988), pp. 288–94; Curtis Seltzer, *Fire in the Hole: Miners and Managers in the American Coal Industry* (Lexington, Ky., 1985), pp. 89–91; James Vowell to Director's Office, July 14, 1967, United Mine Workers of America Health and Retirement Funds Archives, ser. II, Investigation of Fund, box 3, folder: Disabled Miners, West Virginia and Regional History Collection, West Virginia University Library,

Morgantown; Jeanne M. Rasmussen, "On the Outside Lookin' In," *Mountain Life and Work*, Sept. 1969, p. 9.

6. Robinson, interview; Bank, interview.

7. *Charleston Gazette* (W. Va.), June 4, 1968, p. 13, May 28, 1968, p. 15, May 29, 1968, p. 17, June 7, 1968, p. 21, July 22, 1968, p. 13, Sept. 25, 1968, p. 15; *Sunday Gazette-Mail* (Charleston, W. Va.), June 2, 1968, p. 6A; Bank, interview; Frances Fox Piven and Richard A. Cloward, *Poor People's Movements: Why They Succeed, How They Fail* (New York, 1979), pp. 264–361; David J. Garrow, *Bearing the Cross: Martin Luther King, Jr., and the Southern Christian Leadership Conference, 1955–1968* (New York, 1986), pp. 574–618.

8. Lee, "Catalyst," p. 207; Bank, interview; Robinson, interview; Union Members to W. A. Boyle, July 26, 1968, HRFA, ser. II, Investigation of Fund, box 3, folder: Disabled Miners; E. P. Thompson, "The Moral Economy of the English Crowd in the Eighteenth Century," *Past and Present* 50 (1971): 76–136, esp. 78, 95; George Rude, *Ideology and Popular Protest* (New York, 1980), pp. 27–38; Herbert G. Gutman, "Protestantism and the American Labor Movement: The Christian Spirit in the Gilded Age," *American Historical Review* 72 (1966): 74–101.

9. *Charleston Gazette*, May 28, 1968, p. 15, July 23, 1968, p. 11; Philip Trupp, "Doctor Buff versus the Black Lung," *Reader's Digest*, June 1969, pp. 102–3.

10. Trupp, "Buff versus Black Lung," pp. 102, 102–4; *Charleston Gazette*, Sept. 11, 1968, p. 13; Brit Hume, *Death and the Mines: Rebellion and Murder in the United Mine Workers* (New York, 1971), pp. 99–104; Rasmussen, interview. On the politics of simplifying scientific knowledge, see Stephen Hilgartner, "The Dominant View of Popularization: Conceptual Problems, Political Uses," *Social Studies of Science* 20 (1990): 519–39.

11. Rasmussen, interview; *Charleston Gazette*, July 23, 1968, p. 11, Sept. 17, 1968, p. 12, Sept. 25, 1968, p. 26, Oct. 23, 1968, p. 7; *Sunday Gazette-Mail*, Sept. 1, 1968, p. 4B; *New York Times*, Jan. 7, 1969, p. 24; Robinson, interview.

12. *Charleston Gazette*, Aug. 27, 1968, p. 4, Sept. 17, 1968, p. 12, Sept. 18, 1968, p. 23.

13. Rasmussen, interview; Robinson, interview; McAteer, interview; Donald L. Rasmussen, et al., "Pulmonary Impairment in Southern West Virginia Coal Miners," *American Review of Respiratory Disease* 98 (1968): 658–67.

14. Robinson, interview; Rasmussen, interview; Barbara Ellen Smith, *Digging Our Own Graves: Coal Miners and the Struggle over Black Lung Disease* (Philadelphia, 1987), pp. 109–13.

15. Rasmussen, interview; Ken Hechler, "Coal Mine Health and Safety," [1986], pp. 4–5, Ken Hechler personal papers; *Charleston Gazette*, Nov. 22, 1968, pp. 1, 10; William N. Denman, "The Black Lung Movement: A Study of Contemporary Agitation" (Ph.D. diss., Ohio University, 1974), pp. 53–59; McAteer, interview; Murray Hunter, interview with author, Feb. 15, 1992, Ann Arbor, Mich. (tape in author's possession).

16. McAteer, interview; Rasmussen, interview; Hume, *Death and the Mines*, pp. 108–10.

17. Lee, "Catalyst," pp. 208–9; Robinson, interview; Bank, interview.

18. *Charleston Gazette*, Oct. 16, 1968, p. 17, Oct. 15, 1968, pp. 1–2, Oct. 19, 1968, p. 1, Oct. 22, 1968, p. 17.

19. Robinson, interview; Bank, interview; *Charleston Gazette*, Dec. 23, 1968, p. 3, Jan. 11, 1969, p. 6.

20. *Sunday Gazette-Mail*, Jan. 26, 1969, p. 10A; *New York Times*, Jan. 7, 1969, p. 24; *Charleston Gazette*, Jan. 10, 1969, pp. 9, 22, Jan. 16, 1969, p. 32, Jan. 21, 1969, p. 8; Rasmussen, interview; Robinson, interview. On chronic bronchitis and emphysema as "a classic example of disorders that may mainly be occupational in origin or partly work-

related," see World Health Organization, *Identification and Control of Work-Related Diseases*, Technical Report Series 714 (Geneva, 1985), pp. 25, 25–30. See also A. G. Heppleston, "The Pathological Anatomy of Simple Pneumokoniosis in Coal Workers," *Journal of Pathology and Bacteriology* 66 (1953): 235–46; G. W. H. Schepers, "Industrial Asthma and Bronchitis," *Industrial Medicine and Surgery* 24 (1955): 53–61, esp. 58–59; Medical Research Council, "Chronic Bronchitis and Occupation," *British Medical Journal* 1 (1966): 101–2; John Pemberton, "Chronic Bronchitis, Emphysema, and Bronchial Spasm in Bituminous Coal Workers: An Epidemiologic Study," *Archives of Industrial Health* 13 (1956): 529–44; compare George W. Wright, "Emphysema—Terminology and Classification," *Archives of Industrial Health* 13 (1956): 140–43.

21. *Sunday Gazette-Mail*, Jan. 5, 1969, p. 5A, Jan. 12, 1969, p. 8C, Jan. 26, 1969, p. 10A; *Charleston Gazette*, Jan. 13, 1969, p. 2, Jan. 21, 1969, p. 8; Robinson, interview; Bank, interview; Rasmussen, interview; Denman, "Black Lung Movement," pp. 60–64.

22. *Washington Post*, Jan. 27, 1969, pp. C1, C3; *Charleston Gazette*, Jan. 27, 1969, pp. 1, 8.

23. Hechler, "Coal Mine Health and Safety," pp. 18, 17–18; Ken Hechler, interview with author, July 25, 1991, Charleston, W. Va. (tape in author's possession); Ralph Nader, "Message from Ralph Nader to the Coal Miners of West Virginia," Jan. 26, 1969, Hechler personal papers; *Charleston Gazette*, Jan. 27, 1969, p. 1; *New York Times*, Jan. 27, 1969, p. 30. For Nader's earlier commentary, see Ralph Nader, "They're Still Breathing," *New Republic*, Feb. 3, 1968, p. 15; *Charleston Gazette*, Jan. 8, 1969, p. 13.

24. Bank, interview; Rasmussen, interview; Hechler, interview; *Washington Post*, Jan. 27, 1969, p. C3; *Charleston Gazette*, Jan. 27, 1969, p. 8.

25. *Sunday Gazette-Mail*, Feb. 2, 1969, p. 12B, Feb. 9, 1969, p. 9A; *Charleston Gazette*, Feb. 4, 1969, p. 11, Feb. 10, 1969, p. 4

26. *Charleston Gazette*, Dec. 12, 1968, p. 13, Feb. 8, 1969, p. 4, Feb. 10, 1969, pp. 1, 4; Spindletop Research, *Coal Workers' Pneumoconiosis (CWP): A Summary of Medical Views* (Lexington, Ky., [1969]); *Sunday Gazette-Mail*, Feb. 2, 1969, p. 6M; Rasmussen, interview; William Keith C. Morgan, "Coalworkers' Pneumoconiosis: The Clinical Features," in West Virgina Coal Mining Institute, *1969 Proceedings* (Morgantown, 1970), pp. 77–84.

27. Hunter, interview; Kerr, interview, 1990.

28. *Charleston Gazette*, Feb. 12, 1969, p. 1; *New York Times*, Feb. 12, 1969, p. 36; Rasmussen, interview.

29. West Virginia Senate, Judiciary Committee, and West Virginia House of Delegates, Judiciary Committee, partial transcript of joint hearing, Feb. 11, 1969, pp. 1, 1–3, Murray Hunter personal papers; Hunter, interview.

30. West Virginia Judiciary Committees, transcript, Feb. 11, 1969, esp. pp. 12, 25, 5–6, 10, 12–14, 16, 19; *Charleston Gazette*, Feb. 12, 1969, pp. 1–2; Hume, *Death and the Mines*, p. 131. For Rasmussen's position on disability from simple CWP, see Rasmussen et al., "Impairment in Southern West Virginia," pp. 658–67, esp. 665.

31. West Virginia Judiciary Committees, transcript, Feb. 11, 1969, pp. 14, 15, 18–23, 28, 29; Rasmussen, interview.

32. Hume, *Death and the Mines*, pp. 128–33; Rasmussen, interview; *Charleston Gazette*, Feb. 12, 1969, p. 2.

33. *Charleston Gazette*, Feb. 19, 1969, p. 13, Feb. 21, 1969, p. 1; *New York Times*, Feb. 24, 1969, p. 16; Hume, *Death and the Mines*, pp. 134–35; Bank, interview.

34. Hume, *Death and the Mines*, pp. 138, 134–40; *Charleston Gazette*, Feb. 22, 1969, p. 1, Feb. 20, 1969, p. 1, Feb. 24, 1969, p. 1, Feb. 26, 1969, p. 13; Lee, "Catalyst," pp. 208–9; Rasmussen, interview; Robinson, interview; Robert G. Sherrill, "West Virginia Miracle: The Black Lung Rebellion," *Nation*, April 28, 1969, p. 529. On the intricate dy-

namics of such maneuverings, see Alvin W. Gouldner, *Wildcat Strike: A Study in Worker-Management Relationships* (1954; New York, 1965), pp. 89–95; Rick Fantasia, *Cultures of Solidarity: Consciousness, Action, and Contemporary American Workers* (Berkeley, 1988), pp. 75–120, esp. 116–17 for a discussion of wildcats as the essence, not rejection, of the spirit of unionism.

35. *Charleston Gazette*, Feb. 21, 1969, p. 10, Feb. 20, 1969, p. 1, Feb. 26, 1969, p. 4.

36. *Charleston Gazette*, Feb. 25, 1969, p. 10, Feb. 27, 1969, pp. 1, 2, 5; Hechler, interview; Bank, interview.

37. *Charleston Gazette*, Feb. 27, 1969, p. 1, March 1, 1969, p. 2, Feb. 28, 1969, p. 6.

38. *New York Times*, March 2, 1969, p. 30; *Charleston Gazette*, March 4, 1969, p. 2, March 8, 1969, p. 3; Sara Kaznoski, interview with author, June 6, 1994, Fairmont, W. Va. (tape in author's possession).

39. Bank, interview.

40. West Virginia, *Acts, 1968–69* (Charleston, n.d.), pp. 1271, 1267–96; *Charleston Gazette*, March 10, 1969, p. 2.

41. West Virginia, *Acts, 1968–69*, p. 1271; Rasmussen, interview.

42. West Virginia, *Acts, 1968–69*, pp. 1283–87.

43. Robinson, interview; *Charleston Gazette*, March 10, 1969, p. 1, March 11, 1969, p. 2.

44. Lorin E. Kerr, "Statement," May 6, 1969; Murray B. Hunter, "Statement," May 6, 1969; Milton D. Levine, "Statement," May 6, 1969; W. A. Boyle to Josephine Roche, May 1, 1969; Thomas A. Williams and R. C. Owens to Theodore M. Gray, July 28, 1969; all in UMW Archive, President's Office Files, Subject Files, folder: MA Pneumoconiosis, Ohio. *Times-Leader* (Bellaire, Ohio), March 13, 1969, p. 1; *UMWJ*, May 1, 1969, p. 7, June 1, 1969, pp. 6, 11; Hunter, interview. On developments in Tennessee, see William J. Turnblazer to W. A. Boyle, March 14, 1969, UMW Archive, President's Office Files, Subject Files, folder: Tennessee Occupational Disease Law; Tennessee, *Public Acts, 1969* (Nashville, n.d.), pp. 224–25. On the abortive campaign in Illinois, see *UMWJ*, May 15, 1969, p. 18, July 1, 1969, p. 9, Aug. 15, 1969, p. 18.

45. Hunter, "Statement," May 6, 1969; Kerr, "Statement," May 6, 1969; both in UMW Archive, President's Office Files, Subject Files, folder: MA Pneumoconiosis, Ohio. Hunter, interview; *UMWJ*, Sept. 1, 1969, p. 5; Ohio, *Legislative Acts, 1969–70*, 3 vols. (Columbus, 1970), vol. 1, pp. 2477–93, esp. 2490.

46. *UMWJ*, May 15, 1969, p. 17; Rasmussen, interview; *Charleston Gazette*, April 28, 1969, p. 4, May 17, 1969, p. 6, May 19, 1969, p. 3, June 9, 1969, p. 15, July 28, 1969, p. 2.

47. Lorin E. Kerr, interview with author, Sept. 6, 1990, Chevy Chase, Maryland (tape in author's possession); *Charleston Gazette*, May 5, 1969, p. 2, June 26, 1969, p. 30, Aug. 22, 1969, p. 17; Kentucky, *Acts, 1970* (Louisville, 1970), pp. 68–78; *UMWJ*, May 15, 1969, p. 18, July 1, 1969, p. 8, Oct. 1, 1969, p. 10, Nov. 15, 1969, p. 7, Jan. 15, 1970, pp. 7–8, April 15, 1970, p. 9.

48. George Rosen, *A History of Public Health*, expanded ed. (Baltimore, 1993), pp. 261–62; Charles E. Rosenberg, *The Cholera Years: The United States in 1832, 1849, and 1866* (Chicago, 1962), pp. 193–94.

49. American Mining Congress, *Report of the Proceedings of the Twenty-Fifth Annual Convention, 1922* (Washington, D.C., 1923), pp. 422–35; *Coal Age*, Sept. 26, 1914, p. 513; *Mining Congress Journal*, July 1924, pp. 298–99; *Coal Age*, Jan. 1941, pp. 62–63; James L. Weeks, "From Explosions to Black Lung: A History of Efforts to Control Coal Mine Dust," *Occupational Medicine: State of the Art Reviews* 8 (1993): 10–14.

50. Mark Aldrich, "Preventing 'the Needless Peril of the Coal Mine': The Bureau of Mines and the Campaign against Coal Mine Explosions, 1910–1940," *Technology and Culture* 36 (1995): 483–518; O. W. Morgan, "Dust Suppression in Coal Mines," *National Safety News*, Jan. 1941, pp. 30–31, 67; *Coal Age*, Nov. 1941, pp. 63, 89–91, March 1942,

p. 86, July 1942, pp. 58–59, Jan. 1948, pp. 77–79, Aug. 1951, pp. 100–2, July 1956, pp. 56–59; *Mining Congress Journal*, Dec. 1969, p. 77.

51. Daniel Harrington, "The Engineering-Hygienic Aspects of Dust Elimination in Mines," *Journal of Industrial Hygiene* 7 (1925): 207–14; *Mining Congress Journal*, Jan. 1934, p. 22; J. J. Forbes and Alden II. Emery, "Sources of Dust in Coal Mines," *Transactions of the American Institute of Mining and Metallurgical Engineers* 75 (1927): 645–63; BOM, *Some Preliminary Data on Methods for Controlling the Dust Hazards in Mechanical Mining*, by C. W. Owings, Information Circular 7151 ([Washington, D.C.], 1941); Lawrence B. Berger, "Some Considerations on Dust Control in Coal Mining," *Archives of Industrial Health* 15 (1957): 499–504.

52. *UMWJ*, July 15, 1946, p. 20, Jan. 15, 1953, p. 11, Feb. 15, 1957, p. 11; UMW, *Proceedings of the Fortieth Consecutive Convention, 1948*, 2 vols. (n.p., n.d.), vol. 1, p. 327, vol. 2, pp. 69–70, 103; UMW, *Proceedings of the Forty-First Consecutive Constitutional Convention, 1952*, 2 vols. (Washington, D.C., n.d.), vol. 1, p. 156, vol. 2, p. 277; UMW, *Proceedings of the Forty-Second Consecutive Constitutional Convention, 1956*, 2 vols. (n.p., n.d.), vol. 1, pp. 137–80, esp. 140, vol. 2, p. 23; UMW, *Proceedings of the Forty-Third Consecutive Constitutional Convention, 1960*, 2 vols. (Washington, D.C., n.d.), vol. 2, pp. 32–33; UMW, *Proceedings, 1964*, vol. 1, pp. 113–25; Maier B. Fox, *United We Stand: The United Mine Workers of America, 1890–1990* (Washington, D.C., 1990), pp. 447–49, 465; Joseph E. Finley, *The Corrupt Kingdom: The Rise and Fall of the United Mine Workers* (New York, 1972), p. 232.

53. Michael Encrapera, Tim Jenkins, and S. A. Leaghty, "Vesta No. 4 Safety Committee Report from September 28, 1946, to February 19, 1947," box 9, folder 9; William Bain, et al. (Local 3436), "Safety Committee Report, Montour #9 Mine," April 19, 1951, box 9, folder 31; both in District 5, UMW, Collection, Special Collections, Stapleton Library, Indiana University of Pennsylvania, Indiana, Penn. UMW, *Proceedings, 1952*, vol. 1, p. 380, vol. 2, pp. 51–52, 153–54, 170; Alan Derickson, "Participative Regulation of Hazardous Working Conditions: Safety Committees of the United Mine Workers of America, 1941–1969," *Labor Studies Journal* 18 (1993): 30–36.

54. Nader, "They're Still Breathing," p. 15; *Charleston Gazette*, July 4, 1968, p. 19, Sept. 25, 1968, p. 26, Nov. 26, 1968, p. 1; Trupp, "Doctor Buff," p. 105.

55. American Conference of Governmental Industrial Hygienists, *Transactions of the Tenth Annual Meeting, 1948* (n.p., n.d.), p. 32; American Conference of Governmental Industrial Hygienists, *Transactions of the Twenty-Seventh Annual Meeting, 1965* (n.p., n.d.), p. 123; W. Roy Cunningham, "Dust Study Program, Pennsylvania Department of Mines and Mineral Industries," in National Safety Council, *Transactions, 1961*, 26 vols. (Chicago, n.d.), vol. 1, pp. 24–28; Henry N. Doyle, "Importance of Dust Control," in National Safety Council, *Transactions, 1967*, 28 vols. (Chicago, n.d.), vol. 7, p. 5; T. E. Jones to H. B. Charmbury, Nov. 28, 1966, District 5 Collection, box 13, folder 2. On the ACGIH and its voluntary standards, see Jacqueline K. Corn, *Protecting the Health of Workers: The American Conference of Governmental Industrial Hygienists, 1938–1988* (Cincinnati, 1989); Barry I. Castleman and Grace E. Ziem, "Corporate Influence on Threshold Limit Values," *American Journal of Industrial Medicine* 13 (1988): 531–59; Jeffrey M. Paull, "The Origin and Basis of Threshold Limit Values," *American Journal of Industrial Medicine* 5 (1984): 227–38. On the many difficulties of converting dust counts into weight, see Philip Drinker and Theodore Hatch, *Industrial Dust: Hygienic Significance, Measurement, and Control*, 2d ed. (New York, 1954), p. 121. In 1966, the ACGIH changed its threshold limit value for "inert dusts" to either fifty million particles per cubic foot of air or fifteen milligrams of dust per cubic meter of air, "whichever is less." Although for coal dust this reformulation should have led to adoption of the gravimetric value, it does not appear that such a conversion was widely applied. See ACGIH, *Documen-*

tation of Threshold Limit Values, 2d ed. (Cincinnati, 1966), p. 107; U.S. Senate, Committee on Labor and Public Welfare, Subcommittee on Labor, *Coal Mine Health and Safety: Hearings . . . on S. 355, S. 467, S. 1094, S. 1178, S. 1300, and S. 1907*, 91st Cong., 1st sess., 1969, 5 parts (Washington, D.C., 1969), pt. 2, p. 580; Doyle, "Importance of Dust Control," p. 5.

56. *New York Times*, Dec. 10, 1968, p. 38; *UMWJ*, Jan. 15, 1969, p. 11; Ken Hechler, news release, Dec. 13, 1968, Hechler personal papers; Ken Hechler, "Coal Mine Health and Safety," pp. 14, 15; *Washington Post*, Sept. 12, 1968, p. A7.

57. *Charleston Gazette*, Jan. 15, 1969, p. 10, Jan. 20, 1969, pp. 4, 13; Hechler, "Coal Mine Health and Safety," pp. 22–23; Hume, *Death and the Mines*, p. 82.

58. Rasmussen, interview; *Charleston Gazette*, March 4, 1969, p. 11; Senate, *Coal Mine Health and Safety*, pt. 1, p. 451, pt. 2, pp. 648–49.

59. U.S. House of Representatives, *Federal Coal Mine Health and Safety Act of 1968: Communication from the President*, 90th Cong., 2d sess., 1968 (Washington, D.C., 1968), pp. 2, 1–2; *Congressional Record*, 90th Cong., 2d sess., 1968, 114, pt. 20: 26400, 26405, 26513; Senate, *Coal Mine Health and Safety*, pt. 1, pp. 522, 521–22, pt. 2, pp. 744, 658.

60. Senate, *Coal Mine Health and Safety*, pt. 1, pp. 450–51, pt. 2, pp. 574–75, 594–95, 729–30, 816; Henry N. Doyle, "Pneumoconiosis in Bituminous Coal Miners," in PHS, *Pneumoconiosis in Appalachian Bituminous Coal Miners*, by William S. Lainhart, et al., PHS Publication 2000 (Washington, D.C., 1969), p. 19. Not surprisingly, Stewart's historical review of federal epidemiological work overlooked Meriwether's study in Alabama and Kentucky. See Senate, *Coal Mine Health and Safety*, pt. 2, p. 720. For another instance of PHS amnesia on this subject, see Doyle, "Pneumoconiosis in Bituminous Coal Miners," pp. iii, 15–16.

61. U.S. House of Representatives, Committee on Education and Labor, General Subcommittee on Labor, *Coal Mine Health and Safety: Hearings . . . on H.R. 4047, H.R. 4295, and H.R. 7976*, 91st Cong., 1st sess., 1969 (Washington, D.C., 1969), pp. 312, 311–13, 315, 319; Ralph Nader to Ralph Yarborough, April 26, 1969, HRFA, ser. II, Investigation of Fund, box 1, folder: Ralph Nader Statements; Senate, *Coal Mine Health and Safety*, pt. 2, pp. 641, 670, 674.

62. House, *Coal Mine Health and Safety*, pp. 97, 94, 99, 93–104, esp. 98; Ken Hechler, "Statement," Jan. 26, 1969, Ken Hechler, "Statement," April 1, 1969; both in Hechler personal papers. Senate, *Coal Mine Health and Safety*, pt. 2, pp. 772, 774.

63. Senate, *Coal Mine Health and Safety*, pt. 2, p. 645; *Sunday Gazette-Mail*, April 27, 1969, p. 5A; *Charleston Gazette*, May 24, 1969, p. 5; House, *Coal Mine Health and Safety*, pp. 313–14; *UMWJ*, June 1, 1969, p. 9.

64. House, *Coal Mine Health and Safety*, pp. 71, 71–73, 245–46; *Charleston Gazette*, Feb. 25, 1969, p. 11.

65. House, *Coal Mine Health and Safety*, pp. 498, 118–35, 493–95; *Congressional Record*, Jan. 24, 1969, p. S889; Herbert E. Jones, Jr., to Ken Hechler, March 19, 1969, Hechler personal papers; *Charleston Gazette*, Aug. 30, 1969, p. 4; *Coal Age*, Sept. 1969, p. 43; Denman, "Black Lung Movement," pp. 119–22. On the reviving health and bright prospects of the coal industry in the sixties, see McAteer, *Coal Mine Health*, pp. 3–12; Seltzer, *Fire in the Hole*, pp. 83–84.

66. Senate, *Coal Mine Health and Safety*, pt. 2, pp. 778–79; Hechler, interview.

67. Ken Hechler, "Coal Mine Health and Safety," pp. 44, 43–44, 48, 67–68, 79–82; Hechler to W. A. Boyle, July 8, 1969, Hechler personal papers; Hume, *Death and the Mines*, pp. 173–74. On the Yablonski campaign and the broader reform movement within the UMW, see Paul F. Clark, *The Miners' Fight for Democracy: Arnold Miller and the Reform of the United Mine Workers* (Ithaca, 1981); Finley, *Corrupt Kingdom*, pp. 258–96. In 1995, federal authorities recommended reducing the permissible exposure limit to one milligram of respirable dust per cubic meter of air. See U.S. National Institute

for Occupational Safety and Health, *Criteria for a Recommended Standard: Occupational Exposure to Respirable Coal Mine Dust*, DHHS (NIOSH) Publication 95–106 (Washington, D.C., 1995).

68. John O'Leary, "Panel Discussion on Mine Safety at the NCA Convention," p. 3, June 16, 1969, UMW Archive, Health and Safety Files, folder: 1969 Health and Safety Act, Conferences on Coal Mine Health and Safety.

69. U.S., *Statutes at Large*, vol. 83 (Washington, D.C., 1970), pp. 760, 760–61.

70. *Charleston Gazette*, March 22, 1969, p. 7; Rasmussen, interview; Senate, *Coal Mine Health and Safety*, pt. 2, pp. 776–77, 784–85.

71. Hechler, "Coal Mine Health and Safety," p. 14; Senate, *Coal Mine Health and Safety*, pt. 1, pp. 107–10; Hechler, news release, Feb. 24, 1969, Hechler personal papers. On Hechler's flexibility on this issue, see U.S. House of Representatives, Committee on Education and Labor, Select Subcommittee on Labor, *Benefits to Employees in the Mining Industry: Hearings . . . on H.R. 11476*, 91st Cong., 1st sess., 1969 (Washington, D.C., 1969), pp. 135–54, esp. 139.

72. *Charleston Gazette*, March 22, 1969, p. 7, March 28, 1969, p. 5, Jan. 20, 1969, p. 13; *UMWJ*, April 1, 1969, pp. 16, 21; Senate, *Coal Mine Health and Safety*, pt. 2, pp. 822–23. The UMW resolution of September 1968 called for compensation initiatives at the state level only; see UMW, *Proceedings, 1968*, vol. 1, pp. 432, 462.

73. House, *Coal Mine Health and Safety*, pp. 262, 262–68; John Jacobs, *A Rage for Justice: The Passion and Politics of Phillip Burton* (Berkeley, 1995), pp. 187, 178–97; Hume, *Death and the Mines*, pp. 159–60, 217; *New York Times*, Oct. 31, 1969, p. 44; Rasmussen, interview; Hechler, interview; W. E. Chilton III to Sala [Burton], April 11, 1983, Phillip Burton Papers, box 44, folder: Special, Bancroft Library, University of California, Berkeley, House, *Benefits to Employees*, pp. 2, 19–22, 25–29.

74. Senate, *Coal Mine Health and Safety*, pt. 1, p. 522; House, *Coal Mine Health and Safety*, p. 261; *Charleston Gazette*, June 4, 1969, p. 1; House, *Benefits to Employees*, pp. 18–20, 24.

75. House, *Coal Mine Health and Safety*, pp. 363–65; Rasmussen, interview; Hunter, interview; *New York Times*, Sept. 14, 1969, p. 73; Great Britain, Medical Research Council, *Lung Function in Coalworkers' Pneumoconiosis*, by J. C. Gilson and P. Hugh-Jones, Special Report 290 (London, 1955); John C. Gilson, "The Disability of Coal Workers in South Wales," *Archives of Industrial Health* 15 (1957): 487–93.

76. Senate, *Coal Mine Health and Safety*, pt. 2, pp. 842, 837–42, 760–63; House, *Coal Mine Health and Safety*, p. 275; House, *Benefits to Employees*, p. 246.

77. Senate, *Coal Mine Health and Safety*, pt. 2, pp. 696–97, 851, 854, 857, 859; House, *Coal Mine Health and Safety*, pp. 357, 366.

78. Senate, *Coal Mine Health and Safety*, pt. 2, pp. 662–63; *Charleston Gazette*, May 7, 1969, p. 2, May 12, 1969, p. 20, July 1, 1969, p. 2.

79. U.S., *Statutes at Large*, vol. 83, pp. 793, 792–93.

80. U.S., *Statutes at Large*, vol. 83, p. 793. For Phillip Burton's role in extending benefit eligibility to victims of simple pneumoconiosis, see Jacobs, *Rage for Justice*, pp. 193–94.

81. Ken Hechler, "Statement," Dec. 30, 1969, Hechler personal papers; U.S., *Statutes at Large*, vol. 83, pp. 793–95; *New York Times*, Sept. 30, 1969, p. 18, Oct. 1, 1969, p. 20; Jacobs, *Rage for Justice*, p. 191; Senate, *Coal Mine Health and Safety*, pt. 2, p. 826. For proposals that employers pay for black lung benefits, see House, *Coal Mine Health and Safety*, pp. 333–34; *Charleston Gazette*, March 28, 1969, p. 5; Ken Hechler, "Medievalism in the Coal Mines," p. 11, April 9, 1969, Hechler personal papers.

82. U.S., *Statutes at Large*, vol. 83, pp. 763–64.

83. Ibid., p. 763.

84. Ibid., pp. 799, 798–99. On the National Study, see, among others, W. K. C. Morgan, et al., "The Prevalence of Coal Workers' Pneumoconiosis in U.S. Coal Miners," *Archives of Environmental Health* 27 (1973): 221–26; Michael D. Attfield and Robert M. Castellan, "Epidemiological Data on U.S. Coal Miners' Pneumoconiosis, 1960 to 1988," *American Journal of Public Health* 82 (1992): 964–70; Michael D. Attfield and Noah S. Seixas, "Prevalence of Pneumoconiosis and Its Relationship to Dust Exposure in a Cohort of U.S. Bituminous Coal Miners and Ex-Miners," *American Journal of Industrial Medicine* 27 (1995): 137–51.

85. Bank, interview.

86. For an analysis of mining injuries that similarly emphasizes competitive considerations and unionism, see Michael Wallace, "Dying for Coal: The Struggle for Health and Safety Conditions in American Coal Mining, 1930–82," *Social Forces* 66 (1987): 336–64.

87. For varied cross-class configurations contributing to disease recognition, see Allard Dembe, *Occupation and Disease: How Social Factors Affect the Conception of Work-Related Disorders* (New Haven, 1996); Christopher C. Sellers, *Hazards of the Job: From Industrial Disease to Environmental Health Science* (Chapel Hill, 1997); Claudia Clark, *Radium Girls: Women and Industrial Health Reform, 1910–1935* (Chapel Hill, 1997); Laura Pulido, *Environmentalism and Economic Justice: Two Chicano Struggles in the Southwest* (Tucson, 1996), pp. 57–124; David Rosner and Gerald Markowitz, *Deadly Dust: Silicosis and the Politics of Occupational Disease in Twentieth-Century America* (Princeton, 1991); David Rosner and Gerald Markowitz, "Safety and Health as a Class Issue: The Workers' Health Bureau of America during the 1920s," in *Dying for Work: Workers' Safety and Health in Twentieth-Century America*, ed. Rosner and Markowitz (Bloomington, 1987), pp. 53–64. For a movement that drew directly on the experience in coal, see Robert E. Botsch, *Organizing the Breathless: Cotton Dust, Southern Politics, and the Brown Lung Association* (Lexington, Ky., 1993).

88. U.S. Social Security Administration, *Social Security Bulletin: Annual Statistical Supplement, 1995* (Washington, D.C., 1995), p. 351; U.S. Department of Labor, *Black Lung Benefits Act: Annual Report on Administration of the Act during Calendar Year 1979* (Washington, D.C., 1980), p. 34; Attfield and Castellan, "Epidemiological Data, 1960 to 1988," pp. 964–70; Michael D. Attfield, et al., "The Incidence and Progression of Pneumoconiosis over Nine Years in U.S. Coal Miners: I. Principal Findings," *American Journal of Industrial Medicine* 6 (1984): 407–15; Smith, *Digging Our Own Graves*, pp. 145–204; Alan Derickson, "Down Solid: The Origins and Development of the Black Lung Insurgency," *Journal of Public Health Policy* 4 (1984): 35–38.

INDEX